D1570797

Pharmaceutical Skin Penetration Enhancement

DRUGS AND THE PHARMACEUTICAL SCIENCES

A Series of Textbooks and Monographs

edited by

James Swarbrick
School of Pharmacy
University of North Carolina
Chapel Hill, North Carolina

Pharmaceutical Skin Penetration Enhancement

edited by

Kenneth A. Walters
An-eX Analytical Services, Ltd.
Cardiff, Wales

Jonathan Hadgraft
University of Wales
Cardiff, Wales

Marcel Dekker, Inc.   **New York • Basel • Hong Kong**

Library of Congress Cataloging-in-Publication Data

Pharmaceutical skin penetration enhancement / edited by Kenneth A.
Walters, Jonathan Hadgraft.
     p. cm — (Drugs and the pharmaceutical sciences : v. 59)
     Includes bibliographical references and index.
     ISBN 0-8247-9017-0 (alk. paper)
     1. Transdermal medication. 2. Skin—Permeability. I. Walters,
Kenneth A. II. Hadgraft, Jonathan.
III. Series.
     [DNLM: 1. Administration, Cutaneous. 2. Dermatologic Agents.
3. Skin Absorption—physiology. W1 DR893B v. 59 1993 / WR 102 P536
1993]
RM151.P48   1993
615'.6—dc20
DNLM/DLC
for Library of Congress
                                        92-48507
                                            CIP

This book is printed on acid-free paper.

Marcel Dekker, Inc.
270 Madison Avenue, New York, New York 10016

Current printing (last digit):
10 9 8 7 6 5 4 3 2 1

PRINTED IN THE UNITED STATES OF AMERICA

Preface

Over the past decade, the interest in skin penetration has blossomed, primarily as a result of the developments in transdermal drug delivery systems and their perceived advantages over conventional drug therapy. To optimize the formulation of such systems, and also those used in topical therapy, it has been necessary to gain a better understanding of the mechanisms of skin penetration. This has been facilitated by the advent of more sophisticated physicochemical instrumentation such as Fourier transform infrared spectroscopy, nuclear magnetic resonance spectroscopy, electron spin resonance, and other spectroscopic techniques that now have the precision and sensitivity to probe the complex nature of the skin. The mechanistic evaluation at a molecular level has resulted in a better understanding of the route of drug penetration through the stratum corneum and the physicochemical factors that control the rate of transport through this complex membrane.

Penetration enhancers have been examined for several years and, again, their significance has become greater with the developments of transdermal delivery. Two decades ago the most significant penetration enhancers were probably the dipolar aprotic materials, such as dimethyl sulfoxide and dimethyl acetamide. The former is a very potent enhancer of many drugs, and our understanding of its precise mechanism of action has still not been fully clarified. The spectroscopic techniques mentioned have been used extensively in trying to establish precise mechanisms of action for the many enhancers that have now been identified.

Because of their widely differing chemical structures, it is apparent that they act by more than one mechanism and that their precise enhancer activity will depend on the physicochemical properties of the penetrant. Owing to the application of fundamental physicochemical concepts to the skin transport process, it is becoming possible to identify the features that an enhancer should possess to have optimal activity.

In this book, contributions have been sought to represent the different types of enhancer that have been identified. Not only has the use of chemical enhancers been addressed, chapters have also been contributed on the use of physical enhancement using the processes of iontophoresis and phonophoresis. Authors have been chosen who are at the forefront of research in their individual areas and who, where possible, put a mechanistic interpretation on the ways in which enhancers act. We feel that it is only with an understanding, at a molecular level, that significant advances can be made in the future development of enhancer strategies for transdermal and topical therapy. The book has been written both to answer specific questions and to highlight the ways in which our future research can be directed in a fruitful and challenging fashion. In the future, our ability to probe the skin will become more refined, and it may be possible to use molecular graphics to design drugs that act as their own enhancers. This book lays the groundwork for this promising future.

Kenneth A. Walters
Jonathan Hadgraft

Contents

Contributors

Geoffrey Allan Whitby Research, Inc., Richmond, Virginia

Brian W. Barry School of Pharmacy, University of Bradford, Bradford, West Yorkshire, United Kingdom

Heather A. E. Benson Department of Pharmacy, University of Queensland, Queensland, Australia

J. Gordon Black Colworth Laboratory, Unilever Research, Sharnbrook, Bedford, United Kingdom

Harry E. Boddé Leiden-Amsterdam Center for Drug Research, Leiden University, Leiden, The Netherlands

Joke A. Bouwstra Leiden-Amsterdam Center for Drug Research, Leiden University, Leiden, The Netherlands

Keith R. Brain Welsh School of Pharmacy, University of Wales, Cardiff, Wales

Adrian F. Davis OTC Medicines Applied Research Group, SmithKline Beecham Consumer Brands, Weybridge, Surrey, United Kingdom

Michael Flanagan   Department of Research, CIRD Galderma, Valbonne, France

Michael L. Francoeur   Pharmetrix, Inc., Menlo Park, California

Edward J. French   R. P. Scherer, Swindon, United Kingdom

David R. Friend   Controlled Release and Biomedical Polymers, SRI International, Menlo Park, California

Philip G. Green   Department of Pharmacokinetics and Toxicology, Zyma SA, Nyon, Switzerland

Richard H. Guy   School of Pharmacy, University of California–San Francisco, San Francisco, California

Jonathan Hadgraft   The Welsh School of Pharmacy, University of Wales, Cardiff, Wales

Jorge Heller   Controlled Release and Biomedical Polymers, SRI International, Menlo Park, California

Thomas Hille   Department of Research and Development, LTS-KG, Lohmann Therapie Systeme GmbH & Co., Neuwied, Germany

A. Janet Hoogstraate   Leiden-Amsterdam Center for Drug Research, Leiden University, Leiden, The Netherlands

Ad P. IJzerman   Department of Medicinal Chemistry, Centre for Biopharmaceutical Sciences, Leiden University, Leiden, The Netherlands

Hans E. Junginger   Leiden-Amsterdam Center for Drug Research, Leiden University, Leiden, The Netherlands

Ron Kadir   Laboratory for Development and Manufacture of Skin Care Products, Baselstreet, Tel Aviv, Israel

Gary P. Martin   Department of Pharmacy, King's College, University of London, London, United Kingdom

James C. McElnay   School of Pharmacy, The Queen's University of Belfast, Belfast, Northern Ireland

Birgitte Møllgaard*   Pharmacia AS, Hillerød, Denmark

T. Maria Murphy   Serono Pharmaceuticals, Geneva, Switzerland

David W. Osborne   Calgon Vestal Laboratories, St. Louis, Missouri

Carl C. Peck   Department of Health and Human Services, Center for Drug Evaluation and Research, Food and Drug Administration, Rockville, Maryland

Maria Ponec   Department of Dermatology, University Hospital, Leiden University, Leiden, The Netherlands

Russell O. Potts   Cygnus Therapeutic Systems, Redwood City, California

Colin W. Pouton   School of Pharmacy and Pharmacology, University of Bath, Bath, United Kingdom

Michael S. Roberts   Department of Medicine, University of Queensland, Queensland, Australia

M. A. Ineke Salomons   Centre for Biopharmaceutical Sciences, Leiden University, Leiden, The Netherlands

Vinod P. Shah   Center for Drug Evaluation and Research, Food and Drug Administration, Rockville, Maryland

Braham Shroot   Department of Research, CIRD Galderma, Valbonne, France

Harry L. G. M. Tiemessen   Sandoz AG Pharma Division, Basel, Switzerland

Michael Walker   Department of Biological Development, ConvaTec Wound Healing Research Institute, Deeside, Clwyd, United Kingdom

---

Current affiliation: Department of Pharmaceutical Development, H. Lundbeck A/S, Copenhagen-Valby, Denmark

Kenneth A. Walters   An-eX Analytical Services, Ltd., Cardiff, Wales

Anthony J. I. Ward   Department of Chemistry, Clarkson University, Potsdam, New York

Adrian C. Williams   The School of Pharmacy, University of Bradford, Bradford, West Yorkshire, United Kingdom

Dafydd G. Williams   The Welsh School of Pharmacy, University of Wales, Cardiff, Wales

Roger L. Williams   Center for Drug Evaluation and Research, Food and Drug Administration, Rockville, Maryland

1

Water

The Most Natural Penetration Enhancer

Michael S. Roberts

University of Queensland, Queensland, Australia

Michael Walker

ConvaTec Wound Healing Research Institute, Deeside, Clwyd, United Kingdom

The state of hydration of the stratum corneum (SC) is one of the most important factors in determining the rate of percutaneous absorption of a given solute. The level of hydration is a function of the water concentration gradient between the dermis and the surface of the skin as well as on the ability of the stratum corneum to "bind" the water. Many of the environmental, physiological, and pharmacological factors modifying skin hydration can be related to their effects on the water concentration gradient across the stratum corneum

In a practical sense, hydration of the skin is an important determinant of the skin texture ("softness") and appearance. Many dermatological disorders affect the extent to which stratum corneum binds the water for hydration.

I. WATER CONCENTRATION GRADIENT IN THE STRATUM CORNEUM

The SC represents a distinct phase between the environment and the epidermis. Transfer of water at the SC–environment and SC–lower epidermis interface (i.e., *absorption*) occurs much faster than diffusion through the SC (1,2). The overall water gradient in the SC, therefore, is determined by the diffusivity of water in the SC and the thickness of the SC.

The SC water content, at normal relative humidities, is between 15 and 20% of dry weight. Soaking, occlusion and high humidities may increase the water content further—up to 300–400% of the dry weight after extensive soaking. An increase in water content results in an increased elasticity and permeability of SC, whereas reducing the water content will lead to an opposite effect. Very dry SC loses its elasticity and fissures under stress, as observed in many dry skin conditions.

The transepidermal water loss (TEWL) reflects the continuous diffusion of water from within the body through the SC to the ambient environment. With an increase in the environmental humidity, the concentration difference of water between the inner and outer surface of the SC is diminished and the TEWL is reduced. The normal TEWL is about 0.5 $\mu L \cdot cm^{-2} \cdot hr^{-1}$. The SC water content decreases when the percentage relative humidity (RH) is decreased, and the skin flexibility is reduced at RH values below 60% (3). The amount of water per gram of dry tissue in human SC is 0.2 g and 0.7 g for relative humidities of 40 and 70%, respectively (4). The skin will become brittle when the water content is less than 10% (3). Increased water loss also occurs as the temperature is increased or when air flows over the skin. These observations, deduced using isolated skin specimens (3), have also been confirmed in clinical studies (5). Singer and Vinson (6) have suggested that the water content of neonatal rat skin varied with RH in a logarithmic manner and was independent of the absolute humidity (Fig. 1).

In the in vivo situation, the SC is sandwiched between the aqueous lower layers of the skin and the ambient environment, which may be very dry. As a consequence, the lower layers adjacent to the granular layer are highly hydrated, whereas the surface layers contain less water. The cell layer of SC in equilibrium with the viable epidermis is expected to contain between 5 and 6 g water per gram of dry tissue (4). Given a water content of 0.2 g/g dry SC for 40% RH, Scheuplein and Blank suggest that the average SC water content in vivo from a 40% RH is 0.92 g/g dry tissue (4). An increase in the ambient or atmospheric water content results in a reduction in the water gradient across the SC so that if a completely occlusive aqueous vehicle is applied to the SC surface, it should eventually yield a uniform water concentration throughout the SC. A similar SC water–distance profile would be anticipated for a side-by-side diffusion cell. However, in both cases, water uptake and swelling continues for about 3 days (4).

II.   STATE OF WATER IN THE STRATUM CORNEUM

An increase in hydration of the skin is associated with a swelling of the stratum corneum and a softening of its texture. Consistent with its low diffusion coefficient in SC, water does not ooze from the surface of freshly excised skin. Most studies have used direct-weighing techniques to define the "water holding" capacity of the SC (6,9). Figure 2a shows the topography of the skin before and Figure 2b shows it after hydration following the application of a plastic occlusive

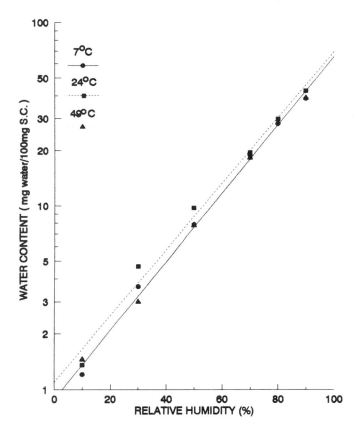

Figure 1 Semilogarithmic plot of water humidity versus relative humidity. (Adapted from Ref. 6.)

dressing—Saran Wrap. After a 16 h application the skin has swollen quite markedly, as illustrated by scanning electron microscopy (SEM) (Fig. 2b). This has also been demonstrated by Harris, who suggests that SC not only swells, but develops multiple folds, resulting in a 37% increase in surface area (10).

Few workers have attempted to differentiate between water that is chemically or physically "bound" with the SC and that which exists as free of "bulk" water (10–12). *Bound water* has been defined as "that part of the total which is not available to dissolve water soluble nonelectrolytes" (13). It is generally accepted that the unbound or free water accounts for 70–80% (11,12) of the total water in the SC (i.e., 20–30% of the water is bound).

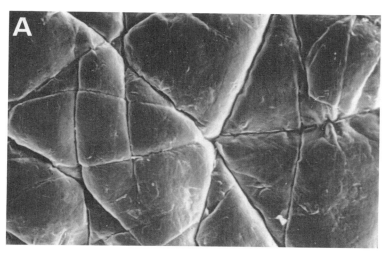

Figure 2a   SEM (×100) demonstrating the microtopography of normal human skin.

Water is strongly bound to the keratin in the SC. Only 35 and 55% of the water is removed from fresh sheep skin and soaked sheep skin, respectively, when subjected to a centrifugal force of 10,000 g (14). At low moisture levels, water is held to high-energy-binding sites of wool keratin by groups such as –OH, –COOH, or NH_3 (15). The initial differential net heat of sorption is very high and consistent with high-binding energy for water. When more water is absorbed, the heat of sorption falls, indicating weaker-binding energies. It has been demonstrated that peptide groups are responsible for a considerable part of the water uptake from the vapor phase in proteins (16). Hence, at a low-water content the equilibrium absorption of water by SC may occur as a single water molecule–keratin interaction, whereas at high-water content there are also water–water interactions or a "condensation" in the SC cells. The affinity of the SC for water may be due to hygroscopic components, collectively known as *the natural moisturing factor* (NMF), as suggested by Jacobi (17).

The relative importance of the free and bound water in the SC has been studied by several techniques (10–12,18). Bulgin and Vinson (10) used differential thermal analysis (DTA) on human and neonatal rat skin and suggested that free water produced a peak near 100°C in hydrated samples. Bound water was thought to be responsible for the transition at 115°C and possibly at 135°C. However, the transition near 135°C appeared independent of water content, whereas the transition at 115°C increased with sample water content. More recent work suggests these transitions are due to protein denaturation (19).

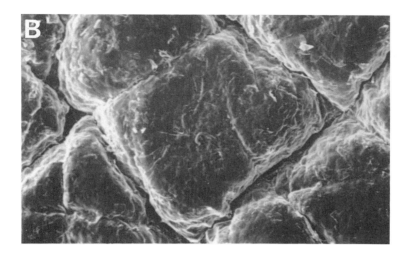

Figure 2b SEM (×100) demonstrating the microtopography of normal human skin following 16 h application of Saran Wrap.

Thermomechanical analysis (TMA) measures the water melting transition in hydrated SC and is based on the linear displacement in a sample caused by viscoelastic or dimensional changes occurring because of increases in temperature. Wilkes and Wildnauer observed a softening between −20° and 60°C and a high modulus value at either temperature. Figure 3 shows the modulus plotted against temperature in human samples hydrated to 10%. Two transitions occur: near 14° and 40°C (20). A transition near 0°C would be anticipated for free water (i.e., not bound to protein) to be consistent with unpublished differential scanning calorimetry (DSC) data. The discrepancy suggests bound water in the SC and that the water content may act as "a plasticizer molecule with respect to mechanical behavior" (20).

A Cahn microbalance has been used by Scheuplein and Morgan (18) to study the desorption of water from SC membranes. The corneum was initially soaked in water for periods of up to 24 h so that the first stage of desorption was a rapid loss of surface water (Fig. 4). After this first phase, the desorption slowed abruptly and remained fairly constant, whereas the bulk of its water content (600%) was lost over several hours. The slow phase is attributed to the loss of bound water— accounting for as much as five times the dry weight of the tissue. A further transition in the desorption curve (not shown in the figure) also occurs and can be attributed to the desorption of "5–10% of water strongly bound to the polar groups

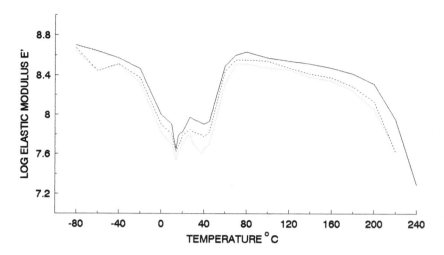

Figure 3   Human stratum corneum hydrated to 10%. (Adapted from Ref. 20.)

of the side chains of keratin" (19). However, the method does have limitations and may underestimate the actual bound water content (18).

Other estimates of the strongly bound water are about two to three times higher. DSC yields a relative amount of bound water in both guinea pig foot pad and human SC of 29 and 34%, respectively (12). Hansen and Yellin (11), using infrared spectroscopy and deuterated water, found a similar bound water fraction of between 30 and 35%. Three optical density (OD) vibrations were identified in spectra between −50° and 30°C: a free water peak at 2432 cm⁻¹, a strongly bound water peak at 2360 cm⁻¹ (which they attributed to primary hydration of polar protein sites), and a less lightly bound water peak at 2481 cm⁻¹. The free water peak (2432 cm⁻¹) was not apparent until the water content had exceeded about 38%, in agreement with other studies (12).

Solvent extraction of the corneum lipids has produced contrasting results (12,18). Walkley, in his studies of the guinea pig foot pad, extracted the lipids with ether/water, and reported that the bound water increased by 41% (12). The increase was attributed to the exposure of water–protein-binding sites on removal of the lipids. However, lipid extraction studies with either hexane or chloroform/ methanol (2:1) have suggested that SC retains essentially no bound water (see Fig. 4D) and behaves like wet filter paper (18).

Proton nuclear magnetic resonance (¹H-NMR) spectroscopy results suggest that the solvent used in SC extraction is of vital importance (21). A decrease in the

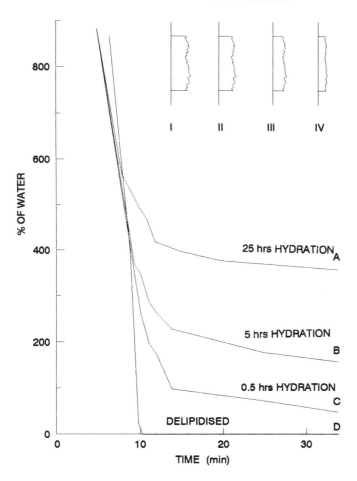

Figure 4 Water desorption curves for human stratum corneum. (Adapted from Ref. 18.)

bound water content of hairless rat SC is observed following extraction with water, chloroform/methanol (2:1), or 1% sodium dodecyl sulfate (SDS) aqueous solution. However, no changes in the bound water content occur with acetone/ether (1:1) extraction (Fig. 5). A 15% reduction in dry weight is observed following acetone/ether extraction, whereas a 40% reduction is observed with the remaining treatments. It is suggested that the natural moisturing factor (NMF) components, such as amino acids and pyrollidone carboxylate contribute to the enhancement of bound water. The two lipid solvent extractions probably extracted

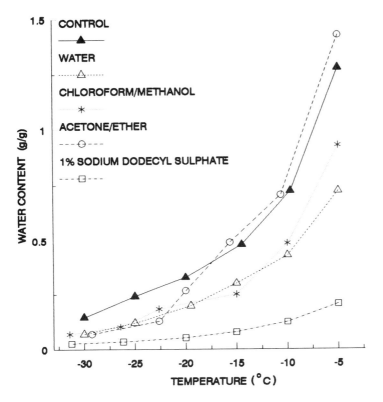

Figure 5 Hairless rat stratum corneum following various extraction procedures. Estimation of bound water content. (Adapted from Ref. 21.)

these components, whereas the acetone/ether fraction did not—given that the extract from the latter contained minimal amino acids. Therefore, it is suggested that most of the protein and possibly NMF components are still present and, consequently, the number of binding sites available increase (21). In contrast, the chloroform/methanol extraction contained large amounts of free amino acids and the more polar lipids, such as sphingomyelin (21). Hence, structured polar lipids and moisturing factors are crucial to the water-holding properties of the SC.

It has been suggested that anionic surfactants may alter the physical state of water in the skin by greatly reducing the amount of bound water, as demonstrated in desorption experiments (11,22). This allows easier movement of charged hydrophilic substances across the SC (23). They appear to have the ability to bind strongly to protein, causing a reversible denaturation and uncoiling of the filaments. This leads to gross expansion of the tissue, making the diffusion of water easier through the unbound water region (24). An alternative mechanism has been proposed by Walters, who suggests that the surfactant acts on the intercellular corneum lipids. He showed that, following hydration of hairless mouse for up to 72 h with both saline and surfactants, the enhancing effect of the surfactant on the penetration rate of methyl nicotinate was not evident beyond 24 h hydration. This data suggests "that the mode of action of the surfactant and that of hydration is similar and primarily on the lipid phase of the membrane" (25).

III. DRY SKIN

The hydration of the skin can be affected by both the ambient environmental conditions and by the effects of applied agents on the properties of the SC. Dry skin, for instance, arises mainly from a lack of the natural moisturizing factor, which is either deficient or has been removed chemically (6). It is exacerbated by a low humidity and lack of sebum (26). Although dry skin is a very common skin complaint, it is very difficult to reproduce experimentally. Singer and Vinson have tried to experimentally produce "housewive's eczema" by immersion of human forearms in water three times daily over an extended period. They succeeded in producing only erythematous reactions on the volar surfaces of the arms, with no irritation observed on the hands and wrists (6).

Some of the earliest clinical observations of dry skin were performed by Gaul and Underwood (5). They demonstrated that chapping could be related to changes in temperature and humidity. They observed that during the colder winter months, with skin temperatures reaching 20°C or below, chapping occurred.

Similar observations have been observed in vitro by the classic experiments of Blank (3,22,27), showing that the water content varied with RH. Pliability was reduced below 60% RH, and he postulated that a minimum of 10% water content was critical to maintain pliability and flexibility. Other workers have subsequently confirmed these earlier studies in a variety of mammalian skin types. These include human (28), neonatal rat (6), and guinea pig foot pad (8). The functional state of the cutaneous barrier also indicates the insensible transepidermal water loss to the atmosphere. There have been many excellent reviews on this subject (29–31), and the interested reader is referred to these for further information.

It has been suggested that sebum, in the presence of insensible perspiration and secretory perspiration, may not act simply as an impervious lipid layer at the skin surface, preventing water evaporation, but may act as an emulsifying agent, allowing the skin to extract water as and when required (27). This hypothesis was put forward by Sulzberger, who indicated that a lipid emulsifier of water-in-oil and possibly oil-in-water is present at the skin surface. This "watery phase" presents the skin with its own hydration reservoir. He further suggested that this reservoir is likely to be greater in the warmer summer months and, therefore, may reduce the instances of chapping (27).

Studies performed by Potts and Buras (33) and Tagami and co-workers (33) have also demonstrated that the SC is more hydrated during the summer months. The former workers measured moisture content changes by monitoring the dynamic mechanical properties as a function of frequency. They showed that under ambient conditions there was a lower moisture content measured because of lower RH values found indoors in winter and that this was age-dependent (32). They suggest that skin aging is accompanied by a decrease in the moisture content of the SC. The latter group, using a similar noninvasive method, assessed hydration by electrical impedance measurements. They also concluded the SC had higher levels of hydration in the summer (33).

Downing and coworkers comment that "there is an intuitive belief that low sebum secretion is a cause, or at least a predisposing factor, in dry skin" (26). However, they have argued that at both ends of the human age span [i.e., under 6 years and in elderly subjects (aged 65–97)] there is no relation (lowest sebum levels) or correlation (sebum secretion rate), respectively, with dry skin conditions (26). These authors also stress that human sebum does not resemble any other mammalian species, a fact that must be borne in mind if performing animal experiments.

Other methods to examine skin's flexibility and pliability under different environmental conditions have included measurements of the corneum's rheological properties. A definition of a plasticizer has already been put forward by Van Duzee (34) whereby he suggests that if water actually plasticizes skin, this may not necessarily be a function of its thermodynamic activity, but may be dependent on its total content. By treating the skin with 3 M lithium bromide, he showed that this had no effect on the transition temperature of either the lipid or protein components, yet increased the water content above that of the controls. This he ascribed to lithium bromide's ability to increase hydration owing to its hygroscopicity (i.e., water is absorbed onto the skin surface). He also studied NMF-extracted skin (treated for 5 min with ether, followed by 24 h water extraction) and observed that this had no effect on SC transition temperatures. These results imply that NMF does not bind or significantly interact with protein, as confirmed by Yamamara and Tezuka (21), but because of its natural hygroscopicity, allows water to be absorbed into the SC.

Rheologically, SC appears to perform in a manner similar to fibrous proteins, over a temperature range of approximately 0°–50°C (35). Studies on elastin, fully swollen over a similar temperature range, have shown a similar invariant change in modulus (35). More recently, Takahashi (36) has demonstrated that as the RH increases, the elastic modulus decreases, with an abrupt decrease at 60% RH (Fig. 6). The loss modulus was also reduced. Dielectric constant values also rose

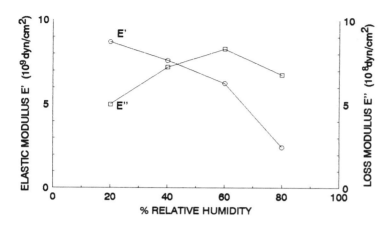

Figure 6 Elastic (E') and loss (E'') modulus for human stratum corneum at 25°C. (Adapted from Ref. 36.)

sharply above 50% RH. According to Takahashi, these results suggest that water is strongly bound, with little freedom of movement. He has applied a clustering theory, proposed by Zimm (37), to determine the extent that water molecules may cluster at sorption equilibrium. If the value of the function is positive, he suggests that there is a tendency for water molecules to cluster; a negative value indicates local sorption between functional groups of keratin and water. Apparently, there was a change from a negative to positive value observed at 60% RH. This suggests that free water may break hydrogen bonds in keratin, which leads to the skin becoming plasticized. At reduced RH values, keratin is immobilized by hydrogen bonding, yet with increasing RH, clusters of water break the hydrogen bonds within the keratin.

IV. CLOTHING EFFECTS

Clothing may also influence SC hydration. The body temperature varies by 1.5°C during the day, in spite of clothing and ambient temperature (38) as a result of (a) heat production from chemical reaction, (b) heat loss by physical routes, and (c) thermoregulation (i.e., sweating, shivering, muscular activity).

Below 25°C the ambient nude body loses more heat than it produces. This stimulates peripheral receptors and thermoregulates and reduces blood flow, as well as induces piloerection, to reduce air movement, trap any residual air, and insulate the body. In the temperature range 25–29°C, vasomotor control is predominant. With sweating and reduced convection, heat loss increases as the temperature is increased to 35°C. Above 35°C, heat is lost almost entirely by evaporation. Both protective and cosmetic clothing influence the levels of water or water vapor at or around the skin surface, dependent on the degree of water resistance of the clothing. When clothing absorbs water, there is a tendency for the material to collapse and "attach" itself to the skin surface. It is our experience that the wearability of protective gloves is probably of more concern than the barrier properties of the skin itself.

V. WATER TRANSPORT

The permeability constant of water through the SC is approximately 0.5×10^{-3} cm·hr^{-1}, which corresponds to a flux from pure water of 0.2 mg·cm^{-2}·h^{-1} (27). Given an SC thickness of 27 μm after 24 hr, the diffusion constant is about 3.0×10^{-10} cm^2·sec^{-1} (4). The self-diffusion coefficient for water is about five orders of magnitude lower at 2×10^{-5} cm^2·sec^{-1} (39). At lower or higher degrees of SC hydration, both the thickness of the SC and the diffusion coefficient of water are affected. After 3 days of hydration, the SC thickness is about 40 μm and the permeability constant 0.5×10^{-3} cm·hr^{-1} (4). However, comparing human SC water permeability with that of hairless mouse SC, it has been demonstrated that the permeability coefficient for human SC remains relatively constant over 3 days. In comparison, hairless mouse SC showed marked improvement after 24 hr (Fig. 7; 60-62). In contrast, the dry SC is about 8 μm thick, and the permeability constant is 1.17 cm·hr^{-1}. The high permeability constant for dry SC reflects the very affinity of dry SC for water, yielding a stratum corneum–water partition coefficient (K) of 2560. The value for K for water when the SC is fully hydrated is 0.88 (4). If one uses the relation: permeability coefficient = partition coefficient × diffusion coefficient/thickness, the diffusion coefficient (D) can be estimated for each condition by appropriate rearrangement and substitution of values. The values obtained for D are 1×10^{-10}, 3×10^{-10}, and 6.3×10^{-10} cm^2·sec^{-1} for nil, 1 day, and 3 days hydration of human SC.

Further insight into the effect of varying hydration on water permeability through SC is provided by Blank (40). In his experiments, only water vapor came in contact with both sides of SC mounted in a diffusion cell. He suggests that the diffusion coefficient and permeability coefficient increase by factors of 2 and 3, respectively, between the relative humidities of 46 and 93%. The SC thickness changes from 11.1 to 15.6 μm and the SC–water partition coefficient from 0.135 to 0.413 over this range (40). Of interest is the relation between thickness and the water content in the SC generated both in vitro and in vivo by different relative humidities (Fig. 8).

The mechanism by which water moves across the SC is still the subject of debate. Scheuplein reported a similar permeability for water, methanol, and

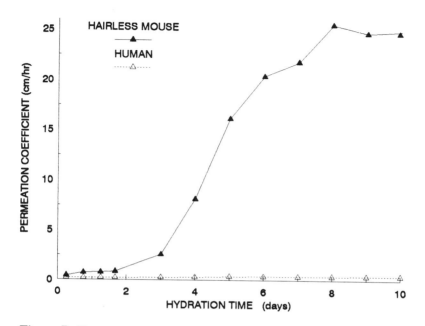

Figure 7 Human and hairless mouse stratum corneum hydration over 10-day period of hydration. (Adapted from Ref. 60 and 62.)

ethanol across SC. He suggested that these solutes may be rate-limited in their transport by the hydrated intercellular keratin (4). The activation energy for these solutes is $16.5 \pm 2 \text{ kcal·mol}^{-1}$. In contrast, the activation energies for the lipophilic alcohols decrease to $10 \pm 2 \text{ kcal·mol}^{-1}$, leading Scheuplein to propose a lipid pathway (4). Roberts and co-workers (41) suggested that a more likely explanation of this phenomenon was a single, more polar lipid barrier with aqueous diffusion layers contributing to the overall resistance when the solute becomes more lipophilic. Potts and Guy (42) have suggested that the constant permeability coefficient of water, methanol, and ethanol is accounted for by a lipid barrier, provided the dependence of the solute diffusion coefficient on molecular volume is considered. Correction for this effect has led to the conclusion that the mechanism for transport of most solutes through SC and other lipid membranes is by the tortuous intercellular lipid pathway.

Given that water is the SC plasticizer (4), the amount of water in a bilayer and its distribution are important determinants of water permeability. Within the intercellular spaces, the presence of water is associated with the polar head groups. The binding of water to these groups may lead to an expansion of the

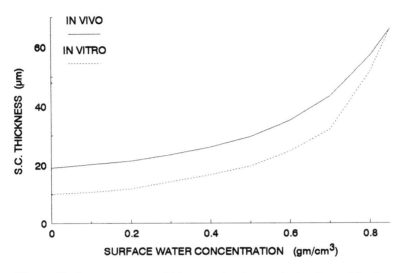

Figure 8 Stratum corneum thickness estimations under in vitro and in vivo conditions. (Adapted from Ref. 40.)

lateral packing, relative to that of the hydrocarbon chain, and an increase in the surface area that each lipid molecule occupies within the bilayer (43,44). Bouwstra and co-workers have recently used x-ray diffraction and shown that there is no apparent swelling of the lipid bilayers in the presence of water (45,46). Thus, it is possible that there may be an increase in the mean interfacial area of the headgroup, if water incorporates itself into the polar head group region, but this does not necessarily change the alkyl (hydrocarbon) chain length. The increase in surface area may result in lateral swelling, or expansion, of the headgroup region relative to that of the hydrocarbon chains (47). If the overall density does not change, then there may be some shortening of the chain length as the chains become possibly more fluid. It, therefore, follows that if there is swelling of the head groups with increasing hydration, they may be compensated for by a reduction in overall chain length, possibly by bending, allowing the overall distance of the bilayer to remain constant. Seddon, has suggested that "the hydrocarbon chains do not passively fill any volume accessible to them, rather they maintain nearly identical conformational state at a given temperature, independent of the shape of the aggregate" (47).

Hence, one theory is that hydration causes an increased permeability by aqueous solvation of the intercellular lipids, in particular the glycosphingolipids and ceramides. The demonstration that hydration was less marked in the nail plate, in which the lipid content is less than 1% compared with 10% lipid in SC (48), has been used in support of this proposal.

An alternative theory could also be proposed on the rapid and extensive uptake of water into the SC. Clearly, much of the water is binding to the keratin in the cells. A general swelling of the bricks in a bricks-and-mortar model will cause a loosening of the mortar and an increased movement through the intercellular route. Changes in lipid mobility would also be anticipated in this process. This theory is not in contradiction with either the tortuous lipid pathway or hydrated intracellular keratin route. It simply argues that hydration may be a general plasticization of the SC, increasing the diffusion of water by whatever route the solute permeates through the SC.

VI. SOLUTE TRANSPORT AND HYDRATION

Scheuplein and Blank have presented data for the diffusion coefficients of alcohols in SC after absorption of a vapor into dry SC, from aqueous solutions through SC, to an aqueous receptor, and from pure solutions through SC, to aqueous solutions (4, 76). Their results are shown in Figure 9. The diffusion coefficient of alcohols through fully hydrated SC is more than ten times that for dry SC for all solutes, and twice that for partially hydrated SC (carbon number >3). There is no apparent change in diffusion coefficient with hydration for alcohols with carbon numbers between 1 and 16.

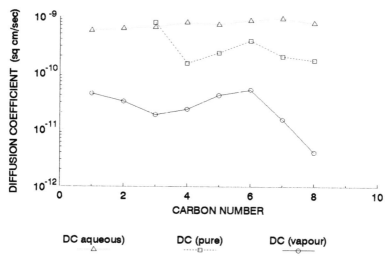

Figure 9 Diffusion coefficients in stratum corneum from vapor, pure and aqueous solutions: Δ, DC aqueous; ▫, DC pure; ○, DC vapor. (Data adapted from Ref. 4 and 76.)

More recently, Roberts (49) reported the relation between the permeability coefficients of several phenols and various vehicles, in terms of the effects of hydration. Given that the SC water content could not be measured directly, he expressed the vehicles in terms of the relative humidities generated and plotted by permeability as a function of percentage RH (Fig. 10). If the relation shown in Figure 1 is valid (6), his relation suggests that the permeability coefficient is directly related to SC water content. In reality, a convex relation between diffusion coefficient and SC water concentration probably exists, as suggested by Blank (40).

Other authors have suggested that penetration rates can be related to relative humidity, for other solutes could be related to the RH. Fritsch and Stroughton (50)

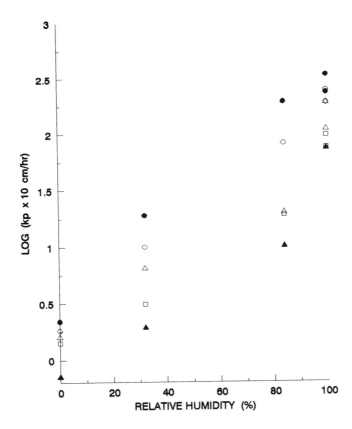

Figure 10 Phenolic compound permeability as a function of relative humidity: ●, benzyl alcohol; ○, phenol; Δ, O-chlorophenol; ▲, chlorocresol; ☐, p-ethyl phenol. (Adapted from Ref. 49.)

and Vickers (51) suggested increased permeability for aspirin and sodium fusidate, respectively, at higher relative humidities. Other studies on hydration include those of Wurster on methyl ethyl ketone, in which he showed a high penetration rate in hydrated SC in vivo, relative to normal or dehydrated SC (52). In general, an increase in the relative humidity from 50 to 100% increases the penetration of substances, such as triamcinolone acetonide, fluocinolone acetonide, and hydrocortisone, by about tenfold (53).

It is also apparent from Figure 10 that hydration appears to increase the penetration of all phenols by a similar magnitude. McKenzie (54), in a study of the effect of hydration on the percutaneous absorption of steroids, concluded that hydration produced no preferential absorption of highly water-soluble compounds. Hawkins and Reifenrath (55) have suggested that an increase in relative humidity promotes the penetration of polar solutes [N,N-diethyl-m-toluamide, caffeine, and malathion]. The changes, however, are very small (Fig. 11). Less or no change is

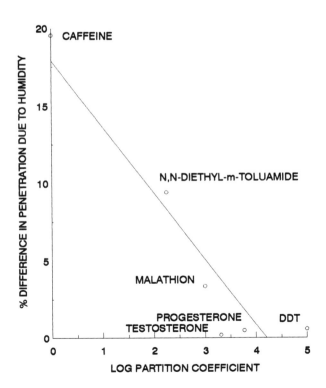

Figure 11 Plot of percutaneous penetration percentage difference versus log P. (Adapted from Ref. 55.)

observed for the penetration of the more lipophilic compounds (progesterone, testosterone, and DDT; 55).

In addition to affecting the diffusivity of solutes, hydration will affect the partitioning and solubility of solutes in the stratum corneum. It could be anticipated, for instance, that polar substances would have a greater solubility (relative to nonpolar substances) in hydrated stratum corneum than in dehydrated stratum corneum. The observation by Wurster and Kramer (56) that hydration aided the absorption of pure glycol salicylate to a greater extent than methyl or ethyl salicylate (Fig. 12) would be consistent with effects of hydration on solubility.

The results obtained for the alcohols and phenols for human SC can be compared and contrasted with results reported for rat skin. Behl and coworkers have suggested that hydration had little effect on the permeation of water, methanol, and ethanol through hairless mouse skin (57). An increased permeability of the more lipophilic alcohols is associated with an increase in the hydration time. A change of about twofold in the lipophilic alcohols is, however, consistent with the

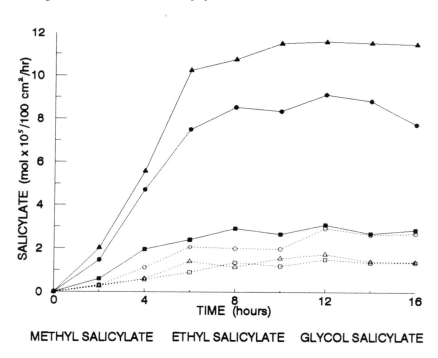

Figure 12   Effect of hydration on the absorption of salicylate esters. Methyl salicylate: ●, hydrated systems, ○, anhydrous system. Ethyl salicylate: ■, hydrated system, □, anhydrous system. Glycol salicylate: ▲, hydrated system, Δ, anhydrous system. (Adapted from Ref. 56.)

twofold increase in permeability of butyric acid through human SC, as reported by Scheuplein and Blank (4).

Behl concludes "there may be a pronounced molecular size sensitivity to hydration" (58). Later work by Behl (58), using Swiss mouse skin, reported that hydration induced increases in the permeability coefficients for water, methanol, and ethanol. As stated by Behl, "it is difficult to interpret these collective observations" (58). In contrast with these observations, Barry suggests that hydration of human cadaver skin by occlusion had little effect on the permeation of mannitol, ibuprofen, and flurbiprofen (53). Although explanations, such as enhanced transfollicular penetration, may be put forward to explain the animal data, the work also raises the dilemma of whether animal skin can ever be an appropriate model for human skin. Several workers have demonstrated the fragility of hairless mouse skin (59–62) to a wide range of compounds. Bond and Barry have suggested, following long-term hydration studies, that any experiment beyond 72 hr should not be conducted on hairless mouse skin. By comparison, human skin maintains its integrity and strength for approximately 200 hr under the same experimental conditions (60).

They also showed that the permeability of the hairless mouse skin was increased 50-fold by hydration, the effects being similar to tape-stripping of the SC barrier. In contrast, human SC was relatively unaffected (62).

Hence, in conclusion, the effects of hydration on the penetration rate of solutes with varying molecular size and polarity remains equivocal. The major sources of this variation appears to be the type of skin used. Some work suggests hydration facilitates the penetration of lipophilic solutes through hairless mouse skin (57) and may be due to a size effect. However, this work contrasts with their later work through fuzzy rat skin (58), for which hydration increased the penetration rate of the polar compounds. In contrast, the work of Wurster and Kramer (56) suggests that the penetration of pure polar compounds through human skin is facilitated by hydration. In general, the available data on human skin permeability are consistent with hydration causing a significant increase in permeability in the relatively solute-structure independent fashion. A major consideration in resolving the role of hydration on structure–permeation relation is the relative contributions of the partition coefficient and diffusion coefficient.

VII. VEHICLE EFFECTS

Probably the most widely investigated external method of affecting hydration is that of occlusion with plastic films, especially for steroids. McKenzie and Stoughton (63) showed that a plastic film over applied steroids leads to a 100-fold increase in absorption, compared with simple topical application.

With the introduction of more sophisticated analytical equipment, in particular Fourier transform infrared spectroscopy, it is now possible to quantitatively determine SC water concentration both in vivo and in vitro (64,65). By occluding the skin with hydrocolloid adhesive dressings having a range of water-uptake properties, it has been demonstrated that dressings with low water vapor measurements cause greater SC hydration in vivo (Fig. 13; 65).

Topical vehicles may also act as "occlusive dressings," if they contain fats and oils, reducing water loss to the atmosphere. This increases the water content of the SC and can promote drug penetration. Often skin commercial products promote "skin-softening" capabilities based on the presumption that these formulations actually increase the moisture content. These formulations often contain humectants, such as glycerol or propylene glycol, which are distinctly hygroscopic and may actually withdraw water from the skin. Powers and Fox demonstrated that one such product resulted in a water loss of up to 56% (66).

Recent studies by Friberg and coworkers have suggested that at low ambient humidity (i.e., 6% RH) glycerol does not act as a humectant, but maintains intercellular lipids in a liquid crystalline state. With use of an in vitro mixture of SC lipids, he proposed that glycerol, being a small polar molecule, interacts with the polar head groups of the bilayer, rather than by penetrating the alkyl chains (67). In vivo studies have demonstrated similar improved skin conditioning, under which glycerol was found to penetrate and accumulate in SC (68). Washing with

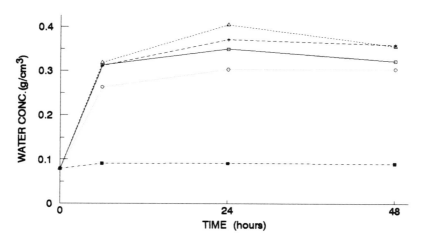

Figure 13   A plot of stratum corneum hydration against time following occlusion with adhesive dressings: □, Actiderm; Δ, prototype B; ○, prototype A; *, Blenderm; ■, control.

soap and water did not remove it, and long-term benefits included both a visible improvement and reduced skin surface roughness.

Skin keratin has an isoelectric point between 3.7 and 4.5, indicating that alteration of the pH of the vehicle may alter skin hydration. However, studies performed on neonatal rats (6), hairless mouse skin (69), and human fingernails and skin (70), have demonstrated that only at pHs above 10 was there evidence of increased water penetration. Therefore, vehicle pH does not appear to affect skin hydration under the normal physiological conditions encountered (i.e., those that do not cause skin irritation and obvious damage).

More recent work by Loden and Lindberg suggests that different types of moisturizers (petroleum and three oil-and-water creams containing humectant agents) increased the skin capacitance by the same magnitude 2 hr after application (71). Removal of the excess product reduced the capacitance for the cream sites, but not for the petrolatum-treated sites. This work contrasts with that of Dempski (72) in which oil-in-water emulsions were less occlusive than a polymer film, petrolatum, or isopropyl myristate gel. Oil baths increase the skin surface lipids for about 3 hr and result in an increased binding of water (12–27%) to the SC (73).

In general, as summarized in Table 1, greases or oils or impermeable plastic induce the greatest occlusion and hydration. Water-in-oil emulsions are less occlusive, whereas volatile solvents (e.g., alcohol) may dry. A humectant will dehydrate the SC and decrease penetration in a low RH environment. Powders increase the surface area and evaporation rate of water, effectively reducing the extent of hydration (74).

Any evaluation of vehicle effects on SC permeability should separate drug–vehicle interactions from vehicle–skin interactions. Roberts and Anderson have suggested that the contribution of the drug–vehicle component may be assessed from the permeability coefficient of the solute through an inert membrane, such as polyethylene (75). The ratio of the permeability coefficient of the solvent through skin to that through polyethylene will be at a constant "baseline" value if the vehicle does not affect the skin. In studies with phenol as a solute, a baseline of 2 was obtained for light liquid paraffin, arachis oil, and glycerol. A ratio of 4 for water corresponds to a twofold increase in permeability because of hydration. The high values for ethanol, dimethyl sulfoxide (DMSO), and dimethyl formamide correspond to the known enhancement in permeability caused by these vehicles. With ethanol, for instance, the diffusion coefficient from the pure alcohol is 2.9 times that for aqueous solutions (76). Roberts and Anderson have suggested an enhancement of 2 for ethanol, using their method (75). More recently, Roberts has suggested that high concentrations of pentanol decrease its self-penetration flux through human epidermis by hydration, using the ratio of flux: epidermis/inert membrane technique (49). Such a conclusion is consistent with the vehicle effects

Table 1   Expected Vehicle Effects on Skin Permeability and Hydration

Vehicle	Examples	Skin permeability	Skin hydration
Humectant	Glycols, glycerols	+/–	–
Powder	Clays, shake lotions	NE	–*
Oil/water (O/W) emulsion	Aqueous creams	+?	+?
Water/oil (W/O) emulsion	Oily creams	+	+
Emulsifying base	Anhydrous lipid + O/W emulsifiers	++	++
Absorption base	Anhydrous lipid ± W/O emulsifiers	++	++
Lipophilic	Fats, waxes, oils, silicones	++	++
Occlusive dressing	Saran Wrap	+++	+++

–   Decreased effect (*decrease in excessive hydration)
NE No (or little) effect
+?   Slight increase
+   Increase
++ Marked increase
+++ Excessive (total) hydration

of pure alcohols relative to aqueous solutions on alcohol self-diffusion coefficients in human epidermis. The mean diffusion coefficient ratio (aqueous/pure alcohol solution) is 3.4 ± 1.4, based on the data of Scheuplein and Blank (76).

Hence, although vehicle effects on percutaneous penetration are often interpreted in terms of solute availability or the vehicle damaging the skin, the vehicle also affects percutaneous penetration by modulating hydration.

VIII. INTERSUBJECT VARIABILITY

Berardesca has shown the SC water content, skin extensibility, recovery, and elastic modulus differed markedly among races (77). The differences were not accounted for by the site of study or presence of hair. The SC water content and skin elasticity are also affected by *aging* (78). It is suggested that a reduction in blood flow and water supply, together with defective SC water binding, cause a reduced SC water content and TEWL. In elderly patients with dry skin, skin hydration can be increased to the control group by appropriate local treatment (79).

An impaired barrier function can arise in *diaper dermatitis*, as a result of occlusion, which increases skin hydration. Impairment is further enhanced by an increase in skin pH and the effect of fecal enzymes on the SC (80).

Dry-looking skin of unknown etiology also occurs in most patients with *chronic renal failure*. A lower water content in the SC is apparent when pruritus is present, but the hydration of the SC does not account for the differences in skin texture between uremic patients and healthy subjects (81).

Patients with *atopic dermatitis* have a lower preexposure barrier function and higher TEWL following irritant exposure than a group with allergic contact dermatitis and a control group. Clinically, patients with dry skin in this group are more susceptible to irritant damage than the control group (82).

Diseased corneum contain lower levels of water (7). In *senile xerotic* skin and *psoriasis vulgaris*, the water content is 32 and 28%, respectively, compared with about 38% in normal skin (Fig. 14). It is suggested that the maximum amount of secondary (bound) water in normal skin is 20–30% greater than that found in pathological skin (7). Takenouchi also suggests that the free amino acids present in the soluble components are greatly reduced in pathological specimens (7). Associated with the decreased water content of the SC, the TEWL in psoriasis patients is higher than normal (85).

Scoggins and Kliman examined the absorption of several steroids applied to areas of dermatitis, with and without occlusion. They commented that "without an occlusive dressing, systemically significant amounts of these substances are absorbed only if the dose applied is very large" (86).

IX. MODIFYING HYDRATION IN SKIN DISORDERS

The general axiom often presented in the treatment of dermatological disorders is "if it's wet, use a wet dressing and if it's dry, use a salve (ointment)." Hence, baths or wet dressings are frequently used in acute eczema when weeping, vesiculation, and crusting are present. A possible danger is overdrying, as can occur with calamine lotion. In subacute conditions, such as psoriasis, emollient creams are frequently used, with steroids being the most common medicament. Chronic dry skin, such as ichthyosis, is frequently managed using creams or ointments, sometimes containing powders. A slowing of water loss in dry skin conditions by emollients is one means of replenishing and maintaining at least 10% water in the SC so it can remain soft and flexible.

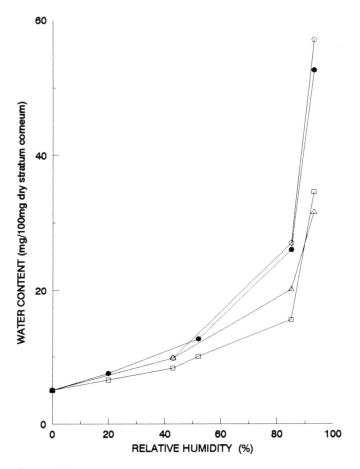

Figure 14   Relation between normal and pathological stratum corneum: •, control SC; ○, plantar SC; □, xerosis senilis; Δ, psoriasis. (Adapted from Ref. 7.)

Although astringents, such as zinc oxide, are commonly used to reduce exudation, we are not aware of studies on their effects on SC water and permeability. A similar concern applies with keratolytics, such as salicylic acid. The changes in the permeation rate of salicylic acid with repeated application have been reported (87).

The decrease in the skin/dimethyl polysiloxane membrane ratio at higher salicylic acid concentrations has been ascribed to "the suspended salicylic acid particles reducing the occlusive properties of the hydrophilic ointment or to a dehydrating effect of the salicylic acid" (87). More work is needed on the effects of astringents, keratolytics, and other agents on SC water content and permeability. More of the type of work, reported in Figure 13, will be expected to be applied to a wider range of "therapeutically active" as well as nonactive vehicles in the future.

X. CONCLUSION

Hydration increases the permeability of the SC to several solutes. One of the proposed mechanisms for the facilitation of transport is by water being absorbed into the SC where it acts as a plasticizer in its bound state. Many of the current therapies for dry skin are based on maintaining water content in the SC by reducing the evaporation rate (e.g., by occlusive dressings).

However, the penetration rates of therapeutically applied solutes through diseased skin are not well-defined in terms of the combined effects of the vehicle and disease on SC water content and permeability. Much of the future experimentation on hydration in percutaneous penetration needs to be directed toward the more difficult, but most clinically pertinent, diseased and dry skin in vivo. Toxicology will also be a more important consideration in the future, especially for environmental or industrial products being used at high humidities with minimal protection.

ACKNOWLEDGMENTS

One of us (MSR) acknowledges the support of the National Health and Medical Research Council (Australia) and the Northern NSW and Queensland Lions Kidney and Medical Research Foundation for their support.

REFERENCES

1. Zwolinski, B. J., Eyring, H., and Reece, C. E. Diffusion and membrane permeability. *J. Phys. Coll. Chem.* 53:1426–1453 (1949).
2. Scheuplein, R. J. Skin as a barrier. In *The Physiology and Pathophysiology of the Skin*, Vol. 5. Jarrett, A. (ed.). Academic Press, New York, pp. 1693-1730 (1978).
3. Blank, I. H. Factors influencing water content of stratum corneum. *J. Invest. Dermatol.* 18:433–440 (1952).
4. Scheuplein, R. J. and Blank, I. H. Permeability of the skin. *Physiol. Rev.* 51:702-747 (1971).
5. Gaul, L. E. and Underwood, G. B. Relation of dew point and barometric pressure to chapping of normal skin. *J. Invest. Dermatol.* 18:9–18 (1951).
6. Singer, E. J. and Vinson, L. J. The water binding properties of skin. *Proc. Sci. Sect. Toilet Goods Assoc.* 46:29–33 (1966).

7. Takenouchi, M., Suzuki, H., and Tagami, H. Hydration characteristics of pathologic stratum corneum—evaluation of bound water. *J. Invest. Dermatol.* 87:574–576 (1986).
8. Middleton, J. The mechanism of water binding in stratum corneum. *Br. J. Dermatol.* 80:437–450 (1968).
9. Harris, D. R., Papa, C. M., and Stanton, R. Percutaneous absorption and the surface area of occluded skin. *Br. J. Dermatol.* 91:27–32 (1974).
10. Bulgin, J. J. and Vinson, L. J. The use of differential thermal analysis to study the bound water in stratum corneum membranes. *Biochim. Biophys. Acta 136*:551–560 (1967).
11. Hansen, J. R. and Yellin, W. NMR and infrared spectroscopic studies of stratum corneum hydration. In *Water Structure at the Water Polymer Interface.* Jellinck, H. H. G. (ed.). Plenum Press, New York, pp. 19–28 (1972).
12. Walkley, K. Bound water in stratum corneum measured by differential scanning calorimetry. *J. Invest. Dermatol.* 59:225–227 (1972).
13. Yates, J. R. Mechanism of water uptake by skin.In *Biophysical Properties of the Skin.* H. R. Eldon (ed.), Wiley Interscience, New York, pp. 485–512 (1971).
14. Yates, J. R. Investigations into the controlled drying of sheepskins II. Effect of drying conditions on various properties of the skins. *J. Am. Leather Chem. Assoc. 61*:235–400 (1966).
15. Watt, I. C., Kennett, R. H., and James, J. F. P. The dry weight of wool. *Textile Res. J. 29*:975 (1959).
16. Mellar, E. F., Korn, A. H., and Hoover, S. R. Water absorption of protein III, contribution of the peptide group. *J. Am. Chem. Soc. 70*:3040–3044 (1948).
17. Jacobi, O. K. About the mechanism of moisture regulation in the horny layer of the skin. *Proc. Sci. Sect. Toilet Goods Assoc. 31*:22–23 (1959).
18. Scheuplein, R. J. and Morgan, L. J. "Bound water" in keratin membranes measured by a microbalance technique. *Nature 214*:456-458 (1967).
19. Potts, R. O. Physical characterisation of the stratum corneum: The relationship of mechanical and barrier properties to lipid and protein structure. In *Drugs and the Pharmaceutical Sciences*, Vol. 35, *Transdermal Drug Delivery.* Hadgraft, J. and Guy, R. H. (eds.). Marcel Dekker, New York, pp. 23–58 (1989).
20. Wilkes, G. L. and Wildnauer, R. H. Structure–property relationships of the stratum corneum of human and neonatal rat. II. Dynamic mechanic studies. *Biochim. Biophys. Acta 302*:276–289 (1973).
21. Yamamura, T. and Tezuka, T. The water holding capacity of the stratum corneum measured by H-NMR. *J. Invest. Dermatol.* 93:160–164 (1989).
22. Blank, I. H. and Shappirio, E. B. The water content of the stratum corneum. Effect of previous contact with aqueous solutions of soaps and detergents. *J. Invest. Dermatol.* 25:391–401 (1955).
23. Sprott, W. E. Surfactants and percutaneous absorption. *Trans. St. John's Hosp. Dermatol. Soc. 51*:56–71 (1965).
24. Scheuplein, R. J. and Ross, L. Effects of surfactants and solvents on the permeability of epidermis. *J. Soc. Cosmet. Chem. 21*:853–873 (1970).
25. Walters, K. A., Walker, M., and Olejnik, O. Non-ionic surfactant effects on hairless mouse skin characteristics. *J. Pharm. Pharmacol. 90*:525–529 (1988).

26. Downing, D. T., Wertz, P. W., and Stewart, M. E. The role of sebum and epidermal lipids in the cosmetic properties of skin. *Int. J. Cosmet. Chem. 8*:115–123 (1986).
27. Blank, I. H. Further observations of factors which influence the water content of the stratum corneum. *J. Invest. Dermatol. 21*:259–271 (1953).
28. Spencer, T. S., Linamen, C. E., Akers, W. A., and Jones, N. W. Temperature dependence of water content of stratum corneum. *Br. J. Dermatol. 93*:159–164 (1975).
29. Rougier, A., Lotte, C., and Maibach, H. I. In-vivo relationship between percutaneous absorption and transepidermal water loss. In *Percutaneous Absorption: Mechanisms–Methodology–Drug Delivery*, 2nd ed. Bronaugh, R. L. and Maibach, H. I. (eds.). Marcel Dekker, New York, pp. 175–190 (1989).
30. Wilson, D. R. and Maibach, H. I. Transepidermal water loss: A review. In *Cutaneous Investigation in Health and Disease, Non-invasive Methods and Instrumentation.* Leveque, J. L. (ed.). Marcel Dekker, New York, pp. 113–134 (1989).
31. Spencer, T. S. Transepidermal water loss: Methods and applications. In *Methods for Cutaneous Investigations.* Reitschel, R. L. and Spencer, T. S. (eds.). Marcel Dekker, New York, pp. 191–218 (1990).
32. Potts, R. O. and Boras, E. M. In-vivo changes in the dynamic viscosity of human stratum corneum as a function of age and ambient moisture. *J. Cosmet. Chem. 36*:169–176 (1985).
33. Tagami, H., Ohi, M., Iwatsuki, K., Kanamuru, Y., Yamada, M., and Ichijo, B. Evaluation of the skin surface hydration in-vivo by electrical measurement. *J. Invest. Dermatol. 75*:500–507 (1980).
34. Van Duzee, B. F. The influence of water content, chemical treatment and temperature on the rheological properties of stratum corneum. *J. Invest. Dermatol. 71*:140–144 (1978).
35. Hoeve, D. A. J. and Flory, P. J. The elastic properties of elastin. *J. Am. Chem. Soc. 80*:6523–6526 (1958).
36. Takahashi, M., Kawasaki, K., Tanaka, M., Ohta, S., and Tsuda, Y. The mechanism of stratum corneum plasticization with water. In *Bioengineering and the Skin.* Marks, R. and Payne, P. A. (eds.). Lancaster, England, pp. 67–73 (1981).
37. Zimm, B. H. Simplified relation between thermodynamics and molecular distribution functions for a mixture. *J. Chem. Phys. 21*:934 (1953).
38. Chao, K. N., Eisley, J. G., and Yang, W. J. Heat and water migration through normal skin: Part 1. Steady state. *Med. Biol. Eng. Comput. 17*:301–310 (1979).
39. Scheuplein, R. J. Mechanism of percutaneous absorption. 1. Routes of penetration and the influence of solubility. *J. Invest. Dermatol. 45*:334–346 (1965).
40. Blank, I. H., Moloney, J., Emslie, A. G., Simon, I., and Apt C. The diffusion of water across the stratum corneum as a function of its water content. *J. Invest. Dermatol. 82*:188–194 (1984).
41. Roberts, M. S., Anderson, R. A., Swarbrick, J., and Moore, D. E. The percutaneous absorption of phenolic compounds: The mechanism of diffusion across the stratum corneum. *J. Pharm. Pharmacol. 30*:486–490 (1978).
42. Potts, R. O. and Guy, R. H. A pore pathway is not necessary to explain skin permeability. *Proc. Int. Symp. Controlled Release Bioact. Mater. 18*:175–176 (1991).
43. Guy, R. H. and Hadgraft, J. Physiochemical aspects of percutaneous penetration and its enhancement. *Pharm. Res. 5*:753–758 (1988).

44. Sadoc, J. F. and Charvolin, J. Frustration in bilayers and topologies of liquid crystals of amphiphilic molecules. *J. Phys. 47*:683–689 (1986).
45. Boustra, J. A., Gooris, G. S., and Bras, W. The lamellar structure of stratum corneum as determined by small angle x-ray scattering. Presented at Surfactants In Solution Congress, Gainsville, Florida. (1990).
46. Bouwstra, J. A., Gooris, G. S., Vander Speck, J. A., and Bras, W. Structural investigations of human stratum corneum by small-angle x-ray scattering. *J. Invest. Dermatol. 97*:1005–1012 (1991).
47. Seddon, J. Structure of inverted (H_{11}) phase, and non-lamellar phase transitions of lipids. *Biochim. Biophys. Acta 1031*:1–69 (1990).
48. Walters, K. A., Flynn, G. L., and Marvel, J. R. Physiochemical characterisation of the human nail. I: Pressure sealed apparatus for measuring nail plate permeabilities. *J. Invest. Dermatol. 76*:76–79 (1981).
49. Roberts, M. S. Structure permeability considerations in percutaneous absorption. In Prediction of Percutaneous Penetration—Methods, Measurement, and Modelling. Scott, R. C., Hadgraft J., and Guy, R. H. (eds.). IBC Technical, 2, pp. 210–228 (1991).
50. Fritsch, W. C. and Stoughton, R. B. The effect of temperature and humidity on the penetration of C^{14} acetylsalicyclic acid in excised human skin. *J. Invest. Dermatol. 41*:307–312 (1963).
51. Vickers, C. F. H. Percutaneous absorption of sodium fusidate and fusidic acid. *Br. J. Dermatol. 81*:902–908 (1969).
52. Munies, R. and Wurster, D. E. Factors influencing percutaneous absorption. II. Absorption of methyl ethyl ketone. *J. Pharm. Sci. 54*:554–556 (1964).
53. Barry, B. W. In *Dermatological Formulations: Percutaneous Absorption*. Barry, B. W. (ed.). Marcel Dekker, New York (1983).
54. Stoughton, R. B. In *Progress in Biological Sciences in Relation to Dermatology*, Vol. 2. Rook, A. and Champion, R. H. (eds.). Cambridge University Press, New York, pp. 263–278 (1964).
55. Hawkins, G. S. and Riefenrath, W. G. Development of an in vitro model for determining the fate of chemicals applied to the skin. *Fundam. Appl. Toxicol. 4*:S133–S144 (1984).
56. Wurster, D. E. and Kramer, S. F. Investigations of some factors influencing percutaneous absorption. *J. Pharm. Sci. 50*:288–293 (1961).
57. Behl, C. R., Flynn, G. L., Kurihara, T., Harper, N., Smith, W., Higuchi, W. I., Ho, N. F. H., and Pearson, C. L. Hydration and percutaneous absorption: 1. Influence of hydration on alkanol permeation through hairless mouse skin. *J. Invest. Dermatol. 75*:346–352 (1980).
58. Behl, C. R., Bellantone, N. H., and Pei, J. Effect of the alkyl length and anatomical site on the alkanol permeability through fuzzy rat skin. *Basic Pharm. Abstr. 10*. Presented at the 130th Annual Meeting of American Pharmaceutical Association, New Orleans, April 19 (1983).
59. Walker, M., Dugard, P. H., and Scott, R. C. In-vitro percutaneous absorption studies: A comparison of human and laboratory species. *Hum. Toxicol. 2*:561–562 (1983).
60. Bond, J. R. and Barry, W. Hairless mouse skin is limited as a model for assessing the effects of penetration enhancers in human skin. *J. Invest. Dermatol. 90*:810–813 (1988).

61. Hinz, R. S., Hodson, C. D., Lorence, C. R., and Guy, R. H. In-vitro percutaneous absorption: Evaluation of the utility of hairless mouse skin. *J. Invest. Dermatol. 93*:87–91 (1989).

62. Bond, J. R. and Barry, B. W. Limitations of hairless mouse skin as a model for in vitro permeation studies through human skin: Hydration damage. *J. Invest. Dermatol. 90*:486–489 (1988).

63. McKenzie, A. W. and Stoughton, R. B. Method for comparing percutaneous absorption of corticosteroids. *Arch. Dermatol. 86*:608–610 (1962).

64. Potts, R. O., Guzek, D. B., Harris, R. R., and McKie, J. E. A non-invasive, in-vivo technique to quantitatively measure the water concentration of the stratum corneum using attenuated total reflectance infrared spectroscopy. *Arch. Dermatol. Res. 277*: 489–495 (1985).

65. Edwardson, P. A. D., Walker, M., and Breheny, C. Quantitative FTIR determination of skin hydration following occlusion with hydrocolloid containing adhesive dressings. *Int. J. Pharm.* (in press; 1992).

66. Powers, D. H. and Fox, C. A study of the effect of cosmetic ingredients, creams and lotions on the rate of moisture loss from the skin. *Proc. Sci. Sect. Toilet Goods Assoc. 28*:21–26 (1957).

67. Froebe, C. L., Simion, F. A., Ohlmeyer, H., Rhein, L. D., Mattai, J., Cagan, R. H., and Friberg, S. E. Prevention of stratum corneum lipid phase transitions in-vitro by glycerol—an alternative mechanism for skin moisturisation. *J. Soc. Cosmet. Chem. 41*:51–65 (1990).

68. Batt, M. D., Davis, W. B., Fairhurst, E., Gerrard, W. A., and Ridge, B. D. Changes in the physical properties of the stratum corneum following treatment with glycerol. *J. Soc. Cosmet. Chem. 39*:367–381 (1988).

69. Matoltsy, A. G., Downes, A. M., and Sweeney, T. M. Studies of the epidermal water barrier. Part II. Investigation of the chemical nature of the water barrier. *J. Invest. Dermatol. 50*:19–26 (1968).

70. Memschel, H. Zur kolloidchemic und pharmakolopie der keratinsubstanzen der menschlichen haut. *Arch. Exp. Pathol. Pharmakol. 110*:1–45 (1925).

71. Loden, M. and Lindberg, M. The influence of a simple application of different moisturisers on the skin capacitance. *Acta Derm. Venereol. (Stockh.) 71*:79–82 (1991).

72. Dempski, R. E., Demasco, J. D., and Marcus, A. D. In vitro study of the relative moisture occlusive properties of several topical vehicles and Saran Wrap. *J. Invest. Dermatol. 44*:361–363 (1965).

73. Stender, I. M., Blickmann, C., and Serup, J. Effects of oil and water baths on the hydration state of the epidermis. *J. Exp. Dermatol. 15*:206–209 (1990).

74. Shelmire, J. B. Factors determining the skin–drug vehicle relationship. *Arch. Dermatol. 82*:24–27 (1960).

75. Roberts, M. S. and Anderson, R. A. The percutaneous absorption of phenolic compounds. The effect of vehicles on the penetration of phenol. *J. Pharm. Pharmacol. 27*:599–605 (1975).

76. Scheuplein, R. J. and Blank, I. H. Mechanism of percutaneous absorption IV, penetration of non-electrolytes (alcohols) from alcohols and from pure liquids. *J. Invest. Dermatol. 60*:286–296 (1973).

77. Berardesca, E., de Rigal, J., Leveque, J. L., and Maibach, H. I. In vivo biophysical characterisation of skin physiological differences in races. *Dermatologica 182*:89–93 (1991).
78. Berardesca, E., Farinelli, N., Rabbiosi, G., and Maibach, H. I. Skin bioengineering in the non-invasive assessment of cutaneous ageing. *Dermatologica 182*:1–6 (1991).
79. Thune, P., Nilsen, T., Hanstad, H. K., Grestaten, T., and Lovig-Dahl, H. S. O. *Acta Derm. Venereol. (Stockh.) 64*:272–283 (1988).
80. Berg, R. W. Etiology and pathophysiology of diaper dermatology. *Adv. Dermatol. 3*:75–88 (1988).
81. Stahle-Backdahl, M. Stratum corneum hydration in patients undergoing maintenance haemodialysis. *Acta Derm. Venerol. (Stockh.) 68*:531–534 (1988).
82. Tupper, R. A., Pinnagoda, J., Censaads, P. J., and Nater, J. P. Susceptibility of irritants: Role of barrier function, ulcer dryness and history of atopic dermatitis. *Br. J. Dermatol. 123*:199–205 (1990).
83. Okhandias, R. P., Sinha, R. I. C., and Sinha, R. K. Study of hydration of stratum corneum in leprosy. *Indian J. Leprosy 58*:395–400 (1986).
84. Fulmer, A. W., and Kramer, G. J. Stratum corneum abnormalities in surfactant-induced dry scaly skin. *J. Invest. Dermatol. 86*:598–602 (1986).
85. Schalla, W., Lambrey, B., Lamaunel, E., and Schaefer, M. Skin pharmacokinetics. In *Therapeutic Variables and Pharmacokinetics in Topical Therapy in Pharmacology and the Skin* Vol. 1. B. Shroot and M. Schaefer (eds.). Karger, Basel (1987).
86. Scoggins, R. B. and Kliman, B. Relative potency of percutaneously absorbed corticosteroids in the suppression of pituitary-adrenal function. *J. Invest. Dermatol. 45*:347–355 (1965).
87. Roberts, M. S. and Morlock, E. Effect of repeated application of salicyclic acid to the skin on its percutaneous absorption. *J. Pharm. Sci. 67*:1685–1687 (1978).

2

Simple Alkyl Esters as Skin Penetration Enhancers

David R. Friend and Jorge Heller

SRI International, Menlo Park, California

I. INTRODUCTION

The success of most transdermal delivery systems will depend on the ability of the drug to permeate skin at a rate sufficient to achieve the desired therapeutic effect from a device of acceptable dimensions. Because many drugs are insufficiently skin permeable to allow formulation into transdermal delivery systems without an absorption promoter, numerous chemicals have been investigated as skin penetration enhancers. One such chemical is ethyl acetate (EtAc).

This chapter focuses on the use of EtAc and other simple alkyl esters as skin penetration enhancers using data derived primarily from in vitro studies. Much of the data described herein are based on the progestin, levonorgestrel (LN). The skin penetration-enhancing effects of EtAc and other alkyl esters have also been evaluated with estradiol, hydrocortisone, 5-fluorouracil, nifedipine, and indomethacin.

II. ALKYL ESTERS AS ENHANCERS FOR LEVONORGESTREL

Levonorgestrel is a potent contraceptive agent capable of suppressing ovulation at delivery rates of 20 µg/day from vaginal devices (1). This agent (mp 242°C) has very low water-solubility (about 1 ppm at 25°C) and a log octanol/water partition coefficient ($\log K_{oct/water}$) of 3.7. Because of its low dose requirement and that contraceptives are administered over a prolonged period, a transdermal route of delivery is advantageous (2). However, preliminary studies indicated that LN alone was insufficiently skin permeable to permit formulation of this drug into a transdermal device without a penetration enhancer. Ethanol (EtOH) was investigated as an enhancer for LN because of its previous use with estradiol (ED) in the Estraderm delivery system (3), in which EtOH is technically an excipient in the formulation. Although EtOH did enhance the flux of LN through rat skin, the enhancement was insufficient to permit formulation of a useful LN transdermal delivery system.

The in vitro flux data obtained using excised rat skin and various EtOH and EtOH/H_2O donor solvents, all saturated with excess solid LN, is shown in Table 1. The maximum flux of LN (J_{LN}) obtained from these enhancers was about 0.06 $\mu g/cm^2 \cdot hr^{-1}$. In this study (4), human cadaver skin was investigated with the enhancer EtOH to obtain an estimate of J_{LN} for humans. The J_{LN} was about 0.016 $\mu g/cm^2 \cdot hr^{-1}$ with a very long lag time (40–50 hr) (4). The target flux of LN through human skin in these studies was 0.2–0.3 $\mu g/cm^2 \cdot hr^{-1}$ so that a small, discrete patch could be formulated. From these preliminary experiments, it was clear that a much more potent enhancer would be required to reach the target flux. For evaluation purposes, rat skin was used as a model for human skin. The target flux, therefore, was adjusted to 1.0 $\mu g/cm^2 \cdot hr^{-1}$ when rat skin was used. This target flux was based on the previous data collected (4) showing that rodent skins are, under most circumstances, more permeable than is human skin (5–7), particularly under the influence of chemical penetration enhancers (8,9). Because EtOH was not a particularly effective enhancer for LN, further experiments were performed with other alkanols. These studies revealed that 1-butanol was capable of enhanc-

Table 1 Flux of LN (J_{LN}) Through Rat Skin From EtOH, EtOH/H_2O, and H_2O Donor Vehicles

Vehicle[a]	J_{LN} ($\mu g/cm^2 \cdot hr^{-1}$)[b]
H_2O	0.01
EtOH/H_2O (0.2:0.8)	0.02
EtOH/H_2O (0.4:0.6)	0.06
EtOH/H_2O (0.6:0.4)	0.06
EtOH/H_2O (0.8:0.2)	0.07
EtOH	0.06

[a]The donor vehicles (3 mL) were saturated with excess LN; the surface area of the diffusion cells was 5 cm^2.
[b]Measured at steady state. The lag times (t_L) under these conditions were approximately 15–20 hr.
Source: Data from Ref. 4.

ing J_{LN} to a level of approximately $0.8~\mu g/cm^2 \cdot hr^{-1}$ (4). Butanol, however, was not pursued further owing to potential irritation and toxicity concerns.

Ethyl acetate was examined as a skin penetration enhancer for LN under infinite dosing conditions using rat skin. Surprisingly, there appears to be no reported use of EtAc as a skin penetration enhancer in the literature. Relative to EtOH, J_{LN} was significantly higher under the influence of EtAc (Fig. 1). The J_{LN} was increased about 13-fold relative to that obtained using EtOH as an enhancer and about 75 times relative to that of water as an enhancer. Again, all the solvent enhancers tested were saturated with excess solid drug in all the experiments discussed herein. Drug-saturated vehicles are used to obtain unit activity; therefore, differences in flux from different vehicles can be attributed to specific solvent–skin interactions (10). Thus, use of saturated solutions allows one to evaluate the relative penetration-enhancing effect of various vehicles by simply observing differences in drug flux. This assumes that dissolution of the drug from the suspended crystals is not rate-limiting (i.e., diffusion through the skin is rate-limiting, as is usually the case). At steady state, J_{LN} was very close to the target value for J_{LN} in rat skin.

Because of these encouraging results, further experiments were performed with EtAc to more fully characterize its skin penetration-enhancing properties.

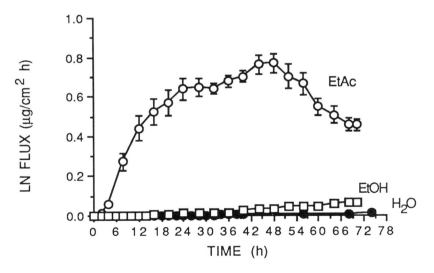

Figure 1 J_{LN} through rat skin in vitro using neat EtAc (n = 3), neat EtOH (n = 4), and neat H_2O (n = 3). Donor vehicles (3 mL) contained excess solid LN; surface area of exposed rat skin was 5 cm^2. Error bars represent the SEM. (From Ref. 11.)

Mixtures of EtAc and EtOH were tested for their penetration-enhancing effect with LN (11). Various volume fractions of EtAc in EtOH were examined: 0.10, 0.18, 0.25, 0.50, and 0.75. The J_{LN} through rat skin from these donor vehicles is shown in Figures 2 and 3. Interestingly, the 0.50 volume fraction donor vehicle gave a higher J_{LN} than did neat EtAc with rat skin. This is easily seen when J_{LN} at steady state is plotted against the volume fraction of EtAc in EtOH (Fig. 4). Similar results were obtained using hairless mouse skin discussed later.

Butyl acetate (BtAc) was also tested as a skin penetration enhancer for LN. The data for the transdermal experiment using neat BtAc as a donor vehicle are shown in Figure 5. The J_{LN} from EtOH and H_2O are also shown in Figure 5 for comparison purposes. In addition to BtAc, several other chemical enhancers were examined for their ability to increase J_{LN} through rat skin. The data collected using the various enhancers tested, including EtAc, are summarized in Table 2. Isopropyl myristate, oleic acid, propylene glycol, and triethanolamine, all were relatively poor enhancers for LN, relative to EtAc and BtAc.

An interesting relation exists between J_{LN} at steady state and the log $K_{oct/water}$ of the enhancing solvents, as shown in Figure 6. The optimum log $K_{oct/water}$ for the penetration enhancer appears to be about 0.8 for the group of solvents tested. The significance of this finding is not yet clear.

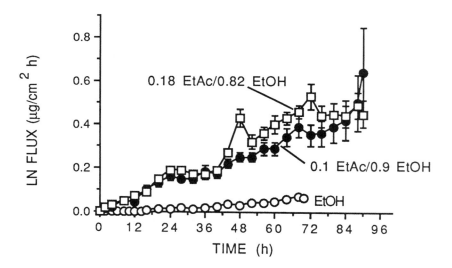

Figure 2 J_{LN} through rat skin in vitro using 0.10 EtAc ($n = 4$), 0.18 EtAc ($n = 4$) volume fractions in EtOH, and neat EtOH ($n = 4$) as donor phase solvents. Donor vehicle (3 mL) contained excess solid LN; surface area of exposed rat skin was 5 cm². Error bars represent the SEM. (From Ref. 11.)

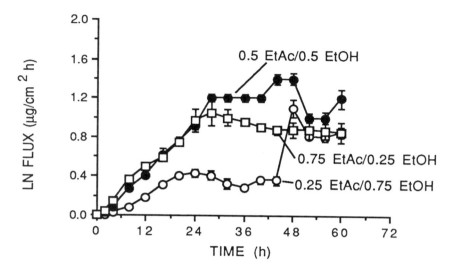

Figure 3 J_{LN} through rat skin in vitro using 0.25 EtAc ($n = 5$), 0.50 EtAc ($n = 3$), and 0.75 EtAc ($n = 3$) volume fractions in EtOH as donor phase solvents. Donor vehicle (3 mL) contained excess solid LN; surface area of exposed rat skin was 5 cm^2. Error bars represent the SEM. (From Ref. 11.)

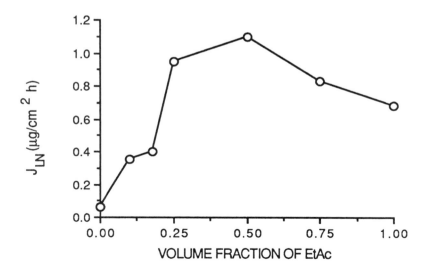

Figure 4 J_{LN} at steady state through rat skin in vitro using various volume fractions (0–1.0) of EtAc in EtOH. (From Ref. 11.)

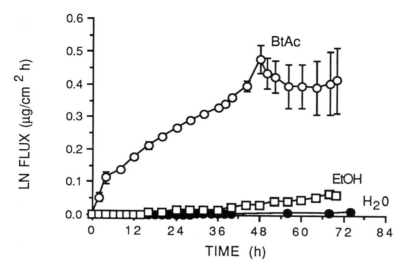

Figure 5 J_{LN} through rat skin in vitro using neat BtAc ($n = 3$), neat EtOH ($n = 4$), and neat H_2O ($n = 3$) as donor phase solvents. Donor vehicle (3 mL) contained excess solid LN; surface area of exposed rat skin was 5 cm^2. Error bars represent the SEM. (From Ref. 11.)

Table 2 J_{LN} at Steady State from Suspensions of LN in Various Solvents (Enhancers) Through Rat Skin in Vitro[a]

Donor vehicle	J_{LN} ($\mu g/cm^2 \cdot hr^{-1}$)	Relative J_{LN}[b]
Water	0.01	1
EtOH	0.06	6
EtAc	0.8	80
BtAc	0.4	40
Isopropyl myristate	0.05	5
Oleic acid	0.02	2
Propylene glycol	0.01	1
Triethanolamine	0.01	1

[a]$n = 3–6$ for each enhancer tested.
[b]Expressed relative to flux from water. These values were obtained from the apparent steady state flux of LN through rat skin. Steady state was generally reached within 24–48 hr.
Source: Ref. 11.

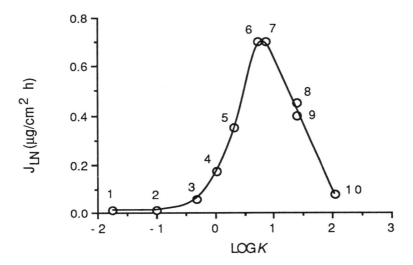

Figure 6 Relation between J_{LN} from the various penetration enhancers and the log $K_{oct/water}$ of those enhancers. 1, triethanolamine; 2, propylene glycol; 3, EtOH; 4, isopropanol; 5, 1-propanol; 6, EtAc; 7, 1-butanol; 8, 1-pentanol; 9, BtAc; and 10, 1-hexanol. Log $K_{oct/water}$ values were obtained from Ref. 12.

These preliminary studies indicated that EtAc was a potent enhancer for LN in rat skin. To gain a better understanding concerning the relation between LN flux, enhancers, and skin type, a series of permeability experiments using hairless mouse, hairless guinea pig, rat, and human cadaver skin were performed (13). This study was useful in determining the relative penetration enhancing effect of EtAc and EtAc/EtOH mixtures between human skin and rodent skins, which are generally more permeable than is human skin, as noted earlier.

The J_{LN} through excised hairless mouse (HM) skin from the EtAc and EtAc/EtOH cosolvents is shown summarized in Table 3. The J_{LN} in some of the experiments exhibited considerable scatter at various times. Such scatter, which is not nearly as evident in cumulative plots, is typical in experiments of this type. The J_{LN} did not reach a steady state condition from either of these vehicles. A peak J_{LN} of about 10 $\mu g/cm^2 \cdot hr^{-1}$ was measured using a donor vehicle of EtAc/EtOH (0.5:0.5 volume fractions). This was the highest flux of LN observed through any of the skins tested. The delivery of solvent through HM skin was also greater and more immediate than was observed for the other skins, as shown in Table 3 for EtAc and EtOH. Solvent delivery through HM skin was relatively constant once steady state was reached.

Table 3 Lag Times and Steady State Fluxes of LN, EtAc, and EtOH Through Rat Skin, Hairless Mouse Skin, Hairless Guinea Pig Skin, and Human Skin

Skin type	Vehicle[a]	Lag time (hr)			Steady-state flux[b]		
		LN	EtAc	EtOH	LN	EtAc	EtOH
Rat	EtOH	16	NA[c]	20	0.06	NA	ND[e]
	EtAc/EtOH (0.3:0.7)	16	16	22	1.2	3	7
	EtAc/EtOH (0.5:0.5)	20	12	14	3.5	5	9
	EtAc/EtOH (0.7:0.3)	20	8	12	3.0	10	9
	EtAc	14	8	NA	1.0	12	NA
HM	EtAc/EtOH (0.3:0.7)	6[d]	6	8	4.4[d]	8	20
	EtAc/EtOH (0.5:0.5)	4[d]	6	4	10[d]	13	16
	EtAc/EtOH (0.7:0.3)	6[d]	6	8	4.1[d]	18	17
HGP	EtAc/EtOH (0.3:0.7)	20	20	22[d]	1.1	1	4[d]
	EtAc/EtOH (0.5:0.5)	12	10	12	1.3	3	4
	EtAc/EtOH (0.7:0.3)	12	8	16	2.3	7	11
Human	EtOH	32	NA	12	0.03	NA	1.5
	EtAc/EtOH (0.3:0.7)	22	18	12	0.08	0.3	1.1
	EtAc/EtOH (0.5:0.5)	22	20	12	0.12	0.5	1.0
	EtAc/EtOH (0.7:0.3)	22	20	12	0.12	0.5	1.1
	EtAc	26	24	NA	0.20	0.5	NA
	EtAc (PEG 400)	26	20	NA	0.25	0.5	NA

[a]Expressed as volume fractions
[b]Expressed as $\mu g/cm^2 \cdot hr^{-1}$ for LN and $mg/cm^2 \cdot hr^{-1}$ for EtAc and EtOH.
[c]NA, not applicable.
[d]Steady state conditions were not reached.
[e]ND, not determined.

The J_{LN} through excised rat skin, using the same donor vehicles, is also summarized in Table 3. The steady state flux from the EtAc/EtOH (0.7:0.3) was 2–3 $\mu g/cm^2 \cdot hr^{-1}$, which was reached in about 20 hr. The J_{LN} from the EtAc/EtOH (0.3:0.7) donor solvent system was about 1.2 $\mu g/cm^2 \cdot hr^{-1}$. The flux of EtAc (J_{EtAc}) from the various donor solvent systems through rat skin is also listed in Table 3. The steady state flux was about 10 $mg/cm^2 \cdot hr^{-1}$ and 3 $mg/cm^2 \cdot hr^{-1}$ from the EtAc/EtOH (0.7:0.3) and EtAc/EtOH (0.3:0.7) donor solvents, respectively. The delivery of EtOH from EtAc/EtOH (0.3:0.7) was still less than that from the EtAc/EtOH (0.7:0.3), despite that there was more EtOH in the EtAc/EtOH

(0.3:0.7) donor solvent. The flux data and lag times for delivery of LN, EtAc, and EtOH are shown in Table 3 for all four skin types tested.

The third rodent skin examined in this study was obtained from the hairless guinea pig (HGP), which has been recently suggested as a good model for human skin (Behl, C., personal communication). The J_{LN} from EtAc/EtOH solvent systems (0.7:0.3 and 0.3:0.7) is shown in Table 3. At steady-state for J_{LN} using HGP skin was reached in about 12–20 hr, depending on the donor phase. The steady state flux of EtAc was about 7 mg/cm^2·hr^{-1} (0.7 EtAc/0.3 EtOH) and about 1 mg/cm^2·hr^{-1} (0.3 EtAc/0.7 EtOH), both of which were close to the measured flux of EtAc and EtOH through rat skin from the same vehicles.

The flux of LN through human cadaver skin using EtAc/EtOH solvent systems (0.7:0.3 and 0.3:0.7) is shown in Figure 7. The lag times for delivery of LN through human skin were longer than those observed with the rodent skins. The lag times with human skin (22–26 hr) are similar to those observed for delivery of LN through human skin in vitro from transdermal devices that use other chemical enhancers (14). The J_{LN} through human skin from the 0.3 EtAc/0.7 EtOH donor vehicle at steady state was about 0.08 µg/cm^2·hr^{-1} and about 0.12 µg/cm^2·hr^{-1} from the 0.7 EtAc/0.3 EtOH donor vehicle. These fluxes were considerably less than was observed through the rodent skins using the same donor solvents (see Table 3). The J_{LN} through human skin using neat EtAc as a donor vehicle

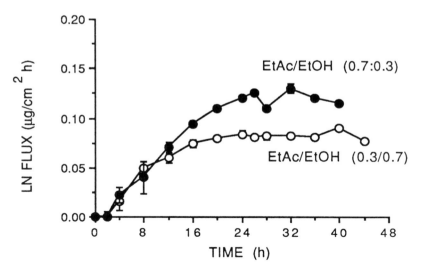

Figure 7 J_{LN} through human skin using EtAc/EtOH (0.7:0.3, *n* = 3) and EtAc/EtOH (0.3:0.7; *n* = 3) as donor vehicles. Error bars represent the SEM. (From Ref. 13.)

was higher than was measured using the EtAc/EtOH cosolvent systems: 0.2 $\mu g/cm^2 \cdot hr^{-1}$. This value is about five times less than that through rat skin from a neat EtAc donor vehicle (see Table 3). The J_{LN} through human skin using neat EtOH as a donor vehicle was about 0.03 $\mu g/cm^2 \cdot hr^{-1}$ close to that reported previously (4).

The permeability of human skin to EtAc (Fig. 8) was considerably less than was observed through the rodent skins for all the EtAc-containing vehicles. J_{EtAc} ranged between 0.3 and 0.5 $mg/cm^2 \cdot hr^{-1}$, depending on the vehicle composition. The flux of EtOH through human skin from these two donor vehicles is shown in Figure 9. The steady state flux (1.0 to 1.5 $mg/cm^2 \cdot hr^{-1}$) was nearly identical for all the EtOH-containing vehicles; lag times (about 12 hr) were about the same as well. The J_{EtOH} through human skin at steady state has been measured by others (15) to be about the same reported here (ca. 1 $mg/cm^2 \cdot hr^{-1}$). It is interesting to note that although rodent skins are more permeable to EtAc than to EtOH, the opposite is true for human skin. All the rodent skins used in these experiments were used within 1 hr of sacrifice, whereas the human skin was removed from cadavers and then frozen before use in the permeability experiments. As discussed further later the human skin was apparently devoid of esterase activity, whereas the rodent skin retained some portion of its activity during the permeability experiment. Esterases can influence the flux of other esters under in vitro conditions (16); therefore, it is

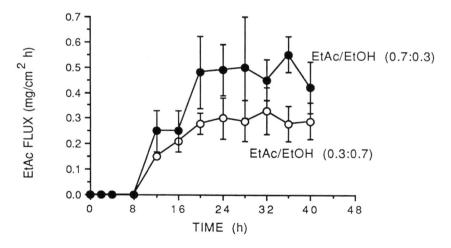

Figure 8 J_{EtAc} through human skin using EtAc/EtOH (0.7:0.3, $n = 3$) and EtAc/EtOH (0.3:0.7; $n = 3$) as donor vehicles. Error bars represent the SEM. (From Ref. 13.)

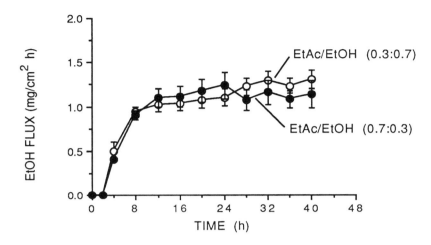

Figure 9 J_{EtOH} through human skin using EtAc/EtOH (0.7:0.3, $n = 3$) and EtAc/EtOH (0.3:0.7; $n = 3$) as donor vehicles. Error bars represent the SEM. (From Ref. 13.)

possible the skin permeability was underestimated in the human cadaver skin experiments.

Polyethylene glycol (PEG) 400 has been used as a solubilizing agent in the receptor solution of in vitro permeability experiments (17). PEG 400 (40% v/v in saline) was used as a solubilizing agent in the receptor phase using neat EtAc as an enhancer with human skin. The J_{LN} was only slightly higher using PEG 400 relative to normal saline as a receptor solution. J_{EtAc} was unaffected by the PEG. Information from this experiment is summarized in Table 3. A further discussion of the use of PEG 400 and other chemicals as additives to the receptor solutions is found in this chapter.

The relation between drug flux and solvent flux was examined by comparing cumulative drug and solvent delivery. This was done for the EtAc/EtOH (0.7:0.3) donor vehicle with all four skin types (Fig. 10). It appears that there is a nearly linear relation between cumulative drug delivered and cumulative solvent delivered regardless of the skin type. Hairless mouse skin permeability deviated from this relation at later time points owing to the drop in J_{LN} after 12 hr without a corresponding drop in J_{EtAc} and J_{EtOH}. The drop in LN flux through HM skin could have been caused by water entering the donor phase from the receptor solution through back diffusion, leading to an alteration of the penetration-enhancing effect of the solvents. Back diffusion of water into the donor chamber

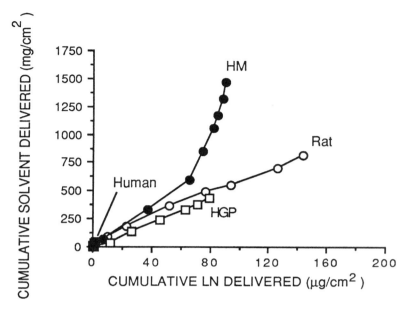

Figure 10 Relation between cumulative LN delivered and cumulative total solvent delivered through hairless mouse skin (HM), rat skin, hairless guinea pig skin (HGP), and human skin using a donor vehicle of EtAc/EtOH (0.7:0.3). (From Ref. 13.)

has been observed by others under conditions used in these in vitro skin permeation experiments (18–20). However, the donor phase was replaced at 24 hr with no change in J_{LN}. This indicates that the change in flux over time may have been due to changes in the skin. For comparison purposes, using HM skin, the flux over the first 12–14 hr was used. After that time, the J_{LN} fell considerably and was not used in comparisons, as this phenomenon was unique to HM skin.

The relative permeability of the skins tested indicated that HM skin is significantly more permeable toward LN, compared with the other rodent skins using combinations of EtAc/EtOH as enhancers. All of the rodent skins were more permeable than was human skin toward LN, EtAc, and EtOH. The permeability of LN through human skin, with neat EtAc as an enhancer, was about five times less than that of rat or HGP skin. Clearly, these results indicate that the three rodent skins tested are not useful for direct comparisons with human skin in permeability experiments using EtAc and EtOH as enhancers. In particular, HM skin appears to considerably overestimate the penetration-enhancing effect of EtAc for LN. Hairless mouse skin has been criticized as a model for human skin, particularly in evaluation of the effect of chemical enhancers (8,9). Another problem with HM is its susceptibility to hydration effects (21). Rat skin and HGP are probably better models for human skin than is HM skin. For example, rat skin does not appear to suffer from hydration effects, as does HM skin (22). Nonetheless, all three rodent skins overestimate absolute drug flux under the influence of the penetration enhancers EtAc and EtOH and, therefore, should be used with caution in making predictions about human skin.

Full-thickness rodent skins (epidermis and dermis) were used in these experiments (13); full-thickness skin, when tested in vitro with hydrophobic compounds, may underestimate the permeability of the same skin in vivo (23,24). This is because compounds of very low water solubility (e.g., LN) do not partition freely from the lipoidal regions of the stratum corneum into the aqueous environment of the viable epidermis or the aqueous receptor fluid. In vivo, the diffusing drugs are absorbed by the blood in the capillaries that lie at a depth of about 200 μm from the surface of the skin (25,26).

A technique used to obviate the problem of poor in vitro–in vivo correlation when using full-thickness skin in vitro to evaluate hydrophobic compounds is to add solubilizing agents to the receptor solution. Examples of solubilizing agents used to increase drug solubility in the receptor solution include PEG-20 oleyl ether, octoxynol-9 (Triton X-100) (23), bovine serum albumin (3% in buffer) (27), Poloxamer 188 (28), and PEG 400 (17). PEG 400 (40% in saline) was used as a solubilizing agent with human skin, using neat EtAc as an enhancer. The results indicated that the percutaneous absorption of LN was increased only slightly by this change. This lack of an apparent effect may have been because the human skin used was relatively thin (100–150 μm thick). Another possibility is that EtAc and EtOH act as solubilizing agents themselves as they enter the skin and pass through the viable epidermis, the dermis, and finally into the receptor solution. Therefore, the addition of PEG 400 to the receptor solution when EtAc and EtOH are used as enhancers might have little or no effect. The flux of EtAc through the human skin using PEG 400 in the receptor medium was unchanged relative to that using saline as a receptor medium, indicating that the PEG 400 did not measurably alter the barrier properties of the skin. However, the concentration of EtAc in the receptor solutions were very close to the detection limits of the high-performance liquid chromatographic (HPLC) technique, making small changes in concentration difficult to measure. Sarpotdar and coworkers observed that PEG 400, when placed in the receptor fluid, can have a significant effect on the penetration barrier of human cadaver skin in vitro (29).

As mentioned earlier, EtAc is hydrolyzed to EtOH and acetic acid in plasma by nonspecific esterases (30). The viable epidermis also contains esterases capable of hydrolyzing ester-containing compounds (31,32). When neat EtAc was used as a donor vehicle with rat, HM, and HGP skins, there were measurable amounts of

EtOH detected in the receptor solutions (13). Ethyl alcohol in the receptor solutions ranged from 5 to 20% by weight of the total EtAc measured in the receptor solutions at steady state. Thus, there appears to be considerable hydrolysis of EtAc as it passes through the viable epidermis and dermis. Ethyl acetate in the donor phase is stable over the course of the experiment. Hydrolysis of EtAc may also be due to esterases released into the receptor medium over the course of the experiment, as has been reported for human skin (33,34). There was no EtOH detected in the receptor solutions when human skin was tested with neat EtAc as a donor vehicle. Esterase activity was probably abolished by the freeze–thaw cycle the human skin was subjected to before the permeability experiments (13). Also, since small amounts of EtAc were found to permeate through human skin, any EtOH generated from hydrolysis was probably below the detection limit for EtOH (less than 200 $\mu g/mL$) (13). The flux values of EtAc and EtOH, as reported in Table 3, were calculated from the measured concentration of EtAc and EtOH in the receptor solutions and are uncorrected for metabolism.

Ethyl acetate has been used in a prototype transdermal delivery system for the delivery of LN. A variety of membranes were tested: ethylene vinyl acetate copolymers were found to possess the appropriate permeability properties to allow preparation of a reservoir-type transdermal patch (35). These membranes were used to prepare devices, which were tested in vitro using a variety of rodent skins (36,37). Several of these devices were evaluated in vivo on rabbits for their ability to deliver LN as well as to evaluate the potential irritation of the devices (38,39).

III. ALKYL ESTERS AS ENHANCERS FOR INDOMETHACIN

The penetration enhancing effects of EtAc and other related alkyl esters were evaluated using indomethacin (INDO) (22). Eight alkyl esters were evaluated as penetration enhancers: EtAc, methyl acetate (MeAc), methyl propionate (MePr), ethyl propionate (EtPr), methyl valerate (MeVal), BtAc, diethyl succinate (DESuc), and ethyl acetoacetate (EtAAc). Also tested as donor vehicles were water (0.05 M sodium phosphate, pH 3.0), EtOH, EtAc/EtOH (0.3:0.7), EtAc in propylene glycol (PG) (0.3:0.7, v/v), Azone (laurocapram) in PG (0.05:0.95, v/v), and dimethyl sulfoxide (DMSO) in PG (0.3:0.7, v/v). The aqueous vehicle was adjusted to pH 3 to suppress ionization of INDO. Each donor vehicle was saturated with excess solid INDO to ensure equal and maximum driving force in all the vehicles tested.

The flux of INDO (J_{INDO}) for several of the donor vehicles tested is shown in Figures 11 and 12. The J_{INDO} at steady state for all the donor vehicles is summarized in Table 4. For most of the vehicles, steady state was reached within 24–48 hr, depending on the vehicle. The J_{INDO} from the Azone/PG mixture reached steady state in about 24 hr (see Fig. 11). Also included in Table 4 are the

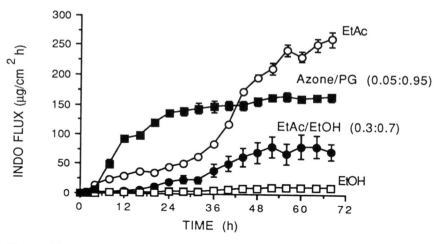

Figure 11 J_{INDO} through rat skin in vitro using EtAc ($n = 3$), Azone/PG (0.05:0.95; $n = 3$), EtAc/EtOH (0.3:0.7; $n = 3$), and EtOH ($n = 3$) as vehicles. Error bars represent the SEM. (From Ref. 22.)

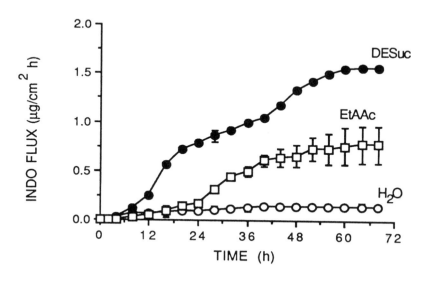

Figure 12 J_{INDO} through rat skin in vitro using DESuc ($n = 3$), EtAAc ($n = 3$), and 0.05 M sodium phosphate, pH 3.0 ($n = 3$) as vehicles. Error bars represent the SEM. (From Ref. 22.)

Table 4   Vehicles, Steady State Fluxes, Solubilities, Partition Coefficients of
Enhancers, Boiling Points, and Enhancement Factors for INDO

Vehicle	J_{INDO} $(\mu g/cm^2 \cdot hr^{-1})^a$	INDO solubility $(mg/mL)^b$	Log K^c	Boiling point (°C)	Enhancement factors[d]
Water (pH 3)	0.15	0.001[e]		100	1
EtOH	12	28	−0.35	78	80
EtAc (30% in EtOH)	80	62			530
EtAc	230	42	0.75	77	1500
MeAc	240	104	0.62	58	1600
MePr	260	47	0.84	79	1700
EtPr	100	28	1.3	99	650
MeVal	19	27	1.8	128	125
BuAc	9	27	1.7	126	60
DESuc	1.6	30	1.2	218	5
EtAAc	0.8	36	0.25	181	0.5
Azone (5% in PG)	165	11			1100
EtAc (30% in PG)	5.5	55			35
DMSO (30% in PG)	3	110			20

[a]Measured at apparent steady state, donor phase: 32°C, receptor phase 37°C.
[b]Measured at 32°C.
[c]Octanol/water, measured at 24°C.
[d]Enhancement factor relative to flux from water, pH 3.
[e]From Ref. 56.

enhancement factors (J_{INDO} in the test vehicle relative to J_{INDO} from aqueous vehicle), the log $K_{oct/water}$ and boiling point of each of the single component vehicles, and the solubility of INDO in each of the vehicles. There was no direct relation between solubility of INDO in the test vehicles and J_{INDO} from those vehicles. Thus, effectiveness of each donor vehicle appears to be the result of specific vehicle–skin interactions.

Ethyl acetate, MeAc, and MePr were the most effective penetration enhancers for INDO. Relative to water, EtAc increased J_{INDO} about 1500-fold at steady state. Relative to EtOH as an enhancer, J_{INDO} was increased over 20-fold. Furthermore, EtAc/EtOH (0.3:0.7) enhanced J_{INDO} over sevenfold relative to EtOH alone.

Although there were no major discernible trends observed in the data, there were several interesting relations noted. Generally, as the alkyl chain length increased, the enhancement effect decreased. Since the alkyl chain length affects the polarity of the esters, the partition coefficients of each ester were measured (see Table 4). When J_{INDO} from the ester vehicle is plotted against log $K_{oct/water}$ of the esters, an interesting relation is observed (Fig. 13). Maximum enhancement was reached with esters having a log $K_{oct/water}$ of 0.6–0.8. A similar relation was noted with LN (see foregoing).

Azone has been an effective penetration enhancer for a variety of drugs (40), including INDO (41,42). Propylene glycol has been used as a cosolvent along with Azone in skin permeation studies with INDO (42). Therefore, a mixture of 5% Azone in PG was tested for its ability to increase the percutaneous absorption of INDO relative to the other enhancers tested. Although J_{INDO} from Azone/PG (0.05:0.95) was about 14 times greater than that from EtOH at steady state, it was somewhat lower than that from EtAc at steady state. However, steady state J_{INDO} was reached earlier with Azone than any of the other enhancers tested.

The EtAc/PG (0.3:0.7) and DMSO/PG (0.3:0.7) combinations were also tested as penetration enhancing vehicles. J_{INDO} from both these vehicles was relatively low (see Table 4). The J_{INDO} from EtAc/PG (0.3:0.7) was much lower than that

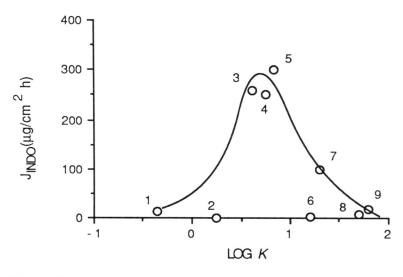

Figure 13 Relation between J_{INDO} at steady state and the log $K_{oct/water}$ for the test vehicles. 1, EtOH; 2, EtAAc; 3, MeAc; 4, EtAc; 5, EtPr; 6, DESuc; 7, EtPr; 8, BuAc; and 9, MeVal. (From Ref. 22.)

from EtAc/EtOH (0.3:0.7) indicating that EtOH is a better cosolvent for EtAc than is PG. The relatively low J_{INDO} from DMSO/PG (0.3:0.7) is not unexpected, since in general, the vehicle should contain at least 80% or more DMSO for effective transdermal flux enhancement (43,44).

Indomethacin appears to be a good transdermal candidate, in that it is used for treatment of chronic inflammatory disorders. A transdermal dose form could improve patient compliance by reducing the number of doses to once-a-day. It is unclear, however, whether gastric side effects would be reduced if INDO were delivered transdermally, as these side effects are largely due to prostaglandin synthesis in gastric mucosa following systemic as well as oral dosing and are probably less due to topical irritation following oral dosing. Perhaps local delivery of INDO to underlying tissues for the treatment of rheumatoid arthritis represents a more realistic use to transdermally applied INDO. Issues related to drug delivery by percutaneous application to muscle and tissues underlying skin has recently been discussed (45).

Penetration of INDO into or through the skin requires a potent skin penetration enhancer, whether the target delivery site is topical, local tissues, or the systemic circulation. Other enhancers tested with INDO are DMSO, isopropyl myristate, diethyl sebacate (41,42), long-chain fatty alkanols, alkanoic acids and esters (46), and calcium thioglycolate (42). Other Azone-like enhancers have been tested as skin penetration enhancers for INDO as well (47). Because of the variety of conditions and skin types, it is difficult to compare the relative effectiveness of the various enhancers tested with INDO.

In the experiments involving EtAc-enhanced delivery of INDO through rat skin, and most other in vitro permeability experiments involving rodent skins, the effects of hydration must be considered. Long-term hydration of HM skin causes increased permeation of solutes (7,8,21). The use of water (pH 3) as a donor vehicle in the INDO permeability experiments with rat skin indicate that there were no appreciable changes in J_{INDO} over the 68-hr-period permeability experiment. This indicates that rat skin is probably not as sensitive as is HM skin to the effects of long-term hydration. The low pH of the aqueous donor vehicle may have had a small effect on J_{INDO}. A pH 3 leads to slightly higher tritiated water flux through excised HM skin relative to pHs in the range of 4–10 (48).

IV. ALKYL ESTERS AS ENHANCERS FOR ESTRADIOL, HYDROCORTISONE, 5-FLUOROURACIL, AND NIFEDIPINE THROUGH RAT SKIN

Ethyl acetate has also been tested for its ability to increase the percutaneous absorption of estradiol (ED), hydrocortisone (HC), 5-fluorouracil (5-FU), and nifedipine (NP) (11). In these experiments, the donor vehicles tested along with EtAc were water, EtOH, EtAc/EtOH. Again, drug-saturated donor vehicles were always used so that the effects of the vehicles could be separated from activity effects. Nifedipine was also tested with methyl propionate (MePr).

It is known that EtOH is an effective enhancer for ED (3). Relative to water, a 0.7:0.3 mixture of EtOH/H_2O increases the percutaneous absorption of ED about 20 times from saturated donor vehicles. To compare the relative skin penetration-enhancing effect of EtAc and EtOH, J_{ED} was measured from donor vehicles of water, EtOH, EtAc/EtOH (0.25:0.75), and EtAc using rat skin. The data collected have been plotted, as shown in Figure 14. As can be seen, J_{ED} was enhanced about fivefold using EtAc as an enhancer relative to that found with EtOH as an enhancer. This indicates that transdermal patches using EtAc could be approximately five times smaller than is possible using EtOH as an enhancer. Whether such a system could be worn for 3.5 days on the same site (a question still unanswered with the current Estraderm patch) is unknown. However, current data suggest that EtAc-containing transdermal devices can probably be worn no longer than 24 hr on the same site, to minimize skin irritation. A

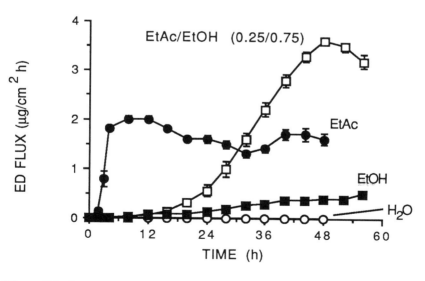

Figure 14 J_{ED} through rat skin using EtAc ($n = 3$); EtOH ($n = 3$); EtAc/EtOH (0.25:0.75) ($n = 3$), and H_2O ($n = 3$) as donor phase vehicles. Error bars represent the SEM. (From Ref. 11.)

Table 5 Steady State J and Relative J for ED, HC, 5-FU, and NP Through Rat Skin from Various Solvents

Drug	Solvent	J ($\mu g/cm^2 \cdot hr^{-1}$)[a]	Relative J[b]
Estradiol	H_2O	0.01	1
	EtOH	0.4	40
	EtAc/EtOH (0.25:0.75)	3.5	350
	EtAc	2.0	200
Hydrocortisone	H_2O	0.09	1
	EtOH	1.7	20
	EtAc/EtOH (0.25:0.75)	30	330
	EtAc	60	650
5-Fluorouracil	H_2O	8.0	1
	EtOH	35	4
	EtAc/EtOH (0.25:0.75)	65	8
	EtAc	590	74
Nifedipine	H_2O	0.07	1
	EtAc	8.4	120
	MePr	8.0	115

[a]J at steady state.
[b]Expressed relative to flux from water. These values were obtained from the apparent steady state J of these drugs through rat skin. Steady state was generally reached within 24–36 hr.

further discussion of the cutaneous effects of topically applied EtAc will be presented later in the chapter.

The transdermal flux of HC from various solvents through rat skin is summarized in Table 5. As with the other drugs tested, EtAc increased J_{HC} considerably: relative to water, J_{HC} was enhanced over 600-fold. Relative to EtOH, J_{HC} was enhanced over 30-fold. Although there is probably little practical use for transdermal HC, the data indicate the potent skin penetration-enhancing characteristics of EtAc.

The two other drugs tested with the alkyl ester enhancers were 5-FU and NP. 5-Fluorouracil is considerably more water-soluble than are the steroids discussed earlier. For 5-FU, the transdermal flux was increased about 75-fold using EtAc as an enhancer relative to water. At steady state, J_{5-FU} was nearly 0.6 mg/cm^2·hr^{-1} through rat skin (see Table 5). The NP flux was also enhanced significantly from about 0.07 $\mu g/cm^2 \cdot hr^{-1}$ (water) up to 8.0 $\mu g/cm^2 \cdot hr^{-1}$ (EtAc), or an increase of about 120 times. The J_{NP} from the solvent MePr was also high relative to water

$(8.4 \ \mu g/cm^2 \cdot hr^{-1})$. For INDO, MePr was the most effective enhancer of all the alkyl esters tested.

V. HOW DO ALKYL ESTERS MODIFY THE BARRIER PROPERTIES OF SKIN?

From the data now collected, it appears that EtAc and several related alkyl esters are potent skin penetration enhancers. There is currently little information concerning how these chemicals are acting on skin to alter its permeability. There is some evidence to suggest that EtAc extracts lipid from the stratum corneum, which would lower the diffusional resistance of the skin (49).

The damage ratio for EtAc-treated HM skin has been determined according to the technique of Matoltsy et al. (48). Briefly, full-thickness HM skins were mounted in Franz-diffusion cells and 4 mL of saline containing 5 $\mu C/mL$ of ^3H_2O were placed into the donor chamber of the cells. Samples were analyzed for appearance of ^3H_2O until an apparent steady state was reached (about 45 min). Next, the tritiated water solution was removed from the donor chamber and the skins were then thoroughly rinsed with saline. The skins were remounted and EtAc was then placed in the donor chamber for periods of 30 min, 2 hr, and 16 hr. After removal of EtAc from the donor chamber, the skins were again rinsed with saline and the ^3H_2O permeability experiment repeated. The steady state flux of ^3H_2O before treatment with EtAc was 0.3 $mg/cm^2 \cdot hr^{-1}$, which was nearly identical with that found by Matoltsy et al. (48) with the same conditions and skin type. Following EtAc treatment, the ^3H_2O flux at steady state was over 20 times higher. Thus, the damage ratio after 30 min treatment with EtAc was 24; at 2 hr and 16 hr exposure times, the damage ratios were approximately the same. In other words, the damaging effect, as measured by an increase in ^3H_2O flux, was complete following 30 min of exposure to EtAc. Longer exposure periods did not result in a further increase in ^3H_2O flux. Interestingly, FTIR and DSC experiments aimed at determining changes in molecular order, by exposing hairless mouse stratum corneum to EtAc for varying periods over 24 hr, indicate that longer exposure periods extract greater amounts of lipid. For example, there was significantly more lipid extracted from the stratum corneum from a 2 hr treatment than from a 30 min treatment (49).

Table 6 shows the damage ratios for HM (HRS/J strain) skin exposed to various solvents, including EtAc. As can be seen, EtOH results in relatively little damage, whereas both acetone and EtAc are more damaging. The more lipophilic solvents, chloroform and diethyl ether, were considerably more damaging than the polar organic solvents. Malten et al. have found that EtAc increases transepidermal water loss to the same extent as does EtOH (50). The role of solvent drag in the enhancement of skin penetration has also been studied (51).

Table 6 Rates of Diffusion of Water Through Hairless Mouse Skin Before and
After Treatment with Organic Solvents for 30 Minutes

Solvent	Flux (mg/cm^{2}hr^{-1})		
	Before	After	Ratio
Chloroform[a]	0.44	160	363
Diethyl ether[b]	0.27	53	197
Dimethyl sulfoxide[c]	0.49	41	83
Acetone[d]	0.50	11	23
Ethyl acetate[e]	0.32	7.4	23
Ethanol[f]	0.63	2.0	3.2

[a]$n = 5$; [b]$n = 3$; [c]$n = 2$; [d]$n = 4$; [e]$n = 3$; [f]$n = 6$.
Source: Data from Ref. 48 with the exception of the ethyl acetate data.

VI. SKIN IRRITATION AND TOXICITY

A major concern with the use of skin penetration enhancers is skin irritation. For
instance, the Estraderm transdermal delivery system, which uses EtOH as an
excipient for its skin penetration-enhancing qualities, is a mild to moderate skin
irritant in a significant number of users (52,53). Although it is not clear that EtOH
is responsible for the irritation, this example typifies the problems encountered in
transdermal delivery systems relying on skin penetration enhancers.

Ethyl acetate has been examined in an occlusive patch test (10% petrolatum) in
humans over 24 hr, during which it was found to be nonirritating and nonsensitiz-
ing (54). Both EtAc and the EtAc/EtOH showed essentially no irritation over the
entire period of a 21-day cumulative closed patch test (Friend, D. R. and Maibach,
H. I., unpublished data). The skin irritation effects have been assessed in rabbits in
transdermal devices designed to deliver LN, EtAc, and EtOH (39). The patches
were mildly, and occasionally, moderately irritating. It was evident that the
adhesive, which was used as a laminate over the entire base of the patch, was
remaining on the site following removal of the patch. This residual adhesive was
found to contribute to the apparent irritation of the devices.

Ethyl acetate is generally recognized as safe (GRAS) by the Food and Drug
Administration (FDA). It has a relatively low toxicity (LD$_{50}$ for acute oral toxicity
of 5.6 g/kg and 3–5 g/kg for subcutaneous toxicity; 54). The joint FAO/WHO
Expert Committee on Food Additives has given EtAc an unconditional acceptable
daily intake (ADI) of 0–25 mg/kg (54). Using the data for EtAc permeability in
Table 3, the maximum amount of EtAc that could be delivered systemically from
a 25 cm^2 device at steady state would be about 300 mg total, or less than 6 mg/kg
for most humans.

VII. CONCLUSIONS

It is clear that EtAc and several related simple alkyl esters are effective skin penetration enhancers for a number of drugs. It is not yet clear how EtAc is modifying the barrier properties of the skin. Thus, there is motivation to improve our understanding of the mechanism of action of this common organic solvent. As with other enhancers, this task will not be simple. It may be that EtAc may be modifying the barrier in several ways simultaneously as suggested in the foregoing.

On a more practical note, it is interesting to consider whether EtAc can indeed be used in commercial transdermal dose forms. Several factors will be important in determining the clinical usefulness of EtAc as a skin penetration enhancer. One factor is skin irritation as well as other topical changes induced by EtAc. It has been noted that EtAc has a certain "drying" effect, probably the result of delipidization of the stratum corneum (55). In fact, EtAc has been used as a delipidizing agent to remove sebum in clinical studies (55). Ethyl acetate was applied neat to the skin repeatedly with no apparent damaging or irritating effects. More studies are required to determine whether EtAc can be used in an occlusive transdermal device in combination with an adhesive and drug. It is highly unlikely that EtAc could be used in a device designed to worn for periods longer than 24 hr. The odor of EtAc, while pleasant under certain conditions, must be considered as well. Wearing the patch on the back will be required to minimize any potential problems concerning the fruity smell of EtAc.

A final consideration is compatibility of EtAc with other patch components as well as stability on storage. As are most esters, EtAc will hydrolyze after long periods of exposure to water; hence, devices will need to remain relatively anhydrous until application. Exposure of EtAc to water once the patch has been applied should not present hydrolysis problems owing to the short exposure period. A second concern is the potential for loss of EtAc through evaporation on storage. Ethyl acetate is considerably more volatile than is EtOH. Hence, design and the packaging of EtAc-based transdermal devices will have to prevent premature loss of EtAc during storage.

REFERENCES

1. Landgren, B. M., Johannisson, E., Masironi, B., and Dicsfalusy, E. Pharmacokinetic and pharmacodynamic investigations with vaginal devices releasing levonorgestrel at a constant, near zero-order rate. *Contraception* 26:567–585 (1982).
2. Friend, D. R. Transdermal delivery of contraceptives. *Crit. Rev. Ther. Drug Carrier Syst.* 7:149–186 (1990).
3. Good, W. R., Powers, M. S., Campbell, P., and Schenkel, L. A new transdermal delivery system for estradiol. *J. Controlled Release* 2:89–97, (1985).

4. Friend, D. R., Catz, P., Heller, J., Reid J., and Baker, R. Transdermal delivery of levonorgestrel I: Alkanols as permeation enhancers in vitro. *J. Controlled Release* 7:243–250 (1988).
5. Scott, R. C., Walker, M., and Dugard, P. H. A comparison of the in vitro permeability properties of human skin and some laboratory animals. *Int. J. Cosmet. Sci.* 8:189–194 (1986).
6. Riefenrath, W. G., Chellquist, E. M., Shipwash, E. A., and Jederberg, W. W. Evaluation of animal models for predicting skin penetration in man. *Fundam. Appl. Toxicol.* 4:S224-S230, 1984.
7. Bronaugh, R. L. and Maibach, H. I. In vitro models for human percutaneous absorption. In *Models in Dermatology*, Vol. 2, *Dermatopharmacology and Toxicology*, Maibach, H. I., and Lowe, N. J. (eds.). S. Karger, Basel, pp. 178–188 (1985).
8. Bond, J. R. and Barry, B. W. Hairless mouse is limited as a model for assessing the effects of penetration enhancers in human skin. *J. Invest. Dermatol.* 90:810–813 (1988).
9. Bond, J. R. and Barry, B. W. Damaging effect of acetone on the permeability barrier of hairless mouse skin compared with that of human skin. *Int. J. Pharm.* 41:91–93 (1988).
10. Theeuwes, F., Gale, R. M., and Baker, R. W. Transference: A comprehensive parameter governing permeation of solutes through membranes. *J. Membr. Sci.* 1:3–16 (1976).
11. Friend, D., Catz, P., and Heller, J. Simple alkyl esters as skin permeation enhancers. *J. Controlled Release* 9:33–41 (1989).
12. Leo, A., Hansch, C., and Elkins, D. Partition coefficients and their uses. *Chem. Rev.* 71:525–616 (1971).
13. Catz, P. and Friend, D. R. Transdermal delivery of levonorgestrel VIII. Effect of enhancers on rat skin, hairless mouse skin, hairless guinea pig skin, and human skin. *Int. J. Pharm.* 58:93–102 (1990).
14. Chien, Y. W., Chien, T.-Y., and Huang, Y. C. Transdermal fertility regulation in females (I) Development of transdermal contraceptive system and in-vitro evaluation. *Proc. Int. Symp. Controlled Release Bioact. Mater.* 15:286–287 (1988).
15. Berner, B., Mazzenga, G. C., Otte, J. H., Steffens, R. J., Juang, R.-H., and Ebert, C. D. Ethanol: water mutually enhanced transdermal therapeutic system II: Skin permeation of ethanol and nitroglycerin. *J. Pharm. Sci.* 78:402–407 (1989).
16. Potts, R. O., McNeill, S. C., Desbonnet, C. R., and Wakshull, E. Transdermal drug transport and metabolism. II. The role of competing kinetic events. *Pharm. Res.* 6:119–124 (1989).
17. Valia, K. H., Chien, Y. W., and Shinal, E. C. Long-term permeation kinetics of estradiol (I): Effect of drug solubilizer-polyethylene glycol 400. *Drug Dev. Ind. Pharm.* 10: 951–981 (1984).
18. Allenby, A. C., Fletcher, J., Schock, C., and Tees, T. F. S. The effect of heat, pH and organic solvents on electrical impedance and permeability of excised human skin. *Br. J. Dermatol.* 81(Suppl. 4):31–39 (1969).
19. Coldman, M. F., Kalinovsky, T., and Poulsen, B. J. The in vitro penetration of flucinonide through human skin from different volumes of DMSO. *Br. J. Dermatol.* 85:457–461 (1971).

20. Ito, Y., Ogiso, T., and Iwaka, M. Thermodynamic study on the enhancement of percutaneous penetration of drugs by Azone. *J. Pharmacobiodyn.* 11:749–757 (1988).
21. Behl, C. R., Flynn, G. L., Kurihara, T., Harper, N., Smith, W., Higuchi, W. I., Ho, N. F. H., and Pierson, C. L. Hydration and percutaneous absorption: I. Influence of hydration on alkanol permeability through hairless mouse skin. *J. Invest. Dermatol.* 75:346–352 (1980).
22. Catz, P. and Friend, D. R. Alkyl esters as skin permeation enhancers for indomethacin. *Int. J. Pharm.* 55:17–23 (1989).
23. Bronaugh, R. L. and Stewart, R. F. Methods for in vitro percutaneous absorption studies III. Hydrophobic compounds. *J. Pharm. Sci.* 73:1255–1258 (1984).
24. Tsuruta, H. Percutaneous absorption of organic solvents (2) A method for measuring the penetration rate of chlorinated solvents through excised skins. *Ind. Health* 15:131–139 (1977).
25. Barry, B. W. *Dermatological Formulations: Percutaneous Absorption.* Marcel Dekker, New York, p. 9 (1983).
26. Schaefer, H., Zesch, A., and Stuttgen, G. *Skin Permeability.* Springer-Verlag, Berlin, p. 549 (1982).
27. Brown, D. W. C. and Ulsamer, A. G. Percutaneous penetration of hexachlorophene as related to receptor solutions. *Food Cosmet. Toxicol.* 13:81–86 (1975).
28. Hoelgaard, A. and Mollgaard, B. Permeation of linoleic acid through skin in vitro. *J. Pharm. Pharmacol.* 34:610–611 (1985).
29. Sarpotdar, P. P., Gaskill, J. L., and Giannini, R. P. Effect of polyethylene glycol 400 on the penetration of drugs through human skin in vitro. *J. Pharm. Sci.* 75:26–28 (1986).
30. Gallaher, E. J. and Loomis, T. A. Metabolism of ethyl acetate in the rat: Hydrolysis to ethyl alcohol in vitro and in vivo. *Toxicol. Appl. Pharmacol.* 34:309–313 (1975).
31. Bucks, D. A. W. Skin structure and metabolism: Relevance to the design of cutaneous therapeutics. *Pharm.Res.* 1:148–153 (1984).
32. Pannatier, A., Jenner, P., Testa, B., and Etter, J. C. The skin as a drug-metabolizing organ. *Drug Metab. Rev.* 8:319–343 (1978).
33. Bundgaard, H., Hoelgaard, A., and Mollgaard, B. Leaching of hydrolytic enzymes from human skin in cutaneous permeation studies as determined with metronidazole and 5-fluorouracil prodrugs. *Int. J. Pharm.* 15:285–292 (1982).
34. Hoelgaard, A. and Mollgaard, B. Dermal drug delivery—improvement by choice of vehicle or derivative. *J. Controlled Release* 2:111–120 (1985).
35. Friend, D. R., Catz, P., Heller, J., and Okagaki, M. Transdermal delivery of levonorgestrel IV. Evaluation of membranes. *J. Pharm. Sci.* 78:477–480 (1989).
36. Friend, D. R., Catz, P., Heller, J., and Okagaki, M. Transdermal delivery of levonorgestrel V. Preparation of devices and evaluation in vitro. *Pharm. Res.* 6:938–944 (1989).
37. Catz, P. and Friend, D. R. In vitro evaluations of transdermal levonorgestrel. *Drug Design Deliv.* 6:49–60 (1990).
38. Friend, D. R., Catz, P., and Phillips, S. J. Transdermal delivery of levonorgestrel VII. In vivo studies. *Contraception* 40:73–80 (1989).
39. Friend, D. R., Phillips, S. J., and Hill, R. J. Cutaneous effects of transdermal levonorgestrel. *Food Chem. Toxicol.* 29:639–646 (1991).

40. Vaidyanathan, R., Rajahyaksha, V. J., Kim, B. K., and Anisko, J. J. Azone. In *Transdermal Delivery of Drugs*, Vol. 2. Kydonieus, A. G. and Berner, B. (eds.). CRC Press, Boca Raton, pp. 63–83 (1987).

41. Sugibayashi, K., Nemoto, M., and Morimoto, Y. Effect of several penetration enhancers on the percutaneous absorption of indomethacin in hairless rats. *Chem. Pharm. Bull.* 36:1519–1528 (1988).

42. Ogiso, T., Ito, Y., Iwaki, M., and Atago, H. Absorption of indomethacin and its calcium salt through rat skin: Effect of penetration enhancers and relationship between in vivo and in vitro penetration. *J. Pharmacobiodyn.* 9:517–525 (1986).

43. Stoughton, R. B. Influence of dimethylsulfoxide (DMSO) on human percutaneous absorption. *Arch. Dermatol.* 90:512–517 (1964).

44. Feldmann, R. J. and Maibach, H. I. Percutaneous penetration of ^{14}C-hydrocortisone through normal skin. *Arch. Dermatol.* 94:649–651 (1966).

45. Marty, J.-P., Guy, R. H., and Maibach, H. I. Percutaneous penetration as a method of delivery to muscle and other tissue. In *Percutaneous Absorption: Mechanisms–Methodology–Drug Delivery*, 2nd ed. Bronaugh, R. L. and Maibach, H. I. (eds.). Marcel Dekker, New York, pp. 511–529 (1989).

46. Chien, Y. W., Heliang, X., Chiang, C.-C., and Huang, Y.-C. Transdermal controlled administration of indomethacin. I. Enhancement of skin permeability. *Pharm. Res.* 5:103–106 (1988).

47. Quan, D., Higuchi, R. I., Takayama, K., Higashiyama, K., and Nagai, T. Promoting effect of 2-*n*-alkylcyclohexanones on the percutaneous absorption of indomethacin. *Drug Design Deliv.* 5:149–157 (1989).

48. Matoltsy, A. G., Downes, A. M., and Sweeney, T. M. Studies of epidermal water barrier. Part II. Investigation of the chemical nature of the water barrier. *J. Invest. Dermatol.* 50:19–26 (1968).

49. Catz, P. and Friend, D. R. Mechanism of skin penetration enhancers: Ethyl acetate. *Pharm. Res.* 6:S108 (1989).

50. Malten, K. E., Spruit, D., Boemaars, H. G. M., and de Keizer, M. J. M. Horny layer injury by solvents, *Berufsdermatosen* 16:135–157 (1968).

51. Friend, D. R. and Smedley, S. I. Solvent drag in ethanol/ethyl acetate enhanced skin permeation of d-norgestrel. *Int. J. Pharm.* (submitted).

52. Utian, W. H. Transdermal oestrogen, a recent advance in oestrogen therapy. *Drugs* 36:383–386 (1988).

53. Utian, W. H. Transdermal estradiol overall safety profile. *Am. J. Obstet. Gyneol.* 156:1335–1338 (1987).

54. Opdyke, D. L. J. Fragrance raw materials monographs: Ethyl acetate. *Food Cosmet. Toxicol.* 12:711–712 (1974).

55. Millns, J. L. and Maibach, H. I. Mechanism of sebum production and delivery in man. *Arch. Dermatol. Res.* 272:351–362 (1982).

56. Inagi, T., Muramatsu, T., Nagai, H., and Terada, H. Influence of vehicle composition on the penetration of indomethacin through guinea pig skin. *Chem. Pharm. Bull.* 29:1708–1714 (1981).

3

Phospholipids as Skin Penetration Enhancers

Gary P. Martin

King's College, University of London, London, United Kingdom

I. INTRODUCTION

It is now well established that many agents, including surfactants, pyrrolidones, dimethyl sulfoxide, propylene glycol, and laurocapram (Azone) can enhance the penetration of coadministered drugs through the stratum corneum (1). Fatty acids of certain structure and sterioisomerism have been shown to act as penetration enhancers. The mechanisms of action of these materials have either been determined or are now being established (2,3). It is perhaps equivocal, however, at the time of writing, whether phospholipids strictly warrant a chapter in a volume entitled *Pharmaceutical Skin Penetration Enhancement*. This is partly due to the relatively few publications that have examined the potential of topical application of phospholipids and also because some of the studies that have been carried out incorporate inappropriate controls against which the test preparation has been compared. It is difficult to determine the precise influence of a phospholipid in the delivery of a drug from a phospholipid-based formulation if, for example, such a formulation is compared with a marketed proprietary formulation of the same drug that has an entirely different and physicochemically complex composition. In some studies, solvents, known to enhance penetration, have been included in the phospholipid formulation. Alternatively, the phospholipid–drug combination has been incorporated into semisolid formulations before topical application to the skin, making real comparisons with appropriate controls very difficult to effect. Another reason to appraise whether it is appropriate to consider phospholipids in

57

a volume entitled thus, is that penetration enhancement, as such, has not frequently been claimed to occur following topical application of phospholipid. Instead, what is often suggested is that phospholipids may enhance the localization of drug within the layers of the epidermis–dermis and, thereby, reduce the amount of drug reaching the systemic circulation. Many of the agents discussed in other chapters are of use in obtaining increased blood levels of a drug and, by inference, increased concentration levels within the skin layers as a result of a reduction in the epidermal permeability coefficient. Should the target receptors lay within the skin layers or within the skin appendages, however, it would have obvious advantages if percutaneous absorption into the blood could be controlled and limited while concomitantly optimizing drug concentrations at the site of action. This goal is particularly desirable for drugs that may be applied over a prolonged period or over extensive areas of the body when systemic toxicity may be a problem. Instances for which localization would be desirable include the topical use of corticosteroids, cytotoxic agents, anesthetics, retinoids, sex hormones, and antifungal, antibacterial, and antiviral agents for a variety of skin disorders. In addition, if exogenously applied lipids can be employed to deliver humectants to the skin layers, they would then have a valuable role in the essentially cosmetic function of moisturization. Therefore, it is perhaps not surprising that there is a section of the cosmetic literature that has described and patented the use of lipids to increase the water content of the skin. Several products from different cosmetic houses based on natural or synthetic lipids have been marketed, and some very enthusiastic claims have been made in commercial literatures for their respective efficacies and efficiencies in fulfilling their declared function. Other agents with intended cosmetic action that have been suggested as suitable candidates for enhanced location within the skin layers include sunscreens, tanning agents, and hair-restoring agents (e.g., minoxidil).

A further complicating feature in attempting to determine whether natural or synthetic lipids per se have application in affecting the localization of drugs within the skin is attributable to the fact that providing the phase transition temperature of the lipids is exceeded, liposomal vesicles are formed in dilute aqueous solutions. In early work (3) it was suggested, without any direct evidence, that such intact liposomal structures penetrate the stratum corneum, carrying payloads of drug with them. It must be remembered, however, that although such vesicles exist in dilute solution, as evaporation of solvent proceeds, perhaps after application to the skin, any liposomes present are likely to be transformed into a liquid crystalline gel. Such a gel, nevertheless, may retain any incorporated drug in an appropriate aqueous or lipid environment within the matrix. In contrast, if excessive concentrations of cosolvents, such as ethanol and propylene glycol, or preformulated lipophilic ointment bases are incorporated into a vehicle that contains liposomes, then any preformed vesicles may be destroyed. Alternatively, if a lipid is incorporated into such cosolvent-based systems, liposomes may never be formed initially. Another difficulty in determining whether lipids may have a function in promoting localization of drug within the skin is that no study has yet been carried out to examine whether the chemical structure of such exogenously applied lipids is of importance. Several studies, for example, have examined systematically the features of molecular structure that determine the effectiveness of fatty acids as percutaneous absorption enhancers (4,5). No equivalent studies have been reported in connection with the topical application of lipids, considering the effects of such factors as chain length, degree of saturation, sterioisomerism, or nature of the headgroup. Different studies have examined the effects of lipids after treatment regimens that have varied from a single application of a "liposomal" preparation through to a twice-daily application for 2 weeks. Considerable variation in composition of the topically applied liposomes, as well as differences in their methods of preparation, have also been features of past investigations that may have had an influence on the resultant drug deposition profiles.

It is thus apparent, even from the foregoing brief introduction, that there are several factors that need to be considered when critically evaluating the results of studies that have involved topical application of lipids. There are others, and these include the influence of lipids on the solubility and, hence, the thermodynamic activity of any coadministered drug; whether the association of the drug with lipid prevents or limits metabolism of the former within the skin; whether applied lipid, by forming a film on the skin surface, provides a more occlusive environment for subsequent drug absorption; and whether lipids may be incorporated into the intercellular matrix of the stratum corneum and, subsequently, modify its fluidity and permeability.

After having established that lipids can potentially modify drug absorption by several different mechanisms, it is intended first to briefly describe the composition and methods of preparation of liposomes that have been employed previously and then to consider, in more detail, the evidence that disposition of topically applied compounds within the skin can be altered by the use of lipids. For convenience of writing, the work pertinent to the field of cosmetic science has been reviewed separately from that which has appeared in the pharmaceutical literature. This is acknowledged to be an artificial division that can be justified only marginally on historical grounds, since even though the use of lecithin in cosmetics was reviewed as early as 1967 (6), it was not until 13 years later that the first scientific paper was published examining the deposition of a corticosteroid after application to rabbit skin as a liposomal suspension (3). The limited number of clinical studies that have employed topically applied lipids will be critically assessed and, finally, the potential benefits will be considered of employing phospholipid matrices, in which interaction of the lipid with the skin is claimed not to occur or is thought not to be the principal controlling mechanism. Finally, current and future prospectives are discussed, with an emphasis placed on the immediate requirements of future research.

II. COMPOSITION AND PREPARATION OF LIPOSOMES

Liposomes have been extensively investigated as potential drug carriers with a view to obtaining selective drug delivery to various internal organs and tissues, usually after administration by the parenteral route. It is beyond the scope of the present review to consider this work in detail, and interested readers are referred elsewhere (7–10). Several reviews have appeared on the preparative procedures that are available to produce liposomes of different structure and type (11–13). Only sufficient detail is included here to enable an understanding of the terminology employed in studies that have considered topical application of lipids.

The liposomes that form after rehydration of lipid films, at temperatures above the phase transition temperature, are termed *multilamellar vesicles* (MLV). These structures have a size range of 0.1–10 µm and consist of concentric bilayers of lipid separated by aqueous channels (Fig. 1). These can subsequently be transformed, if required, by a variety of techniques (Figs. 1 and 2) to smaller vesicles. *Large* (LUV) or *smaller unilamellar* vesicles (SUV) can be produced that, as the name suggests, although different in size (being 150–500 and 20–50 nm, respectively) consist of a central aqueous core surrounded by one lipid bilayer. Water-soluble or lipid-soluble moieties can be incorporated at appropriate stages in the preparation procedure, and partition processes determine their subsequent

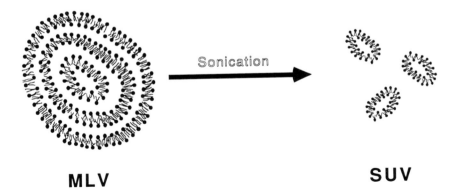

MLV   **SUV**

Figure 1 Multilamellar vesicles (MLV) formed spontaneously from phospholipids in aqueous solution can be transformed to small unilamellar vesicles (SUV) by several different techniques, including sonication.

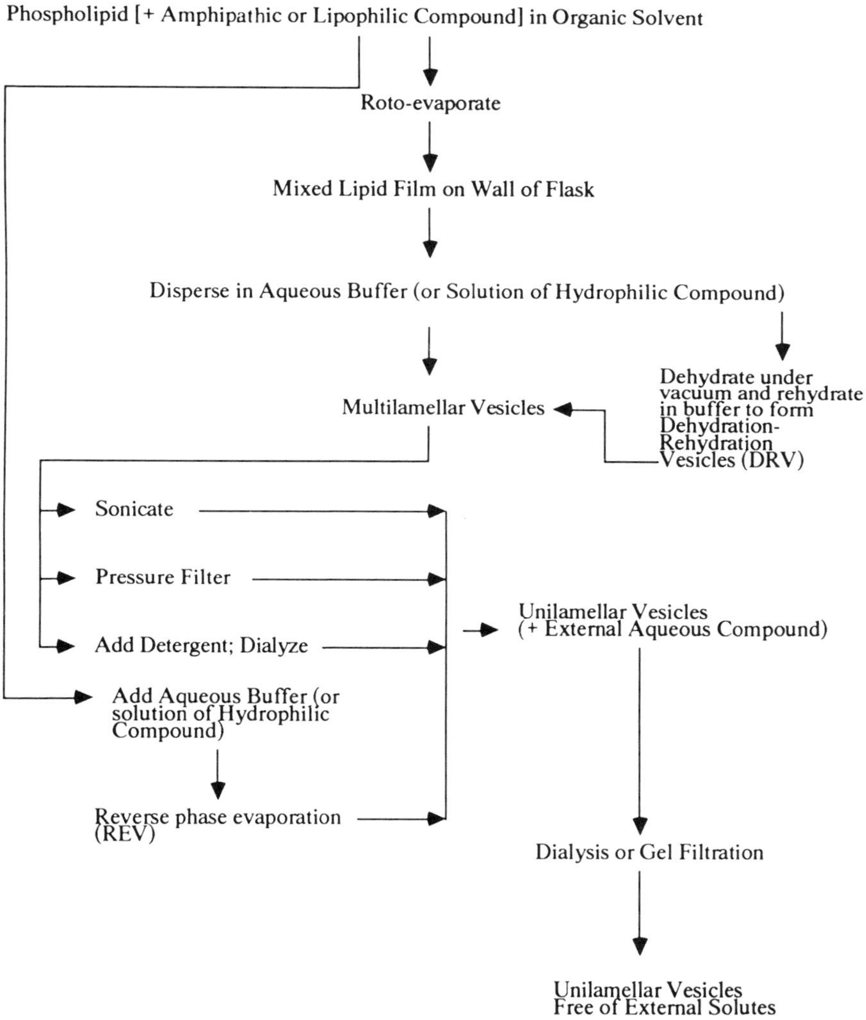

Phospholipid [+ Amphipathic or Lipophilic Compound] in Organic Solvent

Roto-evaporate

Mixed Lipid Film on Wall of Flask

Disperse in Aqueous Buffer (or Solution of Hydrophilic Compound)

Dehydrate under vacuum and rehydrate in buffer to form Dehydration-Rehydration Vesicles (DRV)

Multilamellar Vesicles

Sonicate

Pressure Filter

Add Detergent; Dialyze

Unilamellar Vesicles (+ External Aqueous Compound)

Add Aqueous Buffer (or solution of Hydrophilic Compound)

Reverse phase evaporation (REV)

Dialysis or Gel Filtration

Unilamellar Vesicles Free of External Solutes

Figure 2 Flowsheet for preparing drug- or cosmetic-carrying liposomes (on a laboratory scale).

location within either the aqueous or lipid layers. A dialysis or filtration step may be included to remove any drug that remains unencapsulated at the end of the preparative procedure. Cholesterol is a common component of liposomal membranes, since its inclusion within the bilayer modifies fluidity and permeability. The addition of a charged amphipathic lipid such as stearylamine (SA) or dicetyl phosphate (DCP) enables a positive or negative charge, respectively, to be conferred upon the vesicle. On heating to a characteristic transition temperature (T_c), bilayers undergo a change from a *gel* phase (the lipid chains being ordered and polar headgroups moderately hydrated) to a *liquid crystalline* phase (the lipid chains having liquidlike mobility and the polar headgroups highly hydrated). For bilayers of natural unsaturated phospholipids, T_c lies below room temperature, but some saturated phospholipids [e.g., dipalmitoyl- (DPPC) and distearoylphosphatidylcholine (DSPC)] have T_c well above skin temperature (13,14).

The formation of liposomal structures is not limited to phospholipids, and several synthetic surfactants have been prepared that aggregate in a similar manner (15,16). Indeed, the vesicles formed by certain synthetic nonionic surfactants (Fig. 3) have been termed *niosomes* and employed for cosmetic purposes (17).

Liposomes are formed by certain lipids and surfactants when there is an excess of aqueous phase present. As the concentration of lipid increases, different complex liquid crystalline phases often result (18,19).

III. COSMETIC APPLICATIONS

Lecithin, which consists primarily of a mixture of phosphatidylcholines of different hydrocarbon chain lengths and degree of saturation, is obtained mainly from the commercial extraction of soybeans. It has been incorporated in many different cosmetic formulations, including soaps, lipsticks, shaving creams, deodorants, shampoos, cold creams, moisturizing creams, beauty masks, and hairwaving preparations, since the first half of this century (6). Suggested attributes conferred on such products by incorporation of phospholipids, which are derived primarily from qualitative observations, include useful antioxidant

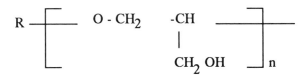

Figure 3 General structure of nonionic lipids that spontaneously form vesicles in solution. n can vary from 1–6; R is an aliphatic, linear or branched, saturated or unsaturated, chain of 12–30 carbon atoms.

function, effective "beard-softening" activity, promotion of lather stabilization, and improved emollient humectant and lubricant properties. The complexity of many of these formulations, which often contain a multitude of materials of natural origin, as well as lecithin from different sources (6), makes the scientific testing and, hence, strict validity of such claims impossible to determine.

The use of liposomes of a specific composition, consisting of 70:20:10 (mole ratio), soybean lecithin/dicetyl phosphate/cholesterol has been claimed to be effective in the delivery of humectants, such as glycerol, urea, ornithine, and sodium pyroglutamate, to the skin (20). The commercial grade soybean lecithin used in these studies (20) is declared to contain choline lecithin, cephalin, and inositol phosphatides, and some evidence is presented to suggest that the cholesterol component could be replaced with other sterols, such as sitosterol, 7-dehydrosterol, and lanosterol, with only slight changes in efficacy. Advantages cited for such "moisturizing units," include the substantivity of the liposomes to keratin, improved absorption of atmospheric water, and enhanced delivery of encapsulated water and moisturizing agent to the skin. The possible function of the applied lipid as having an occlusive effect upon the skin, thereby retarding water loss and leading to increased skin hydration, is also acknowledged.

Studies are presented showing that for solvent-damaged stratum corneum treated with such liposomes in vitro, the water-binding capacity was increased by 110–240% and the water diffusion rate through the membrane decreased by over 100%, compared with controls. Unfortunately, it is unclear whether the control membranes were exposed to the humectants in free solution. Also the amount of humectant that remained encapsulated after a dialysis step to remove unincorporated material is not reported. In addition, the effects of empty liposomes on such damaged membranes were not investigated, an important omission, since phosphatidylcholines are known to bind water tightly (21), an effect promoted by cholesterol. Oleniacz (20) also describes a subjective evaluation carried out on only two individuals when liposomes of the composition just described and containing sodium pyroglutamate were applied to dry, cracked skin of one hand. Visual assessment 18 hr later was claimed to indicate less cracking and scaling than on the control hands.

Vesicles prepared from synthetic nonionic lipids (termed niosomes) having the general formula shown in Figure 3, have also been investigated as possible vehicles for the delivery of cosmetic agents to the skin (17). As with liposomes, dicetyl phosphate and cholesterol can also be incorporated in such vesicles, to modify, respectively, the surface charge and the permeability of the structures to entrapped compounds (22). Niosome particle size would appear to be partially dependent on lipid composition (22), although the specific lipid composition of such structures employed to deliver moisturizing agents to the skin (17) has not been reported, presumably for commercial reasons.

An in vitro comparison of sodium pyroglutamate uptake by isolated stratum corneum from niosomes, with oil-in-water (o/w) and water-in-oil (w/o) emulsions (all of undeclared composition) containing 10% moisturizer, indicated that the niosome formulation after 6 hr delivered 29 times and 14 times the amount of pyroglutamate as the o/w and w/o emulsion, respectively (17). In the same study, a human test panel result (five subjects) indicated that niosomes containing sodium pyroglutamate helped prevent the occurrence of dry skin induced by washing the hands with soap, a similar result being obtained also when empty niosomes were employed. In a later investigation, the same workers used freeze-fracture and electron spin resonance techniques to show that such nonionic synthetic lipids may incorporate into delipidated skin (23,24). Sunscreen, tanning agents, and combinations of these with humectants have also been entrapped in lipid vesicles and suggested to have potential cosmetic advantages over other formulations (22). Somewhat ironically, a review of Japanese patents indicates that liposomes may also have commercial application in the production of skin-whitening lotions (25).

Mammalian stratum corneum is described as consisting of highly cornified cells embedded in a matrix of extracellular lipid lamellae (26). These extracellular lipid sheets, although devoid of phospholipids, are composed primarily of ceramides (50% w/w), cholesterol (25%), free fatty acids (15%), and cholesterol sulfate (CHS) (5%) (27,28). Therefore, it might be thought that if affinity with lipids of the stratum corneum is required, it would be more advantageous to employ lipids in topical applications of the type usually found in the stratum corneum. The suggestion, however, that natural or synthetic glycolipids be employed to delivery compounds topically, although made several years ago (22), has not been investigated until more recently, when ceramides were incorporated either into phosphatidylcholine (PC) liposomes (29) or as the major component of a mixed lipid vesicle (30,31). The potential use of sphingolipid combinations (ceramides, cerebrosides, and sphingomyelins) as *sphingosomes*, in the formulation of cosmetic products, would appear to be under investigation (32).

The composition of the applied liposome dispersion has been claimed to influence skin hydration (33). Three liposome dispersions, containing no moisturizing agent, but consisting of different but complex compositions, were each applied, as well as a control solution consisting of 0.9% sodium chloride, to the flexor surface of the forearms of ten volunteers. Capacitance measurement, obtained using a Corneometer, over the following 3 hr suggested that the liposomes containing the highest proportion of soy-derived PC (SPC) increased hydration to the greatest extent. In contrast, the preparation containing the highest proportion of phosphatidylinositol (PI) and lowest proportion of SPC dehydrated the skin. The authors explain the findings by suggesting that PI, in contrast with SPC, does not penetrate the stratum corneum but remains on the surface of the skin and extracts water from the underlying layers. However, it should be appreciated that because individual, pure phospholipids were not employed in the study, conclusions based on such findings can be regarded as only tentative. There appears to be a clear preference, expressed within the cosmetic literature to employ unsaturated phospholipids within formulations when skin penetration is required, but to use saturated lipids (e.g., hydrogenated phospholipids) when a prolonged residence on the skin is desired (34,35). Scant persuasive evidence is available, however, to support this contention.

The data available in the public domain derived from studies carried out by the cosmetic industry relating to topical delivery of vesicle encapsulated agents do not, in general, bear close scientific scrutiny, because of the omission of important preparative and experimental details and lack of appropriate controls, as discussed earlier and in other reviews (36,37). However, whereas few pharmaceutical topical lipid formulations have been registered (38), it should be acknowledged that there are several cosmetic moisturizing preparations that have been marketed successfully in both the United States and Europe. Some patents assigned to the large cosmetic houses also seek to extend intellectual property rights to encapsulating materials of pharmaceutical relevance such as antibiotics and enzymes (22,39).

It is likely that in the future liposome-containing formulations will be marketed in some countries for what are seen by some as cosmetic problems, such as hair loss prevention, hair growth promotion, deceleration of the skin-ageing process, sunscreening, and changing skin pigmentation (25,40). Empty liposome-containing formulations are available from several companies (25,34) to enable smaller cosmetic manufacturers to produce and market their own "active" products. Whether or not liposome-containing preparations, as opposed to lipid-containing preparations, do confer advantageous properties upon cosmetic formulations, remains to be scientifically validated. However, from the commercial viewpoint, the image that can be portrayed of vesicles, penetrating deeply into the skin and then releasing their contents, is one that is attractive to the advertising industry and one that will undoubtedly be profitably exploited, whether fact or fiction.

IV. DRUG DISPOSITION STUDIES

A number of investigations have now been carried out to examine whether a lipid, concomitantly applied with a topical drug, favorably alters the disposition of the latter within the body and within the skin layers in particular. Table 1 shows some of the lipid combinations that have been applied to the skin of experimental animals and human volunteers, or used in diffusion studies in vitro. The lipids employed have been from a number of different sources and, in many cases, the initial formulation has been liposomal in nature. Therefore, cholesterol has been

Table 1 Drug–Lipid Combinations Examined in Topical Application Studies[a]

Drug	Lipid (lipid ratio)[b]	Vehicle[c]	Applied lipid concentration	Lipid charge	Parameter examined	Species	Ref.
Triamcinolone Acetonide	DPPC/CH(1.1:0.5)	8 mM CaCl$_2$ or Hydrocolloid gel	Not mentioned, constant amount of drug applied	0	Blood, urine, skin; internal organ concentrations in vivo	Rabbit	3, 41
Triamcinolone	EPC/CH(5:2)	Vaseline containing Span 20	0.67% w/w total lipid	0	Transdermal absorption (determined from residual drug remaining on skin in vivo)	Human	42
Triamcinolone acetonide palmitate	DPPC/CH(1.1:0.5)	8 mM CaCl$_2$	Not mentioned, constant amount of drug applied	0	Concentration in cheek pouch ulcers in vivo; internal organ concentrations in vivo	Hamster	43
Hydrocortisone	EPC/CH(3:1, approx.)	Tris buffer (pH 7.0) containing TC	Approx. 800 mM·L^{-1} total lipid; total amount lipid applied varied to ensure constant amount of drug applied	0	Skin concentration determined after diffusion into whole skin in vitro; blood and urine levels in vivo	Human / Guinea pig	44 / 45
5α-Dihydrotestosterone	DPPC/CH(1.1:05)	8 mM CaCl$_2$	Not mentioned, constant amount of drug applied	0	Determination of hormone-induced morphological changes to flank in vivo	Hamster	46

Drug	Lipid	Vehicle	Concentration	Effect	Method	Species	Ref.
Hydrocortisone Clobetasone butyrate Betamethasone valerate Clobetasol propionate	EPC	15 mM Sorensøns phosphate (pH 5.0)	5.0% w/v	0	Assessment of blanching response after pretreatment of skin with lipid in vivo	Human	47, 48
Hydrocortisone Progesterone Glucose	DMPC DPPC DSPC DSPC/CH(2:1) DPPC/DCP(9:1) DPPC/SA(9:1)	Normal saline	65 mM·L⁻¹ total lipid	0 0 0 0 − +	Diffusion through full-thickness abdominal skin in vitro	Hairless mouse	49
Butylparaben	EPC/CH/DCP (4:2:1)	Water	28 mM·L⁻¹ total lipid	−	Whole-body auto-radiography and microautoradiography of excised skin, after topical application in vivo	Guinea pig	50
Butylparaben	EPC/CH/DCP (4:2:1)	Water	Variable (9.3–56 mM·L⁻¹ total lipid)	−	Diffusion through whole skin and through skin stripped of stratum corneum in vitro	Guinea pig	51
Sodium diclofenac	HSP	100 mM PBS (pH 7.4)	0.05–1% w/v	0	Diffusion through whole skin in vitro	Rat	52

Table 1 (Continued)

Drug	Lipid (lipid ratio)[b]	Vehicle[c]	Applied lipid concentration	Lipid charge	Parameter examined	Species	Ref.
Sodium diclofenac	HSP	100 mM PBS (pH 7.4)	0.5%	0	Plasma levels in anesthetized animal in vitro	Rat	52
Sodium diclofenac	HSP	100 mM PBS (pH 7.2) sometimes containing 6.8% TG and 10.0% ethanol	6.8% w/w	0	Plasma levels in anesthetized animal in vivo; plasma levels in vivo	Rat Human	53 53
Indomethacin	EPC	"Gel ointment," sometimes containing benzyl-nicotinate (0.5%)	2%	0	Plasma, urinary, feces, and skin levels in vivo	Rat	54
Flufenamic acid	SPC	Citrate phosphate buffer (pH 3.0); some experiments incorporated either 30% Pg or 30% G Some experiments decreased SPC from 20 to 14 mM·L⁻¹ keeping total lipid constant by replacement with GC	10–60 mM·L⁻¹ 20 mM·L⁻¹	0	Diffusion through abdominal skin in vitro; pretreatment of skin with lipid followed by in vitro diffusion; plasma levels in anesthetized animals in vivo	Rat	29

Drug	Phospholipid	Vehicle	Concentration		Study	Model	Ref.
Bunazocin Theophylline Isosorbide dinitrate	EPC	Pg	1% w/w	0	Diffusion through whole skin in vitro	Rat	55
Bunazocin	EPC	Pg	3% w/w	0	Plasma concentrations in vivo	Rabbit	55
Methotrexate	PC/CH/DCP (10:2:1)	Saline	5% w/v	–	Plasma and skin concentrations	Nude mouse	56, 57
Methotrexate	PC/CH (10:2)	Saline	20% w/v	0	Clinical assessment of improvement in psoriasis in vivo	Human	57
Inulin	PC/CH (10:2)	Saline	10% w/v	0	Skin concentrations in vivo	Rabbit	57
Tetracaine	SPC/StA/CH (7%:0.7%;0.7%)	Water containing 0.65% NaHCO$_3$, 0.45% NaCl, 10.0% ethanol, 7.0% Pg	7% w/w SPC	–	Assessment of topical anesthesia in vivo	Human	58
Interferon	EPC/CH/PS (2:1:0.33) DMPC/CH/PS (2:1/0.33) CM/CH/PA/CHS (4:2.5:2.5:1)	PBS (pH 7.0) containing 1% TC	100 mM·L^{-1} total lipid	– – –	Assessment of herpes lesions in vivo	Hairless guinea pig	30

Table 1 (Continued)

Drug	Lipid (lipid ratio)[b]	Vehicle[c]	Applied lipid concentration	Lipid charge	Parameter examined	Species	Ref.
Interferon Inulin	EPC/CH/PS (1:1:0.5) CM/CH/CHS (4.2:2.8:3) CM/CH/PA/CS	0.05 M HEPES (pH 7.4), containing 1% TC	15 mg·mL^{-1} total lipid	− −	Skin concentration of drugs and lipids after diffusion into whole skin	Hairless guinea pig	31
T4 endonuclease (a DNA repair enzyme)	PC/DCP/CH (7:2:1) PC/SA/CH (7:2:1) DSPC/PC/CH (7:2:1) DMPC/PC/CH (7:2:1) DPPC/PC/CH (7:2:1) PC/DCP (7:3) PG/DCP (7:3) PE/DCP (7:3)	Aqueous solution containing 20 µg·mL^{-1} herring sperm DNA	Total amount applied depended on encapsulation efficiency of DNA	− + 0 0 0 − − −	Survival of UV-mediated cells	Cell culture	59

[a] Abbreviations employed in this table are listed in the chapter Appendix.
[b] Lipid ratio is a molar ratio unless otherwise specified.
[c] Vehicle into which lipid was incorporated for topical application.

included as a component with the view to modifying the permeability of the vesicle, and frequently dicetyl phosphate has been included to impart a negative charge. In some instances, the liposome formulation has been subsequently incorporated either into complex vehicles or other solvent systems before topical application. There has often been no confirmation that liposomes remain intact in such systems. It should be appreciated that even when comparatively simple aqueous liposome formulations are employed, if evaporation is allowed to proceed, the liposomes are likely to fuse to form a liquid crystalline matrix (60). There are large differences in the experimental protocols employed in the amount and concentration of lipid applied, the lipid/drug ratio utilized, dosage regimens, and species of animal employed (see Table 1). When interpreting the significance of data obtained in studies intended to assess the effects of topically applied lipids, it is also important that due consideration be given to the relevance of the control formulation against which the test formulation is compared. Some of these factors will be considered in more specific detail in the following critical review of previous investigations.

One of the first investigations that claimed to show a more favorable deposition of a topically applied drug, after the drug was partitioned within liposomes, was a study carried out by Mezei and Gulasekharam (3). These workers applied a liposomal preparation, consisting of dipalmitoylphosphatidylcholine (DPPC) and cholesterol, containing triamcinolone acetonide, to depilated rabbit skin in vivo twice a day for 5 days. Drug concentrations in the epidermis and dermis were four to five times higher than when an ointment dosage form, containing the same concentration of drug, was similarly applied. In addition, three times less drug was found in the thalamic region of the brain after application of the corticosteroid as a liposomal suspension than as an ointment. A favorable disposition profile for topically applied corticosteroid drugs would be one in which epidermal and dermal concentrations are maintained for as long as possible (being the site of therapeutic activity) while thalamic concentrations are kept to a minimum (being a site of possible adverse effects). When the same liposomal preparation was incorporated into a hydrocolloid gel and tested against a control gel preparation containing free corticosteroid at the same concentration (41), the relative concentration levels between test (liposomal) and control preparations in the skin and the thalamic region were similar to the earlier investigation (3). Approximately five times more triamcinolone acetonide was found in the epidermis and over two times less in the thalamic region after application of the liposomal gel, in comparison with the control gel. In both studies (3,41), the concentration of corticosteroid in the blood after 5 days and the cumulative urinary excretion (Fig. 4) were reduced as a result of liposome encapsulation, suggesting that percutaneous absorption was less if the drug was applied in liposomal form, than in the ointment or gel forms. Kellaway (61), in a critique of the experimental methodology employed by Mezei and Gulasekharem, suggested that swabbing the rabbit skin immediately before sacrifice to remove any preparation still remaining on the skin was likely to destroy liposomal integrity, yield high drug activity at the skin surface and, therefore, partly explain the drug loading of the skin detected after 5 days. It is likely that the thermodynamic activity of the drug in the liposomal and control dose forms differed. Therefore, it could be argued that percutaneous absorption of the drug was reduced purely because the liposomal preparations of the drug were poor formulations that retained the drug in the locality of the skin surface.

The uptake by skin of triamcinolone from a liposome preparation mixed into petrolatum (Vaseline) base has been compared with the same concentration of free drug similarly incorporated after applying both preparations to the arms of human volunteers (42). Residual corticosteroid levels on the skin were determined after 8 hr occlusion by swabbing the application sites with alcohol and, on the basis of the results obtained, "resorption" of triamcinolone was claimed to be threefold greater when the drug was incorporated into the base in liposomal form. No confirmatory evidence is provided to verify that liposomes remain intact in the hydrophobic environment of the vehicle employed.

It has been suggested that liposomes may penetrate the lipid-rich outer skin layers and localize in the more aqueous dermis (3). Accordingly, a long-hydrocarbon–chain corticosteroid ester has been prepared, encapsulated with greater efficiency than the parent drug, within the liposomal bilayer and applied topically with a view to obtaining a more localized action (43). It is argued that one reason for the apparent reduced epidermal and dermal clearance of liposome-entrapped drug is that any encapsulated material, as penetration of the skin proceeds, is unavailable to the metabolizing enzymes within the skin (62). Alternatively, it has been suggested that larger liposomes act as localizers in the dermis, being unable to penetrate to the underlying blood vessels and, therefore, acting akin to localized sustained-release vehicles (38,62). The concept, however, that relatively large lipid vesicles are able to traverse densely packed epidermal tissue to arrive intact within the dermal layers has been received critically (49,63). Results from studies that examined the diffusion of lipophilic and hydrophilic compounds across excised hairless mouse skin in vitro suggested that, within 60 hr, liposomes in solution neither diffused across nor fused with the skin surface (49).

Lipophilic drugs, such as hydrocortisone and progesterone, which when entrapped in liposomes are known to be intercalated within the bilayer, were found to have penetration coefficients through the skin, when applied in liposomes, similar to those determined when applied free in solution. However, the flux of glucose through the skin, entrapped in the aqueous region of the liposome, was markedly slowed. Through the use of supportive theoretical analysis of the results, it was suggested (49,64) that the release of the compound

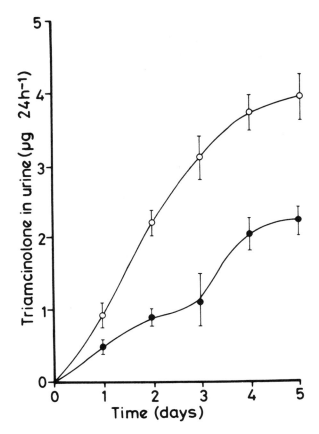

Figure 4 Urinary excretion of triamcinolone 2-[^{14}C]acetonide applied topically in 'free' (o) and in liposomal form (●). The error bars indicate SD ($n = 8$). (From Ref. 41.)

from the liposome was the rate-determining step in the permeation of hydrophilic compounds through skin, whereas a process of direct transfer from liposome to skin was proposed for lipophilic drugs.

A study of the percutaneous penetration of radiolabeled butylparaben through excised guinea pig skin over 30 hr (51) has provided support for the mechanism of direct transfer of drug from liposome to skin, although, in the case of butyl-paraben, this was suggested to occur only to a small extent. The amount of the butylparaben that penetrated the skin decreased as the lipid content of the liposomal suspension was increased, suggesting that release of butylparaben to the aqueous phase, followed by percutaneous penetration, was the major controlling factor in the absorption process. The antimicrobial activity of liposomes containing butylparaben, determined against a range of microorganisms, was also dependent on the free butylparaben concentration, rather than upon total concentration. This finding suggested that the partition of the preservative into the aqueous phase was the rate-controlling factor in its activity. Moreover, on the basis of later experimental in vitro diffusion results obtained in hairless mouse skin (65) it was concluded that progesterone delivery from liposomes did not involve any direct transfer of the drug between liposome and skin. The faster transdermal delivery rate of liposome-entrapped progesterone found in the earlier studies (49,64), in comparison with that obtained later (65), has been suggested to be due to lysophosphatidylcholine (LPC) being present as an impurity. LPC is known to enhance diffusion of compounds through membranes (66), probably as a result of damage (67,68) from interaction with and extraction of endogenous lipids. Pure or well-characterized phospholipids would appear to be a prerequisite before initiating studies involved with the topical application of such materials.

The fate of lipids that are topically applied to the skin has not yet been determined unequivocally. Radiolabeled DPPC from either empty or steroid-containing liposomes could not be detected in the receptor compartment of a diffusion cell, using full-thickness mouse skin as a membrane (49), suggesting that liposomes do not pass intact through such a barrier within the 60 hr time span employed. It can be argued, however, that it is *cutaneous* (into the skin) and not *percutaneous* (through the skin) absorption that is of greater relevance in establishing whether concomitant application of lipid is advantageous to increasing localized drug concentration within the skin. In addition, the lack of metabolic activity within dead skin tissue, which is usually employed in in vitro diffusion studies, is not representative of the situation in vivo during which such reactions may have the potential of providing a destabilizing environment for liposomal membranes and promote the release of entrapped drug to the surrounding tissue (62).

A study, employing microautoradiography, carried out 6 hr after a single application of a dilute liposome suspension containing [^{14}C]DPPC, indicated that most of the phospholipid remained associated with the skin surface (50). Little affinity of the phospholipid with sebum or sebaceous glands was detected, neither was there evidence of transfollicular penetration. A further in vivo study, involving the application of liposomes containing radiolabeled DPPC to rabbit skin, followed by tape stripping (69), led the investigator to conclude that there was no evidence to suggest that liposomes entered the surface layer of the skin, since most of the radiolabel activity was recovered from the surface. In contrast, Wohlrab et al. (70) concluded that radiolabeled egg PC (EPC) penetrated the skin rapidly, with peak epidermal concentrations being attained within 30 min of application. These latter workers examined the diffusion of PC (which was prepared by methylating phosphatidylethanolamine with [^{14}C]methyliodide) from a liposome gel (containing 30 mol% cholesterol) into full-thickness human skin in vitro. The distribution of phospholipid was determined with a microdissection technique followed by scintillation counting of each cut section (44) after 30 and 300 min of application. After both time intervals, a large concentration gradient of PC was found across the stratum corneum, with a much lower, but nearly uniform, distribution across the epidermis and dermis (70). The manipulative processes involved in carrying out such a dissection technique are considerable, and it is obviously essential that rigorous care is exercised when sections are cut to avoid transfer of the radiolabeled species from one location to another. With use of the same methodology, the disposition of hydrocortisone entrapped in liposomes after application to human skin for 30 and 300 min was compared with that obtained from a water-in-oil emulsion (71). The amount of hydrocortisone associated with the stratum corneum was independent of either the dose form or time. However, when the liposomal formulation was compared with the emulsion, epidermal concentrations were reported to be nine and four times higher after 30 and 300 min application, respectively. Similar improved concentration–time profiles were reported to exist in the dermal layers when the liposomal preparation was employed. Moreover, when the same formulations were applied to the dorsal surface of guinea pig ears in vivo, the blood and urine levels over the following 96-hr study period were lower in the liposome- than in the emulsion-treated animals (48,72). From these results, hydrocortisone-loaded liposomes have been claimed, similarly to the triamcinolone acetonide-loaded (3,41), to act as a selective drug delivery system or "drug localizer" and, thereby, provide a means of increasing therapeutic efficacy while concomitantly decreasing adverse systemic effects (45). Similar advantageous disposition profiles have been claimed for other lipophilic drugs, including progesterone in rabbits (73), triamcinolone acetonide palmitate in hamsters (43), and topical anesthetics in guinea pigs (74). In contrast, autoradiographic studies carried out 24 hr after the in vivo application of butylparaben entrapped in liposomes to guinea pigs, suggested that a pattern of distribution was obtained similar to that which resulted after the preservative was applied in an ointment base (50).

Vermoken et al. (46) applied 5α-dihydrotestosterone, encapsulated in the same liposomal formulation as employed by Mezei and Gulasekharam (3), to the female hamster flank for an interrupted period of 20 days out of a 28-day treatment period. The resultant increase in the size of sebaceous structures was compared with that induced by a solution of the same concentration of the drug in acetone. On the basis of changes found in the structures of the untreated controlateral organs, this study showed that the systemic absorption was negligible from the liposome system, but significant from an acetone solution containing the same concentration of drug. The topical biological effect was, however, markedly diminished when the liposome system was used. It is possible, as discussed by Mezei (62), that any liposomes that may have entered the skin did not release the associated drug, rendering it unavailable to the relevant receptor. Alternatively, the relevant receptor may be sited below the dermis in the subcutaneous layer where, after application of the drug in liposomes, localized concentrations may not be increased. Moreover, comparing the activity of a liposomal suspension of a drug against a solution in acetone may be unrealistic because any solvent action of acetone on the skin may promote the biological activity of the control (1). The thermodynamic activity of the drug in the solvent, before evaporation, is also likely to be initially greater in the acetone solution, but this will change as solvent evaporation proceeds. The difficulty in choosing an appropriate vehicle to act as a comparator with a liposome formulation and the resultant problems in data interpretation are clearly exemplified. In addition, the involvement of other factors, such as species differences, and differences in liposome composition, makes interstudy comparisons even more difficult.

Much of the work discussed thus far has been concerned with the disposition of drugs that primarily would be associated or intercalated with the lipid bilayer. The concentrations of radiolabeled methotrexate, a water-soluble drug, has been determined in the skin and blood of nude mice for up to 2 hr after topical application as a liposomally entrapped formulation and compared with those achieved after free drug was applied with empty liposomes (56,57). Entrapped [³H]methotrexate concentration levels were two to three times higher in the skin compared with the free drug, whereas blood levels were up to 40% lower. Penetration of the stratum corneum and localization of liposomes within the epidermis in vivo has also been claimed (57) after the topical application of PC–cholesterol liposomes containing inulin (a sugar that partitions into the aqueous compartments of liposomes). After application of the liposome preparation to shaved rabbit skin, over ten times the amount of inulin was associated with the epidermis 1 hr later, when compared with the same dose of inulin applied in free form. Only 1.27 and 0.17%, respectively, of the doses were recovered from beneath the stratum corneum. In a recent in vitro study (31), inulin could be detected within the lower skin layers when applied in EPC-based liposomes (see Table 1) for 24 hr, whereas, when it was applied as an aqueous solution, no penetration of the skin could be shown.

When lipids are incorporated into a topical vehicle containing a drug, such lipids can modify subsequent topical absorption by two principal means. First, the lipid can interact with incorporated drug and influence drug release from the vehicle. Second, the lipid may modify the absorbing membrane in some manner, such that the resultant barrier to drug diffusion is changed. With this consideration in mind, a study carried out by Jacobs et al. (48) examined the effect of pretreating the skin with phospholipid before the application of any corticosteroid formulation. The human skin-blanching assay (75) was employed to assess the topical bioavailability of four commercially available corticosteroid preparations of different potencies (48). One forearm of each of ten volunteers was treated twice daily for 1 week with EPC presented as a buffered liposomal suspension, while the other arm was treated with buffer alone (Fig. 5). For the following 2 weeks this same treatment regimen was continued, but in addition each of four corticosteroid formulations [containing (a) hydrocortisone 0.1%, (b) clobetasone butyrate 0.05%, (c) betamethasone 0.1%, and (d) clobetasol propionate 0.05%) was applied to sites on both arms. Visual assessments of blanching were made at the time intervals shown in Figure 5. Blanching profiles were derived by expressing blanching at any time point as a percentage of the maximum attainable blanching (i.e., percentage total possible score) and plotting it as a function of time. The resultant profile for clobetasol propionate cream (Fig. 6) was typical of that obtained for all four corticosteroids. On the buffer-treated arm a tachyphylactic response, evidenced by the diminution in peak response between days 1 and 5, is a typical phenomenon associated with continued corticosteroid application (76). Repeated treatment of the skin with EPC caused an alteration in the blanching profile, with the curves diverging with time (see Fig. 6). This effect was clearly shown when the peak response values obtained by combining the results for each corticosteroid formulation (Table 2). Over the course of days 1–5, the difference between the peak response values progressively increased, primarily as a result of the reduction in tachyphylactic response on the EPC-treated arms. The reason for the difference in blanching behavior between phospholipid- and buffer-treated arms is open to speculation. It is possible that exogenously applied EPC incorporates, to a small extent, with the lipid regions of the stratum corneum. Alternatively, after evaporation of the aqueous phase, the applied lipid may form a thin substantive film that remains in intimate contact with the skin. Subsequently applied corticosteroids would partition favorably into such a lipid layer supplement, forming a depot. Therefore, the rate of delivery of corticosteroid to the lower skin layers, at which blanching occurs, may be reduced after pretreatment with phospholipid. This, in turn, may diminish the resultant tachyphylaxis, since arrival of the corticosteroid at the relevant receptor occurs at a more controlled rate than on the buffer-treated arm. It should be acknowledged that any film of phospholipid in contact with the skin could modify transepidermal water loss, which may lead to a greater hydration of the stratum corneum and alter the drug absorption profile.

Since treatment of the skin with a suspension of EPC before and during corticosteroid application sustained blanching activity and reduced tachyphylaxis, this suggested either a change in the delivery or in deposition of the drug, or both. Therefore, a later investigation, using the same assay, examined the effect of applying the corticosteroid as a liposomal suspension over a 1-week interval. A

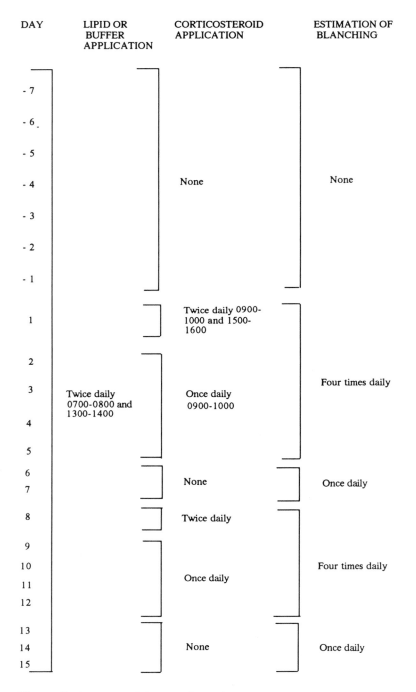

Figure 5 Summary of the experimental protocol employed to examine the effect of pretreating the skin with phospholipid before the application of corticosteroid formulations in vivo. (From Ref. 48.)

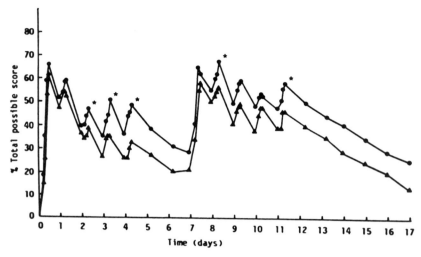

Figure 6 The percentage total possible score values for clobetasol proprionate cream applied to the buffer-treated (▲) and EPC-treated (●) arms with time (*$p < 0.05$). (From Ref. 48.)

similar pattern of corticosteroid application and estimation of blanching was used as that shown in week 1 of the protocol outlined in Figure 5. Three hydrocortisone esters [(a) 21-acetate, (b) 21-hexanoate, (c) 17-butyrate] were formulated either as a EPC–liposomal suspension (containing 5 mg·mL^{-1} EPC; 1% w/w 21-esters, or 0.1% w/w 17-ester) or triturated at the same concentrations into cetomacrogol (polyethylene glycol monocetyl ether) cream (77,78). The resultant blanching profiles for any particular corticosteroid, whether formulated as the cream or in liposomes, were very similar throughout the study, the daily peak blanching usually being observed 6 hr after steroid application. Figure 7 shows the blanching profile of hydrocortisone 17-butyrate produced by the two formulations. Blanching after application of the liposome was nearly always less than that observed when the same steroid was applied as the cream. Statistical analysis of the differences between the daily readings taken 6 hr after corticosteroid application demonstrated few significant differences, but any that were found showed that the cream formulation elicited the better blanching. For both the liposome and cream formulation, the blanching activity of hydrocortisone 17-butyrate was greatest on days 1 and 2 and diminished over the following 3 days because of tachyphylaxis (see Fig. 7). None of the advantages of employing phospholipid in topical application, expected from the results of the first study (47,48), could be shown in the later study (77). It is possible that difference may have become apparent if a longer

Table 2 Peak Blanching Responses (% TPS) Induced by Multiple Steroid Applications; Sum of All Preparations

	Day (% TPS)									
	1	2	3	4	5	8	9	10	11	12
T	27.5	34.5	32.2	34.2	31.4	34.2	41.3	37.2	33.6	34.7
C	26.1	29.8	26.1	23.1	20.0	30.8	31.7	26.7	25.2	25.5
T-C	1.4	4.7	6.1	11.1**	11.4*	3.4	9.6**	10.5**	8.4**	9.2**

*$p < 0.05$
**$p < 0.01$ using a two-tailed t-test.
T, EPC-treated arms
C, Buffer-treated control arms.
T-C, Difference between treatments.
Source: Ref. 48.

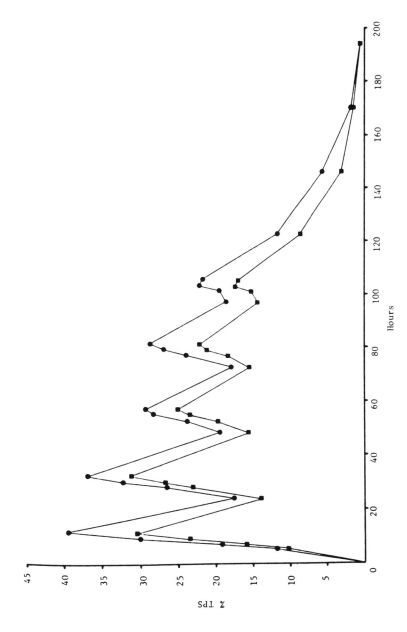

Figure 7 The percentage total possible score values obtained for hydrocortisone 17-butyrate in cetomacrogol cream (●) and liposomal suspension (■) as a function of time. (From Ref. 78.)

application regimen was used, but it should be acknowledged that the choice of cetomacrogol cream as the comparator for the liposomal formulation was purely arbitrary, and that the thermodynamic activity of the corticosteroids in the two formulations was likely to be different. Other workers (72), for example, making a comparison between a water-in-oil emulsion and PC–cholesterol liposomal formulation of hydrocortisone reported the blanching induced by the latter to be greater than that induced by the former. It was suggested that this could be correlated with the increased concentrations of the hydrocortisone that had diffused into human skin in vitro after 30 and 300 min.

So far in this review, only studies that have suggested that incorporation of lipid within a topical dose form may or may not modify subsequent disposition have been considered. There are, however, several investigations that conclude that lipids can enhance absorption. Ganesan et al. (49) acknowledge from in vitro diffusion studies, for example, that more total drug may be delivered through the skin using liposomes, but suggest that the mechanism is solely due to the increased solubility of lipophilic drugs as a result of liposomal incorporation. Kato et al. (55) concluded that the diffusion in vitro through hairless mouse skin of bunazosin, theophylline, and isosorbide from propylene glycol could be enhanced by the inclusion of 1% w/w EPC. Liposomes would not form in this solvent, however, and evidence is presented to show that lipid concentrations of up to 5% w/w EPC had no effect on drug solubility. When 3% EPC was included in a formulation of bunazosin suspended in propylene glycol and topically applied to rabbits, plasma levels of the drug were increased from undetectable (in the absence of lipid) to measurable concentrations.

Diffusion studies carried out in rat dorsal skin in vitro also support the premise that some lipids, when topically applied, can enhance penetration (52,53). Hydrogenated soybean phospholipids [HSP–consisting of approximately 30% PC and 70% phosphatidylethanolamine (PE)] increased the penetration of diclofenac sodium through the skin (within the concentration range 0.05–0.5% w/v when included in phosphate buffer). The HSP also caused a marked accumulation of drug in the subcutaneous tissue. However, when the phospholipid–diclofenac gel was placed in direct contact with subcutaneous tissue, the distribution of the drug into the tissue did not change greatly in comparison with that which resulted in the absence of phospholipid. These observations have been interpreted as providing evidence that the increase in diclofenac accumulation in the underlying skin when HSP is present, occurs as a result of direct surfactantlike action of the latter on the stratum corneum, possibly attributable to the extraction of endogenous lipids (52). Alternatively, the HSP could accumulate in, and modify the order of, the lipid matrix of the stratum corneum (53). Increased percutaneous absorption of diclofenac was also demonstrated in rats in vivo, as evidenced by increased plasma concentrations and increased concentrations attained in the skin (52).

When higher concentrations (6.8% w/v) HSP were applied to rats, sometimes including ethanol and triglyceride in the formulation, increased concentrations of the drug were found in the skin, but plasma levels were also increased (53). However, as with the studies carried out with triamcinolone acetonide in rabbits (3,41), an alcoholic washing of the skin surface before determining skin concentrations (53) could conceivably have artificially increased those concentrations (61). Plasma levels of diclofenac increased gradually after the topical application of a HSP/triglyceride/alcohol-containing formulation to the dorsal skin of four human volunteers (53). It should perhaps be emphasized that no other studies appear to have yet been carried out examining the topical application of lipid consisting of such a high content of PE (see Table 1), and it is likely that no liposomes are present in the applied dose forms, since such a high content of PE is likely to prevent vesicle formation (13). The inclusion of EPC in an ointment–gel of indomethacin has also been reported to increase skin levels and raise plasma concentrations of the drug in rats (54,79). Percutaneous absorption of EPC was reported to occur from the ointment–gel, with almost 30% of the applied EPC being absorbed within 8 hr (79). A gel filtration experiment indicated that the indomethacin was not entrapped in the EPC–liposomes (54), and it has been reported (29) that pretreatment of the skin with the ointment–gel containing EPC for 4 hr increased the subsequent percutaneous absorption of indomethacin applied as the ointment–gel (79). Therefore, it was concluded that the acceleration in percutaneous absorption of this anti-inflammatory drug was due to an alteration in permeability of the skin as a result of interaction of EPC with the membrane (79).

The percutaneous penetration of flufenamic acid (another nonsteroidal anti-inflammatory drug) through rat abdominal skin in vitro was enhanced by SPC (29). The penetration of flufenamic acid from a buffered suspension (pH 3.0) containing no SPC was poor, but was markedly enhanced by the inclusion of SPC in the buffer, up to a concentration of 20 $mM \cdot L^{-1}$. A further increase in lipid concentration to 40 $mM \cdot L^{-1}$ and above apparently reduced the rate of penetration to that achieved when no lipid was present. Enhanced penetration of the drug was obtained also when SPC was included in 30% cosolvent mixtures of buffer (pH 3.0), with either 30% propylene glycol or 30% glycerol. Interestingly, when some of the SPC in the buffered suspension of the drug was replaced with glycosylceramide (GC), penetration was further enhanced. A system containing 18 $mM \cdot L^{-1}$ PC/2 $mM \cdot L^{-1}$ GC increased sixfold compared with the buffer, the cumulative amount of flufenamic acid penetrating the skin in 24 h. When a PC or PC/GC dispersion of flufenamic acid was topically applied to rats in place of a lipid-free dispersion, plasma levels of the drug were elevated. The rationale for including GC within a topically applied formulation was to introduce a lipid, which like PC is not found in the stratum corneum (26,27), into a region that has extremely high contents of acylglycosylceramides (AGC) and acylceramides (AC). It has been suggested that the structurally specific function of AGC and AC is to anchor together the adjacent lipid bilayers of the stratum corneum (80), thereby forming a barrier to water permeation. The lower layers of the epidermis, in contrast, contain no AC and AGC, but have relatively high proportions of more hydrophilic acids such as GC. It was argued, therefore, that incorporation of PC or GC within the stratum corneum may increase the permeability of the principal barrier to diffusion (29). When rat skin was pretreated with drug-free GC/PC dispersions for 12 hr, however, there was no effect upon the subsequent penetration of flufenamic acid from lipid-free suspensions in vitro. A similar finding was also reported when pretreatment of skin with liposomes (EPC/CH/DCP; 4:2:1) (see Table 1) induced only a small change in the penetration of butylparaben (51). Since the inclusion of PC or PC/GC in suspensions of flufenamic acid increased the solubility of the latter by six times (29), it is likely that this phenomenon contributes most to the increases in percutaneous absorption.

As discussed previously, stratum corneum lipids consist primarily of ceramides (CM), cholesterol (CH), free fatty acids [primarily palmitic acid (PA)], cholesteryl sulfate (CHS) in a percentage weight ratio of approximately 50:25:15:5, respectively (26,28). Lipids of similar composition can form liposomes (81,82), and if the transfer of drug from liposomal bilayers is an essential aspect of the mechanism by which lipids facilitate drug transfer to the skin, then liposomes made from "skin lipids" might expedite this process. The concept of employing such liposomes has recently been examined in the topical delivery of encapsulated interferon to cutaneous herpes lesions in guinea pigs (30). The application of several different liposomes containing entrapped interferon caused a reduction of lesion scores, whereas application of interferon formulated as a solution or emulsion was ineffective. Although the skin lipid liposomes appeared to be more efficacious than phospholipid-based liposomes, it was the method of liposomal preparation that appeared to the most important factor for reducing lesion scores. It was concluded that the dehydration–rehydration method (DRV) of preparation (see Fig. 2) facilitated partition of the interferon into the lipid bilayers. Liposomes were ineffective when only free, rather than entrapped, interferon was present; hence, entrapment appeared to provide the correct physicochemical environment in which transfer of interferon could occur to the lipid compartment of the stratum corneum. In a subsequent study (31) the diffusion of interferon from several liposomal formulations (see Table 1) was examined in vitro. Radiolabeled interferon and lipid components were applied as liposome formulations to hairless guinea pig skin for 24 hr, after which it was removed from the diffusion cell and subjected to tape stripping, followed by appropriate radiolabel-counting procedures. The application of skin lipid liposomes resulted in almost twice the amount of interferon in the deeper skin layers than did the application of liposomes prepared from phospholipids. The method of liposomal preparation was also confirmed to be of importance, the DRV method proving to be the technique of choice for delivering most interferon to the skin. Significantly more cholesterol was also distributed to the deeper strata when applied as a component of the skin lipid liposomes, compared with its application within phospholipid liposomes. In addition, the detection of EPC in the deeper skin layers by this technique (31) confirms the earlier findings of Wohlrab et al. (70) and suggests that certain lipids can penetrate the stratum corneum and reach the epidermal and dermal layers.

The technique of one-dimensional electron paramagnetic resonance imaging has been employed to determine diffusion coefficients of a charged hydrophilic spin probe molecule through pig ear skin, after entrapment in a number of different liposome preparations (83). The influence of liposome composition and methods of liposomal preparation were two of the parameters examined, and it was concluded, on incomplete evidence, that both of these affected the diffusion process through the skin. The spin probe molecule was reported to penetrate the skin after it was entrapped in small unilamellar vesicle or reverse-phase evaporation vesicles (REV) composed of unsaturated phospholipids (see Fig. 2). Penetration of the spin probe did not occur from multilamellar vesicles or REV composed of saturated phospholipids. However, the experiments were performed on ear skin that had been soaked for 24 hr in a solution of antioxidant, and whether this modified any barrier to diffusion of molecules from liposome formulations was not reported. In addition, the liposome formulations were applied by soaking a thread in each liposomal gel and then applying the thread to the ear. Any differences in liposomal interaction with or disruption by the fibers of the thread do not appear to have been considered.

The penetration of an electron-dense marker, consisting of colloidal iron, into guinea pig skin was investigated after entrapment within liposomes of unreported composition following multiple-dose treatment (84). The results from this preliminary study are claimed to demonstrate that intact liposomes can penetrate to the dermis, the vesicles and free colloidal iron being identified by using an electron microscopic technique. A recent development has been the apparent success of using liposomes to encapsulate and efficiently deliver a DNA repair enzyme (T4 endonuclease V) to skin cells in culture (59). The active enzyme was encapsulated in several types of liposome (see Table 1), and DNA repair was increased when they were added to both human fibroblasts and keratinocytes. Liposome-mediated delivery of endonuclease V approached the efficiency of laboratory techniques of permeabilization or DNA transfection of cells. It should be appreciated that under cell culture conditions, liposomes are in intimate direct contact with living keratinocytes and do not have to overcome the potential barrier provided by the stratum corneum (85). However, the use of a pH-sensitive liposome containing the foregoing DNA repair enzyme has been reported to enhance the removal of pyrimidine dimers from epidermal keratinocytes of ultraviolet (UV)-irradiated hairless mouse skin within 6 hr of application in a lotion form (86,87). This liposome preparation has received orphan drug from the FDA for treatment of patients with the genetic disease xeroderma pigmentosum, who are deficient in repair of UV-induced DNA damage, and suffer from a very high incidence of skin cancer on sun-exposed skin.

Further potential exploitation of the use of lipids to deliver biopolymers and other drugs to the skin undoubtedly depends on a more thorough understanding of their mechanisms of action. The studies carried out to date, however, do offer certain possibilities for the therapeutic advantages to be gained.

V. CLINICAL STUDIES

Few clinical studies have as yet been carried out to determine the effectiveness of applying drugs topically in formulations containing lipid. In an early investigation involving the treatment of psoriasis in 49 patients, lecithin was added to three fractionated coal tar "cream" formulations (88). Efficacy of each formulation was assessed by a clinician over 6 months in comparison with two different formulations, that did not contain lipid. The author reported that patients found the creams containing lecithin easier "to rub in" and also, in his opinion, "to considerably enhance the penetration and therapeutic effect of the tar functions."

In an uncontrolled study carried out using five or six patients also suffering from psoriasis (57), liposomes containing entrapped methotrexate mixed with white soft paraffin wax or an amphipathic dermatological cream were applied. The patient used one of these preparations once a day. Within a few days, lesions on the skin improved and no complaints of irritation of the skin were reported. There were, however, no attempts made using techniques, such as freeze-substitution (89,90), to confirm that liposomes remain intact within the formulations.

Rowe et al. (91) reported a double-blind crossover study of topical liposomal progesterone as a treatment for hirsutism in four women. Application for 3 months of a 2% lotion of liposomal progesterone to designated areas of terminal hair growth (face or chest) were compared with similar applications of a control lotion containing inert liposomes. It was suggested that liposomal progesterone reduced the rate of hair growth, although in three of four patients the application of inert liposomes also reduced growth and, in one patient, this latter treatment regimen appeared more effective than the application of the progesterone-containing formulation.

After a study that examined the potential of a local anesthetic formulation consisting of liposomal-encapsulated tetracaine, one of the investigators applied the preparation for 1 hr to a superficial skin lesion of his own (58). The investigator underwent surgery for removal of the lesion and reports "feeling no pain." In this same study using 24 volunteers, the induced topical anesthesia evaluated using a pinprick technique, could be demonstrated to last for at least 4 hr after application of a tetracaine–liposomal formulation for 1 hr under occlusion. A comparator cream containing the same anesthetic cream was ineffective after the same time interval.

In three separate clinical studies involving 145 patients, a 1% econazole liposome–gel was highly effective in the therapy of human mycoses when applied daily, and advantages were claimed when this vehicle was compared with the classic econazole nitrate cream (92). The resulting econazole–liposome formulation has since been marketed in Switzerland (Pevaryl lipogel) and has been shown to contain small unilamellar liposomes before application to the skin (90).

VI. LIPID-CONTAINING MATRICES

When a simple aqueous liposomal suspension is applied to the skin, loss of water through evaporation will lead to a structural rearrangement of the liposomal lipid, resulting in the formation of a liquid crystalline matrix. Drugs with high lipid partition coefficients, such as steroids, would be expected to intercalate into the lipid bilayers. High concentrations of hydrocortisone have been achieved, for example, in an ointment vehicle consisting of PC/water liquid crystals (93). Such a preparation was thermodynamically stable, and the diffusion coefficient for hydrocortisone within the liquid crystalline phase was four times higher than the corresponding value for skin.

More recently, a transdermal drug-release device has been described that consists of drug-containing liposomes immobilized within an aqueous-phase matrix (94). Although acrylamide matrices have been suggested (93), a molded matrix system consisting of progesterone-containing liposomes embedded in agarose gel has been examined in detail (65). It is suggested that because the liposomes are immobilized within the gel network, it is impossible for progesterone to be transported across the skin in association with a liposome vesicle. Support for this contention is provided by experimental work that showed that when DPPC liposomes were fabricated within such a gel using a [^{14}C]lipid, no radioactivity was detected in the receptor phase during the 48 hr period postapplication to hairless mouse skin in vitro (14). The claimed advantage of such a liposomal-based reservoir device is that it can modulate drug input into the skin and release the drug at a zero-order rate over a period of 24 hr. Liposomes made from EPC, which contains a mixture of fatty acid chains, approximately half of which are saturated and half *cis*-unsaturated, delivered encapsulated progesterone transdermally from an agarose gel at a faster rate than liposomes made from DPPC, which contains fully saturated hydrocarbon chains (14). Differences in phase transition temperature of the phospholipids did not appear to influence the release rate of progesterone from such a gel system. Differences in the transdermal fluxes of drug from EPC and DPPC liposomes were attributed to the former containing unsaturated fatty acid impurities that can act as penetration enhancers (14). However, an alternative explanation may be that, although saturated phospholipids may not readily penetrate through (49,65) or into the stratum corneum, unsaturated lipids may have this propensity (70,83). The addition of a *cis*-unsaturated fatty acid to saturated acyl chain liposome–gels increased the transdermal delivery rate of progesterone through hairless mouse skin (14), suggesting that such systems could be employed to concomitantly control input of the drug and skin penetration enhancer to the skin.

VII. CURRENT AND FUTURE PERSPECTIVES

The US Food and Drug Administration has given lecithin GRAS status (generally recognized as safe), and it is registered for use in pharmaceutical, cosmetic, and food applications. Indeed, it has been employed in a wide variety of cosmetic products for several years (6) before its recent emergence to prominence as a component of liposomal rejuvenating creams (95,96). However, topical application for 21 days of DPPC/cholesterol (2:1 molar ratio) to hamster cheek mucosae was reported to induce a mild focal immune-type inflammatory reaction (97). Any long-term toxicity of other lipids that may be applied topically remains to be determined. It would seem that, at the very least, the inclusion of lipids within a pharmaceutical formulation can confer advantages that are not unique to this class of compound. For example, it is likely that lipids promote hydration of the stratum corneum (33) probably through partial occlusion, although saturated lipids with transition temperatures above that of skin temperature might be expected to fulfill this function most effectively. Lipids also possess the potential of increasing the solubility and diffusion coefficients of drugs within the vehicle (93), which might be expected, in the absence of any interaction between lipid and stratum corneum, to promote percutaneous absorption (49).

Much work remains to be done and must necessarily be undertaken before it can finally be concluded that the incorporation of lipids within a topical formulation is likely to offer any specific clinical or therapeutic advantage. More experiments need to be carried out involving the pretreatment of skin, for possibly prolonged periods, with lipids of clearly defined structure. The fate of such topically applied lipids and the determination of whether a structure–activity relation controls their incorporation in the stratum corneum is crucial for an understanding of any putative advantageous delivery mechanisms. As discussed earlier, for example, there is evidence to suggest that the degree of saturation of the lipid hydrocarbon chains may determine incorporation efficiency within the skin layers. In addition, recent findings have suggested that the precise composition of applied lipid mixtures may influence the uptake by the skin of concomitantly applied peptide drugs (30,31). There appears to be some advantage in matching the exogenously applied lipids to a composition similar to that found in the lipid bilayers of the stratum corneum if penetration to the deeper skin layers is desired (31), as predicted by Westerhof (98) and Schafer-Korting et al. (38). The influence of the state of the aggregation of the applied lipid, such as the lamellarity of the liposomes, as well as the effects of size and surface charge on drug penetration into the skin are unknown. The changes that occur in the association of lipids after application to the skin as components of the formulation are either absorbed or lost to the atmosphere through evaporation also remain to be investigated. The effects, if any, of incorporating lipid with drugs known to be metabolized by the skin could be usefully evaluated. One suggestion that may have applicability to immobilization of agents, such as sunscreens, to the skin surface is to incorporate lysine or hydrolysine within the lipid bilayer. Addition of the enzyme lysyloxidase during the application of the liposomes would promote the formation of cross links between lysine moieties in the lipid bilayer, with the lysine residues present in the keratinocytes (98). Such immobilized bilayers on the skin surface, possessing inherent resistance to removal by washing, could also be used to provide a reservoir of drug available for subsequent diffusion.

In conclusion, although the inclusion of lipids within topical formulations now appears to offer several advantages, many basic studies need to be initiated before many of the enthusiastic claims relating to the inclusion of such materials in pharmaceutical (99,100) and, in particular, cosmetic vehicles (20,25) can be truly sustained.

ACKNOWLEDGMENTS

I thank Dr. Andrew Lloyd for the provision of Figure 1, Mrs. Chris Leggatt for typing the manuscript and Mr. Bob Seago for preparing photographic material. I also thank Dr. Deborah Ladenheim and Dr. Andrew Lloyd for valuable discussions during the writing of the text.

APPENDIX

AC, acylceramide
AGC, acylglycosylceramide
CH, cholesterol
CHS, cholesteryl sulfate
CM, ceramides
DCP, dicetyl phosphate

DMPC, dimyristoylphosphatidylcholine
DPPC, dipalmitoyolphosphatidylcholine
DSPC, disteroylphosphpatidylcholine
EPC, egg phosphatidylcholine
G, glycerol
GC, glycosylceramide
HEPES, N-2-hydroxyethyl-piperazine-N'-2-ethanesulfanic acid
HSP, hydrogenated soybean phospholipid (composition declared to be 30%
    PC: 70% PE)
LPC, lysophosphatidylcholine
PA, palmitic acid
PBS, phosphate-buffered saline
PC, phosphatidylcholine
PE, phosphatidylethanolamine
Pg, propylene glycol
PG, phosphatidylglycerol
PI, phosphatidylinositol
PS, phosphatidylserine
SA, stearylamine
SPC, soybean-derived phosphatidylcholine
StA, stearic acid
TC, α-tocopherol
TG, triglyceride

REFERENCES

1. Walters, K. A. In *Transdermal Drug Delivery: Developmental Issues and Research Initiatives*. Hadgraft, J. and R. Guy (eds.). Marcel Dekker, New York, p. 197 (1989).
2. Golden, G. M., McKie, J. E., and Potts, R. O. *J. Pharm. Sci.* 76:25 (1986).
3. Mezei, M. and Gulasekharam, V. *Life Sci.* 26:1473 (1980).
4. Cooper, E. R. *J. Pharm. Sci.* 73:1153 (1984).
5. Aungst, B. J., Rogers, N. J., and Shefter, E. *Int. J. Pharm.* 33:225 (1986).
6. Walker, G. T. *Am. Perfum. Cosm.* 82:73 (1967).
7. Juliano, R. L. *Trends Pharm. Sci.* 2:39 (1981).
8. Poste, G. *Biol. Cell.* 47:19 (1983).
9. Gregoriadis, G. (ed.). *Liposomes as Drug: Recent Trends and Progress*. John Wiley & Sons, New York (1988).
10. Nicolau, C. and Cudd, A. *Crit. Rev. Ther. Drug Carrier Syst.* 6:239 (1989).
11. Bangham, A. D. In *Techniques in Life Sciences, Lipid and Membrane Biochemistry*. Elsevier Scientific Publications, Shannon, Ireland, p. 1 (1982).
12. Lichtenberg, D. and Barenholz, Y. *Methods Biochem. Anal.* 33:337 (1988).
13. Szoka, F. and Papahadjopoulos, D. *Annu. Rev. Biophys. Bioeng.* 9:467 (1980).
14. Knepp, V. M., Szoka, F. C., and Guy, R. H. *J. Controlled Release* 12:25 (1990).
15. Kunitake, T. *J. Macromol. Sci. Chem.* A13:587 (1979).

16. Murakami, Y., Nakano, A., and Ikeda, H. *J. Org. Chem. 47*:2137 (1982).
17. Handjani-Vila, R. M., Ribier, A., Rondot, B., and Vanlerberghe, G. *Int. J. Cosm. Sci. 1*:303 (1979).
18. Cullis, P. R. and De Kruijff, B. *Biochim. Biophys. Acta 559*:339 (1979).
19. Small, D. M. In *The Physical Chemistry of Lipids: Handbook of Lipid Research*, Vol. 4. Small, D. M. (ed.). Plenum Press, New York, p. 89 (1986).
20. Oleniacz, W. S. U.S. Patent No 3,957,971 (1976).
21. Lundberg, B., Svens, E., and Ekman, S. *Chem. Phys. Lipids 22*:285 (1978).
22. Vanlerberghe, G. and Handjani-Vila, R. M. U.S. Patent No 4,217,344 (1980).
23. Handjani-Vila, R. M. and Guesnet, J. *Ann. Dermatol. Venereol. 116*:423 (1989).
24. Vanlerberghe, G. and Handjani-Vila, R. M. *Nouv. Dermatol. 5*:259 (1986).
25. Suzuki, K. and Sakon, K. *Cosmet. Toiletries 105*(5):65 (1990).
26. Landmann, L. *Anat. Embryol. 178*:1 (1988).
27. Yardley, H. J. and Summerley, R. *Pharmacol. Ther. 13*:357 (1981).
28. Wertz, P. W., Swartzendruber, D. C., Madison, K. C., and Downing, D. T. *J. Invest. Dermatol. 89*:419 (1987).
29. Kimura, T., Nagahara, N., Hirabayashi, K., Kurosaki, Y., and Nakayama, T. *Chem. Pharm. Bull. 37*:454 (1989).
30. Weiner, N., Williams, N., Birch, G., Ramachandran, C., Shipman, C., and Flynn, G. *Antimicrob. Agents Chemother. 33*:1217 (1989).
31. Egbaria, K., Ramachandran, C., Kittayanond, D., and Weiner, N. *Antimicrob. Agents Chemother. 34*:107 (1990).
32. Brunke, R. *Manuf. Chem. 61*(7):36 (1990).
33. Artmann, C., Roding, J., Ghyczy, M., and Pratzel, H. G. *Perfum. Kosmet. 71*:326 (1990).
34. Lautenschlager, H. *SOFW 114*:761 (1988).
35. Lautenschlager, H. *Cosmet. Toiletries 105*(6):89 (1990).
36. Rieger, M. M. *Cosmet. Toiletries 96*(8):35 (1981).
37. Siciliano, A. A. *Cosmet. Toiletries 100*(5):43 (1985).
38. Schafer-Korting, M., Korting, H. C., and Braun-Falco, O. *J. Am. Acad. Dermatol. 21*:1271 (1989).
39. Redziniak, G. and Meybeck, A. Eur. Pat. 0 087 993 (1983).
40. Lautenschlager, H. *Cosmet. Toiletries 105*(7):63 (1990).
41. Mezei, M. and Gulasekharam, V. *J. Pharm. Pharmacol. 34*:473 (1982).
42. Krowczynski, L. and Stozek, T. *Pharmazie 39*:627 (1984).
43. Harsanyi, B. B., Hilchie, J. C., and Mezei, M. *J. Dent. Res. 65*:1133 (1986).
44. Lasch, J. and Wohlrab, W. *Biomed. Biochim. Acta 45*:1295 (1986).
45. Wohlrab, W. and Lasch, J. *Dermatol. Monatsschr. 175*:348 (1989).
46. Vermoken, A. J. M., Hukkelhoven, M. W. A. C., Vermeesch-Markslag, A. M. G., Goos, C. M. A. A., Wirtz, P., and Ziegenmeyer, J. *J. Pharm. Pharmacol. 36*:334 (1984).
47. Jacobs, M., Martin, G. P., and Marriott, C. *J. Pharm. Pharmacol. 38*:69P (1986).
48. Jacobs, M., Martin, G. P., and Marriott, C. *J. Pharm. Pharmacol. 40*:829 (1988).
49. Ganesan, M. G., Weiner, N. D., Flynn, G. L., and Ho, N. F. H. *Int. J. Pharm. 20*:139 (1984).
50. Komatsu, H., Higaki, K., Okamoto, H., Miyagawa, K., Hashida, M., and Sezaki, H. *Chem. Pharm. Bull. 34*:3415 (1986).
51. Komatsu, H., Okamoto, H., Miyagawa, K., Hashida, M., and Sezaki, H. *Chem. Pharm. Bull. 34*:3423 (1986).

52. Nishihata, T., Kotera, K., Nakano, Y., and Yamazaki, M. *Chem. Pharm. Bull. 35*:3807 (1987).
53. Nishihata, T., Kamada, A., Sakai, K., Takahashi, K., Matsumoto, K., Shinozaki, K., Tabata, Y., Keigami, M., Miyagi, T., and Tatsumi, N. *Int. J. Pharm. 46*:1 (1988).
54. Natsuki, R., Sone, T., Matsuo, R., Takabatake, E., and Nakanishi, M. *J. Pharmacobiodyn. 9*:5 (1986).
55. Kato, A., Ishibashi, Y., and Miyake, Y. *J. Pharm. Pharmacol. 39*:399 (1987).
56. Patel, H. M. *Biochem. Soc. Trans. 13*:513 (1985).
57. Patel, H. M., U.K. Patent, GB 2 143 433A (1985).
58. Gesztes, A. and Mezei, M. *Anesth. Analg. 67*:1079 (1988).
59. Ceccoli, J., Rosales, N., Tsimis, J., and Yarosh, D. B. *J. Invest. Dermatol. 93*:190 (1989).
60. Crowe, J. H. and Crowe, L. M. *Cryobiology 19*:317 (1982).
61. Kellaway, I. W. In *Topics in Topicals. Current Trends in the Formulation of Topical Agents.* Marks, R. (ed.). MTP Press, Lancaster, p. 121 (1985).
62. Mezei, M. In *Liposomes as Drug Carriers: Recent Trends and Progress.* Gregoriadis, G. (ed.). John Wiley & Sons, New York, p. 663 (1988).
63. Ho, N. F. H., Ganesan, M. G., Weiner, N. D., and Glynn, G. L. In *Advances in Drug Delivery Systems.* Anderson, J. M. and Kim, S. W. (eds.). Elsevier, Amsterdam, p. 61 (1986).
64. Ertel, K. D. and Carstensen, J. T. *Int. J. Pharm. 34*:179 (1986).
65. Knepp, V. M., Hinz, R. S., Szoka, F. C., and Guy, R. H. *J. Controlled Release 5*:211 (1988).
66. Illum, L., Farraj, N., Critchley, H., and Davis, S. S. *Int. J. Pharm. 46*:261 (1988).
67. Martin, G. P. and Marriott, C. *J. Pharm. Pharmacol. 33*:754 (1981).
68. Newbery, R. S., Martin, G. P., Turner, N. C., and Marriott, C. *J. Pharm. Pharmacol. 37*:101P (1985).
69. Saket, M. M. PhD Thesis, University of Wales (1986).
70. Wohlrab, W., Lachmann, U., and Lasch, J. *Dermatol. Monatsschr. 175*:344 (1989).
71. Wohlrab, W. and Lasch, J. *Dermalogica 174*:18 (1987).
72. Wohlrab, W., Lasch, J., Taube, K. M., and Wozniak, K. *Pharmazie 44*:333 (1989).
73. Mezei, M., Hilchie, J. C., and Rowe, T. C. *Clin. Invest. Med. 8*:C3 (1985).
74. Gesztes, A., Foldvari, M., and Mezei, M. *Clin. Invest. Med. 11*(6):E5 (1989).
75. Barry, B. W. and Woodford, R. *J. Clin. Pharmacol. 3*:43 (1978).
76. Du Vivier, A. and Stoughton, R. B. *Arch. Dermatol. 111*:581 (1975).
77. Jacobs, M., Martin, G. P., and Marriott, C. *J. Pharm. Pharmacol. 39*:142P (1987).
78. Jacobs, M., M. Phil Thesis, CNAA, Brighton Polytechnic (1987).
79. Natsuki, R., and Takaatake, E. *Yakuguku Zasshi 107*:616 (1987).
80. Wertz, P. W. and Downing, D. T. *J. Lipid Res. 24*:759 (1983).
81. Abraham, W. W., Wertz, P. W., and Downing, D. T. *J. Invest. Dermatol. 90*:259 (1988).
82. Wertz, P. W., Abraham, W. W., Landmann, L., Downing, D. T. *J. Invest. Dermatol. 87*:582 (1986).
83. Gabrijelcic, V., Sentjurc, M., and Kristl, J. *Int. J. Pharm. 62*:75 (1990).
84. Foldvari, M. and Mezei, M. *Clin. Invest. Med. 11*(6):E4 (1989).
85. Bonnekoh, B. and Mahrle, G. *Z. Hautkr. 65*:99 (1989).
86. Yarosh, D. B., Tsimis, J., and Yee, V. *J. Soc. Cosmet. Chem. 41*:85 (1990).
87. Yarosh, D. B. *J. Photochem. Photobiol. B: Biology, 6*:445 (1990).

88. Thorne, N. *Br. J. Dermatol.* 75:422 (1963).
89. Muller, T., Roding, J., and Lautenschlager, H. *SOFW 115*:88 (1989).
90. Singh, M., Falkner, G., Meisner, D., and Mezei, M. *J. Microencap.* 7:77 (1990).
91. Rowe, T. C., Mezei, M., and Hilchie, J. *Prostate* 5:346 (1984).
92. Raab, W. *Arztl. Kosmetol.* 18:213 (1988).
93. Wahlbren, S., Lindstrom, A. L., and Friberg, S. E. *J. Pharm. Sci.* 73:1484 (1984).
94. Guy, R. H., Szoka, F. C., Knepp, V. M., and Wester, R. C. International Patent WP 87/01938 (1987).
95. Strianse, S. J. *Cosmet. Toiletries* 93(4):37 (1978).
96. Strauss, G. *J. Soc. Cosmet. Chem.* 40:51 (1989).
97. Foong, W. C., Harsanyi, B. B., and Mezei, M. *J. Biomed. Mat. Res.* 23:1213 (1989).
98. Westerhof, W. *Med. Hypotheses* 16:283 (1985).
99. Mezei, M. *Pharm. Int.* 7:184 (1985).
100. Mezei, M. In *Topics in the Pharmaceutical Sciences*. Breimer, D. D. and Speiser, P. (eds.). Elsevier, Amsterdam, p. 345 (1985).

4

Terpenes as Skin Penetration Enhancers

Brian W. Barry and Adrian C. Williams

University of Bradford, Bradford, West Yorkshire, United Kingdom

I. INTRODUCTION: TERPENES, TERPENOIDS, AND ESSENTIAL OILS

Essential oils are volatile, fragrant substances residing in the flowers, fruit, leaves, and roots of many plants. Numerous essential oils have been employed as perfumes, flavorings, and medicines for centuries, including oil of turpentine, which was used by the ancient Greeks, and by 1592 some 61 essential oils had been described. Chemical analysis of essential oils has shown that they are a complex mixture of compounds, including nitrogen- and sulfur-containing molecules, aromatic chemicals, and terpenes.

The term *terpene* usually describes a compound that is a constituent of an essential oil and that contains carbon, hydrogen, and may include oxygen, yet that is not aromatic in character. Terpenoid molecules are designated by their chemical structure, being based on isoprene (C_5H_8) units (although exceptions exist such as lavandulol, a component of lavender oil). The terpenes may thus be classified depending on the number of isoprene units they contain: monoterpenes (C_{10}) have two isoprene units, sesquiterpenes (C_{15}) have three, and diterpenes (C_{20}) have four isoprene units. Terpenes may be subdivided as acyclic, monocyclic, bicyclic, and so on.

Terpenes have varied uses. For example, menthol is employed pharmaceutically in inhalations and has a mild antipruritic effect when formulated into emollient preparations. It is also used as a fragrance and can flavor toothpastes and

95

peppermint sweets, as well as mentholated cigarettes. Details of terpenoid biosynthesis, chemistry, and reactions are outside the scope of this chapter, but are well documented in the literature (e.g., 1–9).

Despite the widespread medicinal usage of many terpenes, there are few reports of their skin penetration-enhancing properties. 1,8-Cineole has been used to promote the percutaneous absorption of several drugs (10), including benzocaine (log $P_{octanol/water}$ 1.86), procaine (log P 1.87), bupranolol (log P 2.97), indomethacin (log P 3.08), and dibucaine (log P 4.40). This study thus employed lipophilic drugs and was performed using excised hairless mouse skin, a suspect model for human tissue in permeation studies (e.g., 11–14).

Camphor and eucalyptus oil in a vehicle containing 50% ethanol increased the total flux of nicotine (a lipophilic drug, log P 1.17) permeating hairless mouse skin (15). However, the authors made no comment on the effects the ethanolic vehicle may have on hairless mouse skin; solvents such as ethanol are known to extract stratum corneum lipids (12,16).

The effects of some cyclohexanone derivatives (which show structural similarities to the ketone terpenes discussed later) on percutaneous absorption of ketoprofen (log P –0.01) and indomethacin have been investigated (17); in vitro permeation studies were performed using newborn pig skin, and in vivo studies utilized shaven rats. The authors concluded that the penetration-enhancing effects observed with "bulky" cyclohexanone derivatives (for example those containing butyl chains) were due to a modification of the stratum corneum lipid structure (i.e., leading to an increase in drug diffusivity), as no effect on drug partitioning was observed. However, this study also employed ethanol as a vehicle component and employed animal models.

The effects of a variety of terpenes on percutaneous absorption of indomethacin in rats have been studied (18,19). For the lipophilic drug indomethacin, hydrocarbon terpenes, and particularly limonene, were as effective enhancers as laurocapram (Azone) and limonene was effective at a concentration of 1% in the gel ointment employed. The authors concluded that the terpenes had no appreciable effect on drug partitioning and, hence, that limonene alters the barrier function of the stratum corneum. The cyclic monoterpenes that increased permeation of indomethacin had a lipophilic index of more than zero, and oxygen-containing terpenes (e.g., carvone, α-terpineol, and 1,8-cineole) were ineffective. The opposite trend developed in our work with the polar drug, 5-fluorouracil (see later discussion).

Transdermal permeation of prednisolone, an anti-inflammatory steroid (log P 1.62), has been improved by using the acetone extract of cardamon seed (20). The active constituents of the extract, α-terpineol and acetyl terpineol, were more effective than laurocapram in promoting drug permeation, although this study used excised shaved mouse skin.

Several monoterpenes have been reported to enhance diazepam (log P 2.82) permeation (21). Again, using a lipophilic drug, the authors found that monoterpenes with polar groups (alcohols and ketones) do not act as enhancers, whereas all terpenes tested without polar groups increased diazepam permeation through hairless mouse skin. In an extension of this study (22), propranolol permeation (log P 3.56) was enhanced through hairless mouse skin by cyclic monoterpenes, with or without oxygen atoms (hydrogen-bonding ability), and diazepam transport was increased by menthone and menthol, but to a lesser extent than by the hydrocarbon terpenes tested.

Compounds containing an azacyclo ring (similar to laurocapram) and terpene hydrocarbon chains have been evaluated as accelerants for a variety of drugs (23–26). These studies illustrated that the size of the azacyclo ring had little effect on the potency of the penetration enhancers, whereas the length of the hydrophobic terpene chain had a marked effect on accelerant activity; a chain length of 12 carbon atoms resulted in the most effective enhancers. These studies concluded that the accelerants exerted their action by increasing partitioning of the drugs into the stratum corneum, and they had no effects on diffusivity, although their data suggested that the enhancer effects may vary with the species of animal skin used (hairless mouse skin and rat skin gave different results).

As reviewed in the foregoing, the studies performed using terpenes have employed animal skins and generally lipophilic drugs. Our work has concentrated on the use of a variety of terpenes to enhance transdermal permeation of a model polar drug, 5-fluorouracil, through excised human abdominal skin. The terpenes have been employed neat and in a vehicle (propylene glycol), and the synergism between propylene glycol and terpenes was investigated. The studies have probed the mechanisms of action of the terpenes using thermal analysis, spectroscopy, partitioning, and permeation data as well as investigations of hydration phenomena.

II. NATURE OF TERPENES INVESTIGATED

Our studies to date at Bradford University have predominantly concentrated on monoterpenes and chemically similar compounds selected to provide a related series of molecules. Initial work examined some essential oils. Figure 1 provides the formulas and Tables 1 and 2 list some essential oils that possess high concentrations of the various terpenes, their principal uses, and some toxicity data.

III. ESSENTIAL OILS AS HUMAN SKIN PENETRATION ENHANCERS

The principal barrier to most topical drug delivery is the stratum corneum, the outermost layer of the skin, which comprises keratin-rich cells embedded in

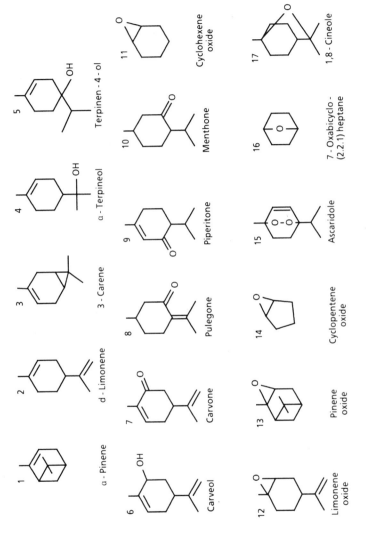

Figure 1 Formulas of terpenes assessed as skin penetration enhancers at Bradford University.

Table 1 Details of Essential Oils Used in Enhancer Studies

Essential oils	Terpenes	Principal use	Toxicity[a]
Ylang–ylang	Geraniol + others	Fragrance	>5 g/kg
Anise	85% anethole	Flavoring	LD_{50} oral rat 2.3 g/kg
Chenopodium	70% ascaridole	Medicinal	0.415 g/kg
Eucalyptus	80% 1,8-cineole	Medicinal	>5 g/kg

[a]Dermal LD_{50} rabbit unless stated otherwise.

multiple lipid bilayers. In recent years, much interest has been focused on methods of increasing stratum corneum permeability, and one approach is the use of *penetration enhancers* (or accelerants). We define these agents as those that partition into, and interact with, the stratum corneum constituents to induce a temporary, reversible increase in skin permeability. We have investigated the penetration-enhancing activities of some essential oils toward the permeation of 5-fluorouracil (5-FU), chosen as a model polar penetrant, in excised human skin (27).

The essential oils selected were chenopodium, eucalyptus, anise, and ylang–ylang. Oil of chenopodium has been used as an effective anthelmintic, and contains approximately 70% ascaridole, as well as *p*-cymene, α-terpinene and *l*-limonene. Eucalyptus oil has been formulated into ointments as a counterirritant and, together with menthol, into inhalations. Its chief constituent is 1,8-cineole (approximately 80%), although it also contains α-pinene and small quantities of other terpenes such as phellandrene. Anise oil provides approximately 85% anethole and is a flavoring agent used in the manufacture of liqueurs and dentrifices. Oil of ylang-ylang yields geraniol and linalool esters of benzoic and acetic acids, together with *p*-cresol methyl ether and other terpenes. It is employed as a delicate fragrance agent and has recently found use in aromatherapy. Because of the popularity of these essential oils, their toxicities are well documented (see Table 1) and are relatively low compared with most synthetic penetration enhancers.

The activities of the essential oils were evaluated using excised human epidermal membranes prepared by a heat-separation technique (28). The skin samples were fully hydrated and placed in stainless steel diffusion cells, comprising stationary donor and flow-through receptor compartments, mounted on an automated diffusion system (29). Aliquots of a saturated, aqueous radiolabeled 5-FU solution were placed in the donor compartments, samples of receptor solution were collected periodically, and the drug concentrations were determined by

Table 2   Details of Terpenes Used in Enhancer Studies

Terpene or terpenoid	Essential oil (example)	Principal use	Toxicity[a]
d-Limonene	Orange	Fragrance	>5 g/kg
α-Pinene	Rosemary	Fragrance	>5 g/kg
3-Carene	Turpentine	Fragrance	>5 g/kg
α-Terpineol	Cajeput	Fragrance	>5 g/kg
Terpinen-4-ol	Cypress	Fragrance	>5 g/kg
l-Caveol	Spearmint	Flavoring	>5 g/kg
Menthol	Peppermint	Medicinal	>5 g/kg
Neomenthol	Japanese mint	Fragrance	>5 g/kg
Carvone	Spearmint	Flavoring	>5 g/kg
Pulegone	Pennyroyal	Flavoring	3.09 g/kg
Piperitone	Peppermint	Fragrance	>5 g/kg
Menthone	Geranium	Flavoring	>5 g/kg
Fenchone	Fennel	Flavoring	>5 g/kg
Cyclohexene oxide	Not natural	Solvent	0.63 mg/kg
Limonene oxide	Lemon grass	Fragrance	Mouse, nonirritant
α-Pinene oxide	Carraway	Fragrance	>5 g/kg
Cyclopentene oxide	Not natural	Solvent	Guinea pig, irritant
Safrole	Sassafras	Fragrance	LD$_{50}$ oral, rat, 1.9 g/kg
Ascaridole	Chenopodium	Medicinal	Mouse, irritant
7-Oxabicyclo[2.2.1]heptane	Not natural	Solvent	Not available
1,8-Cineole	Eucalyptus	Medicinal	>5 g/kg

[a]Dermal LD$_{50}$ rabbit unless stated otherwise.

liquid scintillation counting. At pseudo-steady state, the permeability coefficient (K_p) of the drug in the tissue was evaluated. The drug was then washed from the donor compartments and replaced with samples of the essential oils. After a 12 hr treatment period, the oils were washed from the donor compartments and replaced with the drug solution; the permeability coefficient at steady state was reevaluated. An enhancement ratio (*ER*) may be used to define the activities of the oils:

$$ER = \frac{K_p \text{ after accelerant treatment}}{K_p \text{ before accelerant treatment}}$$

The enhancement ratios reported are mean values, from a minimum of five replicates, using 12 different tissue samples. Human skin permeability shows intersample variations; the experimental technique employed each piece of tissue as its own control, thereby minimizing errors caused by this phenomenon.

Expressing the activities of the oils as the mean of individual enhancement ratios gives a more accurate estimation of penetration enhancement than a simple ratio of the mean membrane permeability coefficients before and after accelerant treatment.

The oils clearly increased drug permeation across the skin, as illustrated in Figure 2.

The most effective oils were eucalyptus and chenopodium, containing primarily 1,8-cineole and ascaridole, respectively. Both these chemicals are polar oxygen-bridged terpenes; 1,8-cineole being a cyclic ether and ascaridole, a cyclic peroxide. Oil of ylang–ylang shows less penetration-enhancing activity toward the polar drug 5-FU, with an enhancement ratio of approximately 8. This oil contains

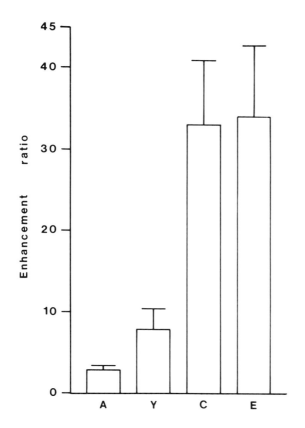

Figure 2 Enhancement ratios (±SEM) for volatile oils; (A) anise, (Y) ylang–ylang, (C) chenopodium, (E) eucalyptus.

oxygen-linked molecules within its terpene ester composition. The least effective essential oil, anise (ER approximately 3), contains primarily anethole, a chemical containing a methoxybenzene structure.

IV. TERPENES AS HUMAN SKIN PENETRATION ENHANCERS

The next stage of our studies (30,31) involved an investigation into a range of terpenes, as shown in Figure 1 and Table 2, using the enhancer ratio technique described in Section III. Figure 3 is a histogram of the relevant enhancement ratios.

The hydrocarbons show a very mild accelerant activity, compared with the oxygen-containing terpenes, with carene increasing the permeability coefficient only threefold—this is the reverse relation shown by other workers using the lipophilic drug, indomethacin (18,19). The alcohols are generally less effective than the ketones, carveol showing an enhancement ratio of 25, whereas methone, the most effective ketone, has a ratio of near 40.

The oxide terpenes provide an interesting series of compounds. The enhancement ratios of the 1,2-oxygen-bridged terpenes (epoxides) are markedly lower than the longer oxygen-bridged terpenes (cyclic ethers), such as cineole which has a 1,8-linkage. The ER differences may be partly due to conformational differences. The six-membered epoxide ring is essentially flat, being in the chair conformation on which the ring is relatively free of angular and torsional strain. The hydrocarbon side chains increase the steric bulk of limonene oxide and α-pinene oxide, both of which are significantly better accelerants for 5-FU than the unsubstituted cyclohexene oxide. The cyclic ethers (ascaridole, 1,8-cineole, and 7-oxabicyclo[2.2.1]heptane) show significantly greater enhancement ratios than the epoxides and exist in the less thermodynamically stable boat conformation. As such, the molecules are under considerable torsional and angular strain. No significant difference was found between the activities of the three cyclic ethers, despite ascaridole containing two oxygen atoms and an unsaturated bond, 7-oxabicyclo[2.2.1]heptane possessing no hydrocarbon side chains, and 1,8-cineole having a 1,8-oxygen bridge instead of the 1,4-linkage of the other two cyclic ethers. The different enhancement ratios observed between cyclohexene oxide (ER 2.4) and cyclopentene oxide (ER 31) may possibly also be explained in terms of molecular conformations; cyclopentene oxide is under considerable torsional strain when planar and, to relieve this strain somewhat, the molecule takes on a slightly puckered conformation. However, whether or not conformational differences are important for rationalizing differences in the enhancement abilities of the terpenes remains to be proved.

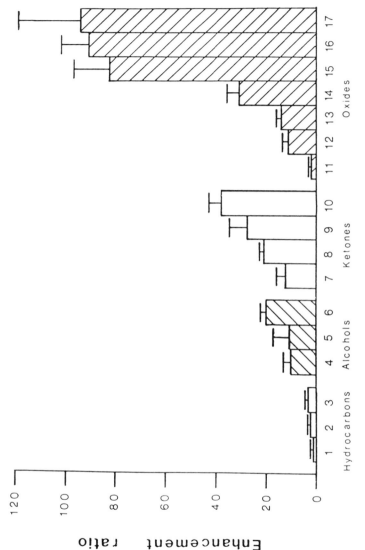

Figure 3 Enhancement ratios (±SEM) for terpenes; numbers refer to terpene molecules shown in Figure 1.

A general theory for the modes of action of penetration enhancers, based on molecular and solvent changes in the stratum corneum, has been proposed (for relevant references, see 32,33). According to this concept, accelerants may act by one or more of the three main mechanisms; disruption of the highly ordered lipid structure between the corneocytes so increasing intercellular diffusivity, interaction with intracellular protein to promote permeation through the corneocyte, and increased partitioning of the drug or a coenhancer into the tissue. This concept is formalized as the lipid–protein–partitioning (or LPP) theory (34), and present results may be rationalized according to this scheme.

The increase in diffusivity of 5-FU in the membranes, calculated from lag time changes following treatment with the terpenes, may be expressed as a diffusivity ratio, D_R^* where:

$$D_R^* = \frac{\text{Diffusivity of 5-FU in membrane after terpene treatment}}{\text{Diffusivity of 5-FU in membrane before terpene treatment}}$$

This ratio may be correlated with the terpene penetration-enhancing activities as illustrated in Figure 4. The equation of the line, by linear regression is:

$ER = 5.83\,D_R^* - 7.24$, correlation coefficient = 0.985.

Figure 4 suggests that the terpenes act, in part, by modifying intercellular lipids, disrupting their highly ordered structure to increase diffusivity. The high log $P_{\text{octanol/water}}$ values of the terpenes imply that there would be little terpene–keratin interaction within the corneocyte, so that possible protein interaction suggested under the LPP theory should be negligible. Despite the deviations from Fickian diffusion laws and unavoidable experimental errors involved in this work (for further detail see 30), it is clear that the permeation lag time decreases, and that the diffusivity of 5-FU through the membrane increases, following terpene treatment of human epidermal membranes.

The role of partitioning phenomena in the increased drug permeation was less clear. Experimentally determined distribution coefficients using human stratum corneum membranes show that the terpenes exert no positive effect in increasing 5-FU partitioning into the tissue; indeed, the reverse may be true. The drug was less soluble in all the terpenes than in water; hence, a decrease in drug–tissue partitioning after terpene treatment may be expected. However, 5-FU is, for example, 100 times less soluble in carvone than in water, yet drug partitioning into the terpene-treated stratum corneum was only half that for the aqueous treated control. With no clear partitioning effects, the terpenes appear to exert their action primarily by increasing the diffusion coefficient of the drug in the membrane.

Clearly, the passage of these terpene accelerants into the lipid domain of the stratum corneum is essential for activity. This feature was well demonstrated when the ERs of the ketone and epoxide terpenes were shown to correlate with the

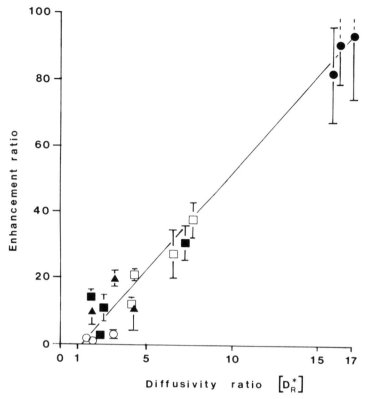

Figure 4 Enhancement ratio (±SEM) as a function of diffusivity ratio for terpenes.

when the ERs of the ketone and epoxide terpenes were shown to correlate with the calculated log partition coefficient (octanol/water) values, albeit that only three and four points were involved. As the partition coefficients of the accelerants increase, so the enhancement ratios increase; the concentration of test agent in the membrane will determine, in part, the scale of lipid disruption and, hence, the increase in diffusivity of 5-FU.

The reversibility of action of the terpenes was verified. Under diffusional conditions, terpene-treated membranes, after prolonged washing, showed no significant increase in the K_p of 5-FU compared with untreated epidermis. This invariance suggests that the terpenes, which are also solvents, do not act by extracting significant amounts of barrier lipid from the tissues. This reversibility is also suggested by the fact that the fluxes of 5-FU in terpene-treated membranes fall with time as the accelerant washes from the skin, producing a tailing-off effect in the permeation profiles.

In summary, our data illustrate the use of naturally occurring terpenes as penetration enhancers in human skin for the polar drug, 5-FU. Of the terpenes evaluated, hydrocarbons were poor accelerants, and alcohols and ketones were more effective. The oxides may be subdivided into two chemical classes, with the epoxides demonstrating mild accelerant activity, whereas the cyclic ethers are very effective; ascaridole, 7-oxabicyclo[2.2.1]heptane, and 1,8-cineole, all induce a near 90-fold increase in the permeability coefficient of 5-FU. The five-membered cyclopentene oxide shows greater penetration-enhancing activity than the six-membered cyclohexene oxide. The terpenes act by disrupting the lipid structure of the stratum corneum, thereby increasing the diffusion coefficient of the polar drug in the membrane, illustrated by the reduced lag time observed and the increased diffusivity calculated from permeation studies. A linear relation may exist between the enhancement ratios and the diffusivity increase caused by the accelerants. The terpenes do not increase the partitioning of drug into human stratum corneum, a reasonable effect, as 5-FU is less soluble in all the terpenes than in water. The high log $P_{octanol/water}$ values of the terpenes imply that the penetration enhancers will not significantly modify corneocyte proteins. The terpene action is reversible. The results of this study show that undiluted terpene penetration enhancers act on 5-FU permeation by increasing diffusivity by stratum corneum *lipid* disruption, provide no significant *protein* interaction, and make no major *partitioning* alterations, the three major features of the LPP theory of penetration enhancer activity.

V. SYNERGY OF PROPYLENE GLYCOL WITH TERPENES

Propylene glycol is a solvent widely used in topical formulations, and it is valuable as a cosolvent for penetration enhancers. Terpenes provide good examples of synergy which delivered to the skin from propylene glycol vehicles (35). Figure 5 compares the enhancement ratios of 5-FU derived by treating human skin with neat terpenes, 0.5 M terpenes in propylene glycol, or saturated solutions (or 90% solutions for miscible terpenes) in the glycol. *If* the propylene glycol were having no effect, and under ideal conditions, we would expect each neat terpene to produce a maximum effect because it is presented to the skin at its greatest chemical potential. On dilution to 0.5 M in propylene glycol we would predict a fall in ER, yet for carvone and pulegone this parameter increased. Saturated solutions (or approximations to saturation for miscible terpenes), being at the same thermodynamic activity as the liquid terpene, should provide ERs equal to pure terpenes. However, these propylene glycol/terpene mixtures increased the

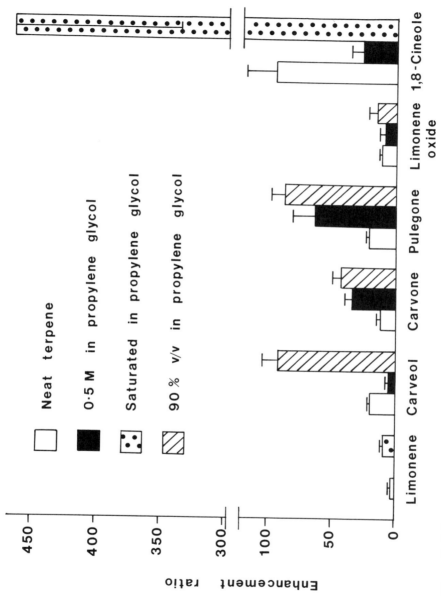

Figure 5 Enhancement ratio (±SEM) for selected terpenes, neat and in propylene glycol.

ERs up to fourfold for carveol, carvone, pulegone, and 1,8-cineole, even though propylene glycol alone had a negligible promoter effect. We explain these results mainly on the basis that propylene glycol is promoting the passage of the terpenes into the stratum corneum where they exert their accelerant activity. Thus, propylene glycol acts by increasing the partitioning of a coenhancer into the stratum corneum (see comments on the LPP concept in Sect. IV).

VI. DIFFERENTIAL SCANNING CALORIMETRY OF HUMAN STRATUM CORNEUM: EFFECT OF TERPENES

Differential scanning (DSC) experiments, together with thermogravimetric and thermomechanical techniques, infrared spectroscopy, and x-ray diffraction, provide evidence on the structure of the stratum corneum and how enhancers modify phase transitions within the tissues (36–43). So far, DSC has been the most fruitful of these techniques for elucidating enhancer mechanisms. With a typical sweep time of 10°C/min, a hydrated sample of human horny layer in hermetically sealed pans usually produces four main peaks, which we can classify as

Endotherm T_1	Lipid melting; from sebaceous lipid/fat contamination?
Endotherm $T_2 + T_3$	Lipid melting
Endotherm T_4	Protein denaturation of intracellular keratin

Endotherm T_1 is of no importance for assessing the mode of action of accelerants. There is some controversy concerning the underlying nature of T_2 and T_3 (36,39). These peaks could arise from the intercellular lipid melting in two stages (36), or the bilayer melting followed by disruption of protein–lipid complexes at cell membranes (39); a third possibility is that the two transitions follow from the changes to asymmetric bilayers, or a fourth suggestion is combination of all three mechanisms (44). The important practical point is that, if an enhancer modifies T_2 and T_3, then the process suggests a lipid interaction and we can use this fact as evidence that the accelerant is working, at least partly, by changing packing in the intercellular lipid domain. It is a reasonable postulate to suggest that we should be able to correlate DSC changes with enhanced activity, and we tested this hypothesis using our terpene data.

The DSC studies were performed using hydrated human stratum corneum. Tissue samples were treated with terpenes for 1 hr (the soaking technique) or 10 sec (the dipping technique) before being hermetically sealed and heated from 10 to 140°C at 10°c/min. A typical thermogram of hydrated stratum corneum is showed together with terpene-treated samples in Figure 6.

After terpene treatment, the lipid peaks shift to lower temperatures as the lipid structure is disrupted (44). However, the lipids appear to be equally affected by both limonene and cineole, despite limonene having little accelerant activity

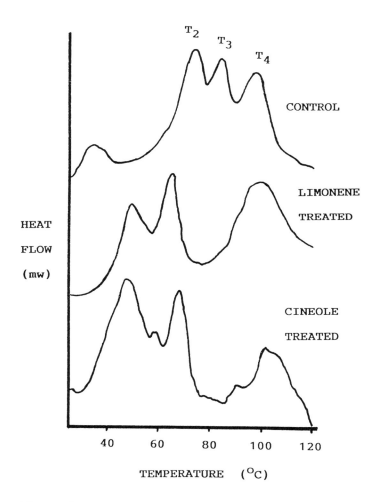

Figure 6 Differential scanning calorimetry traces for hydrated stratum corneum (control), together with limonene-treated and cineole-treated specimens.

(ER = 2), whereas cineole is a very effective accelerant for the polar drug, 5-FU (ER = 94.5). The scale of lipid disruption induced by the terpenes showed no correlation with the experimentally determined enhancement ratios, and terpenes with similar activities, such as carveol (ER = 20) and pulegone (ER = 21), have different peak shifts. An ineffective accelerant (pinene, ER = 1) shows equal lipid disruption to an effective accelerant (e.g., piperitone; ER = 28). The thermogram peak positions are thus unreliable in predicting the magnitudes of penetration enhancer activities, and DSC may best be employed to investigate the mechanisms of action of accelerants the activities of which have been verified by other methods.

REFERENCES

1. Simonsen, J. L. *The Terpenes*. Cambridge University Press, Cambridge (1953).
2. Pinder, A. R. *The Chemistry of the Terpenes*. Chapman Hall, London (1960).
3. Hanson, J. R. In *Chemistry of Terpenes and Terpenoids*, Chap. 1. Newman, A. A. (ed.). Academic Press, London (1972).
4. Whittaker, D. In *Chemistry of Terpenes and Terpenoids*, Chap. 2. Newman, A. A. (ed.). Academic Press, London (1972).
5. Banthorpe, D. V. and Charlwood, B. V. In *Chemistry of Terpenes and Terpenoids*, Chap. 7. Newman, A. A. (ed.). Academic Press, London (1972).
6. Pridham, J. B. (ed.). *Terpenoids in Plants*. Academic Press, London (1967).
7. Goodwin, T. W. (ed.). *Aspects of Terpenoid Chemistry and Biochemistry*. Academic Press, London (1971).
8. Thomas, A. F. In *Terpenoids and Steroids, Specialist Periodical Reports*, Vols. 1–5, Chap. 1. The Chemical Society, London (1971–1975).
9. Yeats, R. B. In *Terpenoids and Steroids, Specialist Periodical Reports*, Vols. 6–9, Chap. 1. The Chemical Society, London (1976–1979).
10. Zupan, J. A. European Patent, 0 069 385 (1983).
11. Bond, J. R. and Barry, B. W. *J. Invest. Dermatol. 90*:486 (1988).
12. Bond, J. R. and Barry, B. W. *Int. J. Pharm. 41*:91 (1988).
13. Bond, J. R. and Barry, B. W. *J. Invest. Dermatol. 90*:810 (1988).
14. Rigg, P. C. and Barry, B. W. *J. Invest. Dermatol. 94*:235 (1990).
15. Nuwayser, E. S., Gay, M. H., De Roo, D. J., and Blaskovich, P. D. Transdermal nicotine—an aid to smoking cessation. In *Proceedings of 15th International Symposium on the Controlled Release of Bioactive Materials*, Basel, Switzerland, pp. 213–214 (1988).
16. Blank, I. H. and Scheuplein, R. J. *Br. J. Dermatol. 81*(Suppl. 4):4 (1969).
17. Nagai, T., Yi, Q. D., Higuchi, R. I., Akitoshi, Y., and Takayama, K. Effect of cyclohexanone derivatives on percutaneous absorption of ketoprofen and indomethacin. In *Proceedings of 15th International Symposium on the Controlled Release of Bioactive Materials*, Basel, Switzerland, pp. 154–155 (1988).
18. Nagai, T., Okabe, H., Ogura, A., and Takayama, K. Effect of limonene and related compounds on the percutaneous absorption of indomethacin. In *Proceedings of 16th International Symposium on the Controlled Release of Bioactive Materials*, Chicago, Illinois, pp. 181–182 (1989).
19. Okabe, H., Takayama, K., Ogura, A., and Nagai, T. *Drug Design Deliv. 4*:313 (1989).
20. Yamahara, J., Kashiwa, H., Kishi, K., and Fujimura, H. *Chem. Pharm. Bull. 37*:855 (1989).
21. Hori, M., Satoh, S., and Maibach, H. I. In *Percutaneous Absorption*, 2nd ed., Bronaugh, R. L. and Maibach, H. I. (eds.). Marcel Dekker, New York, (1989).

22. Hori, M., Satoh, S., Maibach, H. I., and Guy, R. H. *J. Pharm. Sci. 88*:32 (1991).
23. Okamoto, H., Hashida, M., and Sezaki, H. *Chem. Pharm. Bull. 35*:4605 (1987).
24. Okamoto, H., Ohyabu, M., Hashida, M., and Sezaki, H. *J. Pharm. Pharmacol. 39*:531 (1987).
25. Okamoto, H., Hashida, M., and Sezaki, H. *J. Pharm. Sci. 77*:418 (1988).
26. Okamoto, H., Muta, K., Hashida, M., and Sezaki, H. *Pharm. Res. 7*:64 (1990).
27. Williams, A. C. and Barry, B. W. *Int. J. Pharm. 57*:R7 (1989).
28. Kligman, A. M. and Christophers, E. *Arch. Dermatol. 88*:702 (1963).
29. Akhtar, S. A., Bennett, S. L., Waller, I. L., and Barry, B. W. *Int. J. Pharm. 21*:17 (1984).
30. Williams, A. C. and Barry, B. W. *Pharm. Res. 8*:17 (1991).
31. Williams, A. C. and Barry, B. W. In *Prediction of Percutaneous Absorption*, Scott, R. C., Guy, R. H., and Hadgraft, J. (eds.). I.B.C. Technical Services, p. 224 (1990).
32. Goodman, M. and Barry, B. W. In *Percutaneous Absorption*, 2nd ed. Bronaugh, R. L. and Maibach, H. I. (eds.). Marcel Dekker, New York (1989).
33. Barry, B. W. *J. Controlled Release 6*:85 (1987).
34. Barry, B. W. *Int. J. Cosmet. Sci. 10*:281 (1988).
35. Barry, B. W. and Williams, A. C. Human skin penetration enhancement: the synergy of propylene glycol with terpenes. In *Proceedings of the 16th International Symposium on the Controlled Release of Bioactive Materials*, Chicago, Illinois, pp. 33–34 (1989).
36. Golden, G. M., Guzek, D. B., Harris, R. R., McKie, J. E., and Potts, R. O. *J. Invest. Dermatol. 86*:255 (1986).
37. Knutson, K., Potts, R. O., Guzek, D. B., Golden, G. M., McKie, J. E., Lambert, W. J., and Higuchi, W. I. In *Advances in Drug Delivery Systems*. Anderson, J. M. and Kim, S. W. (eds.). Elsevier, Amsterdam, p. 67 (1986).
38. Potts, R. O. In *Transdermal Drug Delivery*. Hadgraft, J. and Guy, R. H. (eds.). Marcel Dekker, New York, p. 23 (1989).
39. Goodman, M. and Barry, B. W. *J. Pharm. Pharmacol. 37*(Suppl.):80P (1985).
40. Goodman, M. and Barry, B. W. *Anal. Proc. 26*:397 (1986).
41. Goodman, M. and Barry, B. W. *J. Pharm. Pharmacol. 38*(Suppl.):71P (1986).
42. Van Duzee, B. F. *J. Invest. Dermatol. 65*:404 (1975).
43. Barry, B. W. *J. Controlled Release 15*:237 (1991).
44. Barry, B. W. and Williams, A. C. *J. Pharm. Pharmacol. 42*:34P (1990).

5

Mechanisms and Prediction of Nonionic Surfactant Effects on Skin Permeability

Edward J. French

R. P. Scherer, Swindon, United Kingdom

Colin W. Pouton

School of Pharmacy and Pharmacology, University of Bath, Bath, United Kingdom

Kenneth A. Walters

An-eX Analytical Services, Ltd., Cardiff, Wales

I. INTRODUCTION

Many topical pharmaceutical formulations and cosmetic products applied to the skin, antiseptics, shampoos, detergents, creams, and lotions, contain surfactants. These are used as emulsifiers, suspending, wetting, solubilizing, and stabilizing agents (1). Of the three major classes of surfactants, nonionics have long been recognized as those with the least potential for irritancy and, hence, have a wider acceptability for use in topical products. Compounds, such as cetomacrogol (polyethyleneglycol monocetyl ether) and cetostearyl alcohol are major components of many nonionic creams. In the formulation of these products, the role of the surfactant is concerned with the physical stability or cosmetic appearance of dispersions; however, nonionic surface active agents may have intrinsic biological activity or may influence the activity of other molecules (2). Nonionic surfactants are known to have effects on the permeability of biological membranes, including skin. Their comparatively low toxicity and irritation potential make these compounds good candidates as potential penetration enhancers for use in transdermal drug delivery systems (3). The purpose of this chapter is to review what is known about the use of nonionic surfactants as enhancers of percutaneous absorption and their mechanisms of action. This will include a consideration of how the effects of these compounds can be predicted and their modes of action elucidated, by reference to surfactant activity on other biological membranes and model systems.

II. THE STRUCTURE OF NONIONIC SURFACTANTS

Molecules that have an amphipathic nature (i.e., they possess both hydrophilic and hydrophobic groups) will often display surface activity. The hydrophobic portion of nonionic surfactants usually consists of alkyl or acyl chains that are attached to a polar headgroup. For many nonionic surfactants, the headgroup is a polyoxyethylene chain (e.g., nonyl phenol ether polyethoxylate). Although there are many types of nonionic surfactants, most studies concerning the penetration-enhancing ability of nonionic surfactants have been limited to five principal series. These are the polysorbates (ethoxylated esters or partial esters of sorbitol); polyoxyethylene alkyl ethers and esters; polyoxyethylene alkylphenols and poloxamers (polyoxyethylene–polyoxypropylene block copolymers). The generalized structures of each of these types of surfactant are given in Figure 1. Commonly, in the literature, industrial-grade nonionic surfactants are referred to by their trade names. Table 1 lists examples of nonionic surfactants that have been investigated for penetration-enhancing activity, quoting the commercial product used in each case. For the Brij series surfactants (straight-chain alkyl ether ethoxylates), a shorthand notation is used to describe their chemical structure. The notation normally used is C_xE_n; where x is the number of carbons of the straight chain alcohol and n is the number of ethylene oxide groups condensed onto the alcohol. The abbreviation $C_{x=}$ refers to an unsaturated alcohol of chain length x, such as the oleyl group.

Nonionic surfactants, such as those of the Brij series or the alkylphenol-based surfactants, are produced by the reaction of ethylene oxide with the hydrophobic alcohol or phenol group. This process produces a polydisperse mixture of molecules of varying ethoxy chain lengths that will be distributed around the mean value quoted by the manufacturer. This situation is further complicated because the alcohols used are often impure, containing mixtures of alkyl chain lengths or, in the alkylphenols, variation in branching of the alkyl group. It is possible to purify these mixtures by various chromatographic methods. However, few, if any, of the studies on the biological properties of nonionic surfactants have been carried out using purified monodisperse surfactants, rendering comparison of work from different laboratories difficult. Also, structure–activity studies carried out with polydisperse surfactants may be subject to some distortion owing to the number of different components present in the industrial mixtures. Structure–activity studies would best be carried out using pure monodisperse surfactants that will have reproducible characteristics and will not suffer from batch-to-batch variability. As the properties of monodisperse surfactants are reproducible and defined, they may be the preferred choice for use as penetration enhancers in transdermal delivery systems.

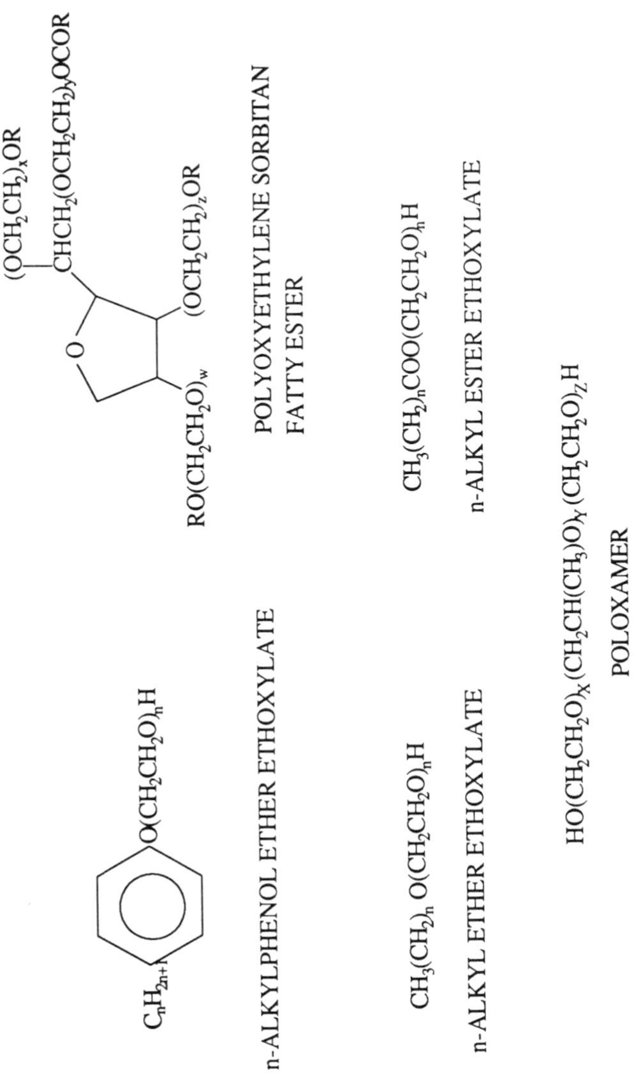

C_nH_{2n+1} —⬡— $O(CH_2CH_2O)_nH$

n-ALKYLPHENOL ETHER ETHOXYLATE

$CH_3(CH_2)_n\, O(CH_2CH_2O)_nH$

n-ALKYL ETHER ETHOXYLATE

RO(CH$_2$CH$_2$O)$_w$

CHCH$_2$(OCH$_2$CH$_2$)$_y$OCOR

(OCH$_2$CH$_2$)$_x$OR

(OCH$_2$CH$_2$)$_z$OR

POLYOXYETHYLENE SORBITAN FATTY ESTER

$CH_3(CH_2)_nCOO(CH_2CH_2O)_nH$

n-ALKYL ESTER ETHOXYLATE

$HO(CH_2CH_2O)_X (CH_2CH(CH_3)O)_Y (CH_2CH_2O)_Z H$

POLOXAMER

Figure 1   The generalized structure of various classes of nonionic surfactant.

Table 1 The Commercial Names and Abbreviated Chemical Structures of Nonionic
Surfactants Investigated for Penetration Enhancing Activity

Commercial name	Abbreviated structure	Ref.
Tween 20	POE(20) sorbitan monolaurate	4,5
Tween 40	POE (20) sorbitan monopalmitate	4,6
Tween 60	POE(20) sorbitan monostearate	4,7,8
Tween 80	POE(20) sorbitan monooleate	9
Tween 85	POE(20) sorbitan trioleate	10
Span 20	Sorbitan monolaurate	4,5
Span 40	Sorbitan monopalmitate	4,6
Span 85	Sorbitan trioleate	4,6,10
Brij 30	$C_{12}E_4$	4,5
Brij 36T	$C_{12}E_{10}$	11
Brij 35	$C_{12}E_{23}$	7,12
Brij 52	$C_{16}E_2$	11
Brij 56	$C_{16}E_{10}$	11,12
Brig 58	$C_{16}E_{20}$	6,11,12
Brij 72	$C_{18}E_2$	12
Brij 76	$C_{18}E_{10}$	11
Brij 78	$C_{18}E_{20}$	12
Brij 92	$C_{18}=E_2$	13
Brij 96	$C_{18}=E_{10}$	10,11
Brij 98	$C_{18}=E_{20}$	12
Triton X-100	POE(10) octylphenol	11
Rewopal HV10	POE(10) nonylphenol	11
Pluronic F68	POE(140) POP(26-31)	4,11
Pluronic L62	POE(15) POP(26-31)	4,11

III. EFFECTS OF NONIONIC SURFACTANTS ON
BIOLOGICAL MEMBRANES

The skin can be considered a very complex biological membrane. It is now widely
accepted that the barrier function of the skin is related to the structure and
character of the intercellular lipid bilayers of the stratum corneum (14–16). This
multiple bilayer structure would be expected to behave in a fashion somewhat
similar to other biological membranes in terms of the general physical phenomena
that will affect membrane permeability characteristics. Accordingly, the large
body of literature concerned with the effect that surfactants have on other natural
or synthetic lipid membranes may provide an insight into the potential of surfactants as skin permeation enhancers.

Nonionic surfactants can have a profound effect on the permeability characteristics of several biological membranes, including intestinal epithelia (17–19), erythrocytes (20), and goldfish gill epithelia (21–23). The effect of nonionic surfactants on the rate of permeation of drug compounds through membranes from a formulation is highly dependent on the physical state of the surfactant and its concentration in the locality of the membrane. In many pharmaceutical and cosmetic preparations, the surfactants incorporated into the formulations will be present in aqueous solution. The net effect of surfactants in solution on membrane permeability is extremely complex, being a function of formulation effects and of direct effects on membrane permeability. Many publications concerning the biological effects of surfactants have noted that there is a concentration-dependent biphasic action on the rate of drug permeation through membranes (see Ref. 1 and references therein). The enhancement of membrane transport occurs at low concentrations of surfactant, but this is seen to decrease at higher concentrations, generally above the critical micelle concentration (CMC) of the surfactant (21,22). The increase in transmembrane flux at low surfactant concentrations is normally attributed to the ability of the surfactant molecule to penetrate the membrane and increase its permeability. This will be discussed in more detail later in this text. Reduction of rate of transport of a drug present in surfactant systems is attributed to the ability of the surfactant to form micelles and is normally observed only if interaction between micelle and the drug occurs. Solubilization of active drug species by surfactant micelles decreases the thermodynamic activity of the drug and, hence, decreases the driving force of drug absorption.

Therefore, the overall effect of a surfactant on the rate of drug permeation across a membrane will be a combination of the influence of these two opposing effects. Thus, there are five possible profiles of surfactant-induced effects upon membrane permeability that can be plotted as a function of surfactant concentration (Fig. 2). Profile A is typical of the situation described previously when permeation is increased at premicellar concentrations, but decreased above the surfactant CMC. Profiles B and C occur if the surfactant increases membrane permeability, but has little or no affinity for the permeant. In B the enhancement of permeability reaches a maximum at the CMC, whereas in C, permeability is increased further above the CMC. Profile D would be obtained if the surfactant did not influence membrane permeability, but was able to solubilize the drug above its CMC, whereas if neither effect was present, profile E would occur.

There is a considerable volume of information available in the literature, including several detailed structure–activity studies, concerning the effects of nonionic surfactants on the permeability of mucous membranes. This work has been extensively reviewed elsewhere (1,2), although certain studies of this type are worth highlighting, as the data they contain provide an insight into the relative potency

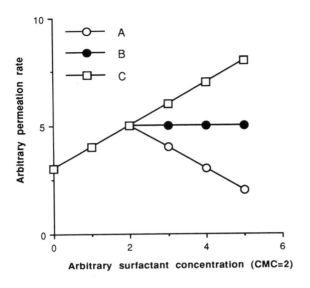

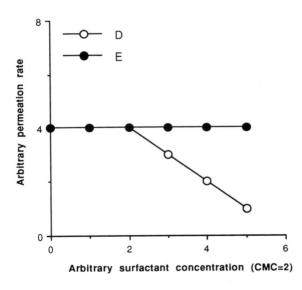

Figure 2 Possible profiles of surfactant-induced alterations in the permeability of biological membranes (see text for details).

of surfactant effects on biological membranes, which is relevant to the enhancement of percutaneous absorption.

Walters et al. (17) studied the effects of a range of alkyl ether ethoxylates of the Brij surfactant series on the diffusion of paraquat from aqueous solutions across isolated rabbit gastric mucosal epithelium. The surfactants used varied in both alkyl and ethylene oxide chain length. The permeability constant (K_p) of paraquat was altered depending on surfactant alkyl chain length, hydrophilic–lipophilic balance (HLB), and concentration. No global structure–activity relation could be proposed relative to a single surfactant property, such as HLB or alkyl chain length. However, for a homologous series of surfactants of given ethoxy chain length at a single concentration, dependency on alkyl chain length could be studied (Fig. 3). Also, for surfactants of given alkyl chain length, the effect of ethoxy chain length could be observed (Fig. 4). From these data it can be seen that, at micellar concentrations, the increase of paraquat flux was greatest for surfactants with an alkyl chain longer than C_9 and possessing ethoxy chains of 10–20 units. Similar findings were reported for the enhanced absorption of various barbiturates through goldfish gill epithelia (23).

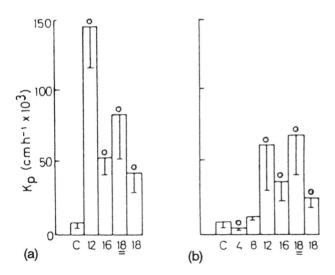

Figure 3 Values of K_p for paraquat obtained at 1.0% w/v surfactant with isolated rabbit gastric mucosa as a function of alkyl chain length: C_{12}, C_{16}, C_{18}, and $C_{18=}$, marked on the abscissa. (a) Compounds with 10 ethylene oxide units and (b) compounds with 20 ethylene oxide units. Results that were significantly different ($p < 0.05$) from the control values without surfactant are marked (o). (From Ref. 17.)

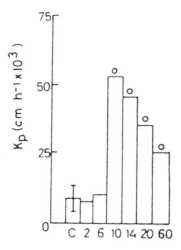

Figure 4 Values of K_p for paraquat obtained at 1.0% w/v surfactant with isolated rabbit gastric mucosa as a function of ethylene oxide chain length. The surfactants all had a C_{16} alkyl chain. Ethylene oxide chain lengths are marked on the abscissa from E_2 to E_{60}. C is the control, paraquat in the absence of surfactant. Results that were significantly different ($p < 0.05$) from the control values without surfactant are marked (o). (From Ref. 17.)

The effect of alkyl ether ethoxylates on the rectal absorption of insulin from corn oil-based suppositories was studied by Ichikawa et al. (24). The authors reported that for a homologous series of C_{12} surfactants the E_9 compound caused the greatest increase in insulin absorption (shown by decrease in blood glucose), whereas, for surfactants with nine ethoxy groups the C_{12} alkyl chain was the most potent (Table 2).

The relative potency of surfactants to act as penetration enhancers may also be related to data obtained from surfactant-induced perturbation of other biological membranes.

Zaslavsky et al. (20) studied the hemolytic activity of homologous series of alkyl ether ethoxylates. As in the foregoing studies, no direct correlation could be made to surfactant HLB, although the strangest effects were observed with molecules that had a C_{12} alkyl chain. In a study on the mobility of the protozoan *Tetrahymena elliotti*, Baillie et al. (25) observed that, for alkyl ether ethoxylates and nonyl phenol ether ethoxylates, as the ethoxy chain length increased, the disruptive potency on the membrane decreased. The most potent alkyl ether ethoxylate was $C_{12}E_4$. The octyl phenol series contained some very hydrophobic

Nonionic Surfactants and Skin Permeability

Table 2 Effects of Polyoxyethylene Fatty Alcohol Ethers in Insulin Suppositories on Blood Glucose Levels in Rabbits[a]

	Decrease in blood glucose (%)			
	Time (min)			
Surfactant	30	60	90	120
C12E3	−8.8 ± 7.7	−3.0 ± 3.5	−11.2 ± 2.3	−9.8 ± 4.1
C12E9	−12.7 ± 8.5	−47.9 ± 5.6	−47.1 ± 7.4	−32.6 ± 11.2
C12E25	+0.6 ± 1.2	−4.2 ± 2.6	−4.0 ± 2.8	−0.9 ± 1.0
C12E40	+17.3 ± 2.9	+18.5 ± 2.5	+14.9 ± 3.1	+13.5 ± 8.2
C8E9	+3.9 ± 5.5	+12.8 ± 8.0	+13.6 ± 9.2	+13.0 ± 6.2
C10E9	−21.6 ± 4.8	−36.2 ± 3.7	−16.2 ± 5.1	−12.6 ± 6.8
C16E9	−28.4 ± 3.6	−43.1 ± 2.6	−35.9 ± 5.7	−16.8 ± 5.4
C18E9	−22.0 ± 6.2	−22.2 ± 3.2	−19.8 ± 4.8	−26.2 ± 7.9

[a]Insulin suppositories contained 0.55% surfactant and 1 $U \cdot kg^{-1}$ of insulin in corn oil. The initial blood glucose concentration was 118.3 ± 6.2 mg·100 mL. Tabulated values represent decrease in the blood glucose level at 30, 60, 90, and 120 min after rectal administration of insulin suppositories (mean of three rabbits ± SEM).
Source: Adapted from Ref. 24.

molecules that had low membrane activity. The structure–activity relation observed was parabolic relative to the degree of ethoxylation, the optimum effect being obtained with the E_5 compound. Structure–activity relation similar to those described in the foregoing were obtained for nonyl phenol surfactants by Gadd and Curtis-Prior (26) working on spermatozoan membranes; Levin (27), who studied effects on rat vaginal membranes; and Cserhati et al. (28), who investigated inhibition of growth in microorganisms. All these workers found maximum activity with surfactants having 6–10 ethylene oxide groups attached to the nonyl phenol moiety. The effects reported in these studies were thought to be explained by fluidization, permeabilization, or destruction of the lipid membrane, and occasionally possible solubilization and extraction of membrane components such as proteins. The membrane protein-solubilizing action of nonionic surfactants is well documented (29).

Levin (27) explained the parabolic relation observed in terms of surfactant solubilities and partitioning. The more hydrophilic surfactants were too water-soluble to attain an effective intermembrane concentration, whereas the more hydrophobic surfactants were so poorly water-soluble that access to the cell membrane was limited by dissolution. A similar hypothesis was proposed by Florence et al. (2). The authors postulated that

[T]he depth of penetration of the hydrocarbon chain may not be equal in a homologous series varying in ethylene oxide chain length, leading to variation in biological activity. When the number of ethoxy groups is lower than optimum, low concentration limits monomer activity, also part of the ethoxy chain may penetrate into the membrane. When the ethoxy chain length is above optimum, high molecular area and decreased surface activity will result in less efficient membrane penetration.

It was also suggested that the relative effectiveness of a particular surfactant will be dependent on the lipophilicity of the target membrane (1).

IV. INTERACTION OF NONIONIC SURFACTANTS WITH MODEL SYNTHETIC LIPID MEMBRANES

A. Lipid Bilayers and Liposomes

Recent studies have shown that increasing the fluidity of the highly structured lipid lamellae of the stratum corneum can be correlated with an increase in stratum corneum permeability (30,31). The fluidization of these lipids is suspected to be one of the major modes of action of many known penetration enhancers (32). Synthetic phospholipid liposomes contain bilayers of structured lipid. These have been used as a simple model for the intercellular lipid lamellae of the stratum corneum to investigate bilayer fluidization by potential penetration enhancers. Physical changes in the characteristics of the lipid bilayers can be quantitatively assessed by a variety of biophysical techniques, such as differential scanning calorimetry (DSC), fluorescence polarization spectroscopy (FPS), nuclear magnetic resonance (NMR), Fourier transform infrared spectroscopy (FTIR), and electron spin resonance spectroscopy (ESR). Such techniques may provide a simple, quick screen for potential enhancers.

Hadgraft and coworkers (33–35) have used a light-scattering technique to determine the gel–liquid crystalline phase transition temperature (T_m) of dipalmitoylphosphatidylcholine (DPPC) liposomes and liposomes treated with several known penetration enhancers, including Brij 36T ($C_{12}E_{10}$). Addition of the surfactant to the liposomes caused a concentration-dependent decrease in T_m. A reduction in the phase transition temperature is indicative of decreased order of packing of the acyl chains of the lipids in the bilayer (36,37). Measurements of changes in gel–liquid crystalline phase transition temperature, transition width, and transition enthalpy provide quantitative information about the fluidity of a lipid membrane. These characteristics can be measured precisely for simple model membranes with use of DSC.

This technique was used to study the effect of a homologous series of pure, single-chain–length dodecyl ether ethoxylates, $C_{12}E_0$–$C_{12}E_8$, upon the fluidity of

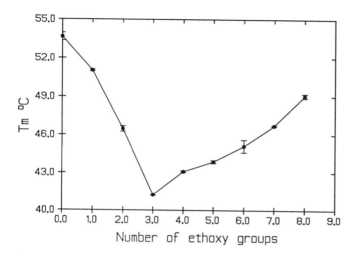

Figure 5 Phase transition midpoint temperature (T_m) of DSPC/surfactant vesicles containing 50 mol% surfactant, plotted against the ethoxy chain length of the incorporated surfactant. Data shown are mean ± SD, $n = 4$. (From Ref. 41.)

distearoylphosphatidylcholine (DSPC) liposomes (38). Figure 5 shows the bilayer phase transition temperature plotted as a function of surfactant ethoxy chain length. Pure DSPC liposomes had a T_m of 54.23 ± 0.37°C (mean ± SD; $n = 27$). As the ethoxy content of the surfactant was increased from $C_{12}E_0$ to $C_{12}E_3$ there was a decrease in T_m to a minimum with $C_{12}E_3$, further increases in ethoxy chain length from $C_{12}E_3$ to $C_{12}E_8$ reversed this trend, the reduction in T_m becoming less pronounced. As described earlier, the lowering of T_m was indicative of bilayer fluidization. The mixture of DSPC C_{18} chains and surfactant C_{12} acyl chains did not pack in as ordered a fashion as pure DSPC molecules, which resulted in a more fluid membrane (39).

Slightly different results, in terms of the structure–activity relation observed, were obtained using the same model membrane system and series of surfactants ($C_{12}E_0$–$C_{12}E_8$), when bilayer fluidization was measured by fluorescence polarization spectroscopy (40,41). This technique differed from DSC in that it was invasive; it required the introduction of fluorescent probe molecules into the membrane. Upon excitation with polarized light, the emission from fluorescent molecules is polarized in the same plane as the excitation. If the fluorophore undergoes rotational motion during the fluorescent lifetime of the molecule—the time between absorption and subsequent emission of a photon—then depolarization of the emission occurs. The degree of depolarization—the anisotropy of the fluorophore—is dependent on the rate and extent of rotational diffusion of the molecule during the fluorescent lifetime. These motions of the molecule depend on its size and shape and more so on the viscosity of its environment. Accordingly, a change in solvent viscosity or in the viscosity of the microenvironment of the fluorophore will result in a change in fluorescence anisotropy (42). The measurement of fluorescence polarization, or anisotropy, is illustrated schematically in Figure 6. The sample is excited with vertically polarized light, and the intensities of emissions are measured through polarizers, oriented parallel to the plane of excitation [i.e., vertically polarized (I_{VV})] and perpendicular to the plane of excitation [i.e., horizontally polarized (I_{VH})]. From these measurements the fluorescence anisotropy (r) can be calculated. The lower the viscosity of the membrane the higher the rate of rotation of the fluorophore and the lower the value of r. From plots of r against temperature, it is possible to calculate the membrane phase transition temperature (43). With use of FPS, it is possible to obtain good estimations of membrane fluidity and the microviscosity of the membrane interior (44).

Several fluorescent probe molecules were used that produced different structure–activity profiles for the fluidization of the DSPC bilayers. The values of T_c measured using cis-parinaric acid (cis-pna) and diphenylhexatriene (DPH) as probes are shown plotted as a function of surfactant ethoxy chain length in Figure 7. With cis-pna as the probe, $C_{12}E_5$ was observed to have had the greatest effect

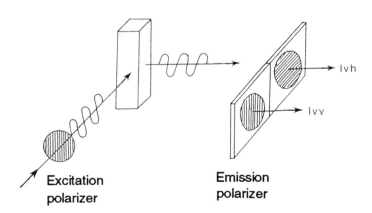

Figure 6 Schematic diagram of the basic principle of the measurement of fluorescence polarization (see text).

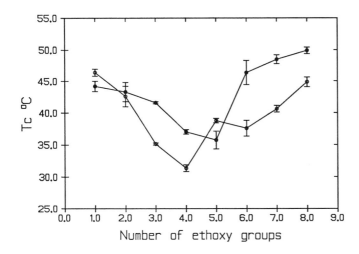

Figure 7   Phase transition onset temperature (T_c) of DSPC/surfactant vesicles containing 50 mol% surfactant, plotted against the ethoxy chain length of the incorporated surfactant. The values were obtained by FPS analysis using either *cis*-pna (○) or DPH (●) as the probe molecule. Data points are means ± SD, $n = 4$. (From Ref. 41.)

both T_c, whereas the results with DPH were slightly different, suggesting maximum reduction in T_c was obtained with $C_{12}E_4$. Figure 8 shows the probe anisotropy, r, at 30°C plotted as a function of surfactant ethoxy chain length for *cis*-pna, DPH, and 1-anilino-8-naphthalene sulfonic acid (ANS) incorporated into DSPC/surfactant vesicles containing 50 mol% surfactant. Little difference was noted between surfactants when *cis*-pna was the probe molecule, $C_{12}E_5$ caused the optimum fluidization; DPH was more greatly affected by $C_{12}E_4$, which was the most active surfactant with this probe. With ANS, however, the shorter ethoxy chain length molecules were less effective fluidizers, optimum activity being observed for $C_{12}E_6$. The observed differences in the surfactant structure–activity relation between probes were thought to be dependent on probe location in the membrane and probe–lipid–surfactant interactions. *cis*-Parimaric acid is a C_{18} fatty acid and was expected to be oriented in the same plane of the membrane as the C_{18} chains of the DSPC molecules with a similar conformation (45). Diphenylhexatriene is a highly hydrophobic molecule and is used to probe throughout the nonpolar membrane interior (46). However, ANS has a negatively charged sulfonate group attached to a hydrophobic naphthalene group. These two groups give the molecule an amphipathic nature, so ANS is thought to adsorb at the bilayer polar–nonpolar interface and is regarded as a good probe for studying the

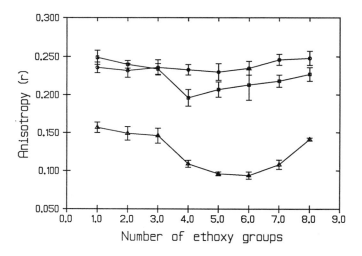

Figure 8 Probe anisotropy (*r*) of *cis*-pna (○), DPH (□), and ANS (Δ) measured at 30°C in DSPC/surfactant vesicles plotted against the ethoxy chain length of the incorporated surfactant. The surfactant concentration was 50 mol%. Data points shown are means ± SD; *n* = 4. (From Ref. 41.)

headgroup vicinity of the membrane (46). From the results of the FPS studies, it would appear that different surfactants in the series affected different parts of the bilayer. The correlation of these results to the surfactants, ability to enhance drug permeation through skin and the validity of the model systems will be discussed later.

A similar method to FPS for membrane fluidization is ESR. In this technique a spin probe (a molecule containing a stable free radical) is incorporated into the lipid bilayers. The local environment of the probe will affect the ESR spectra obtained. From measurements of the hyperfine splitting constraints obtained from the spectra, an order parameter can be calculated (47). The order parameter (*s*) is related to the viscosity of the medium surrounding the probe, a decrease in *s* indicates lower membrane viscosity and a more fluid membrane (48). With this method, it has been shown that dodecyl ether ethoxylate surfactants do fluidize the lipid bilayers of model DSPC liposome systems and the lipid lamellae of isolated porcine stratum corneum (41). Similar results for Brij-36T ($C_{12}E_{10}$) were reported by Gay et al. (35,49), who observed the fluidization of the DPPC bilayers and isolated human stratum corneum by ESR.

The fluidization of lipid bilayers in isolated stratum corneum preparations by penetration enhancers has been studied using DSC by many investigators (50,51).

By use of this technique, it has been shown that lauryl ether ethoxylate surfactants cause lipid bilayer fluidization in situ (34,41).

B. Lipid Monolayers

Insoluble lipid monolayers, spread at a liquid–gas interface, have been widely used as models for the investigation of complex interfacial phenomena. In particular, their usefulness in clarifying processes occurring on or within biological membranes has been established. Insights into the mode of action of several diverse groups of pharmacological agents, including antihistamines (52), narcotic analgesics (53), polypeptide hormones (54), amino acids (55), barbiturates (56), phorbol esters (57), and polyene antibiotics (58), have been obtained using monomolecular lipid films. In addition, several investigators have used monolayer technology to examine the interaction between surfactants and biological membranes (59–61). More recent studies have been designed to evaluate the possible usefulness of monomolecular lipid films in determining the mode of action of skin penetration enhancers (62).

The most common approach to the study of monomolecular lipid films is the use of a Langmuir trough with a film balance. Essentially this involves filling a hydrophobic tank (e.g., Teflon or paraffin-coated glass) with either water or a salt solution and spreading the lipid on the surface as a solution in an organic solvent such as hexane. As the solvent evaporates the lipid is evenly distributed at the air–water interface. Ideally, this lipid is contained between two barriers one of which is mobile. There are several recent refinements to this design, although the essential principle, the ability to compress the lipid film, is retained. The lipid is normally dispensed in such amounts that, in the initial situation, it exists on the aqueous surface in the gaseous phase. Thus, the individual lipid molecules do not interact with each other and the surface tension of the film is equivalent to that of the subphase. In this situation, the surface pressure (π) is zero. As the film is compressed, the area that each lipid molecule occupies is reduced and the aqueous phase changes from the gaseous state through liquid (expanded and condensed) phases to the solid phase. Thus, the *surface pressure*, defined as the difference between the surface tension of the subphase and that of the film, increases. At a finite point, compression is such that the film collapses and the molecules become aligned in some multilayer formation. The phase changes are normally illustrated in a π/A isotherm (Fig. 9) that shows the relation between the surface pressure of the film and the area occupied by each lipid molecule.

The shape of the isotherm is dependent on the lipid used. For example, cholesterol monolayers exhibit a solid film except at low surface pressures, at which they show liquid condensed behavior. On the other hand, films of fatty acids on water show linear solid behavior. Phospholipids generally display liquid

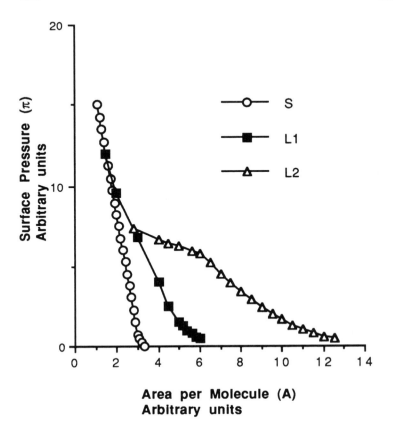

Figure 9 Phases through which lipid monolayers progress during compression: π, surface pressure; A, area per molecule; L1 = liquid condensed; L2, liquid expanded; S, solid.

behavior, which is either condensed or expanded, depending on the state of compression. In general, substances that are not simple straight-chain structures exhibit much less sharply defined behavior.

The picture becomes much more complex with the introduction of mixed monomolecular layer films. Although, very often, simple mixtures will exhibit predictable behavior, interaction between the film constituents can lead to extremely complex alterations in the observed isotherm characteristics (63). This aside, once a pattern has been established for a single or mixed monolayer behavior, the interaction of drugs or pharmaceutical excipients with the monolayer can be investigated. This interaction, which normally involves penetration of the test substance from the subphase into the monolayer, causes alterations in the π/A isotherms, and some correlation between the effect on the monolayer and the biological effect of the substance is often sought.

In typical experiments, the substance under investigation is injected into the subphase of the film, allowed to equilibrate, and the surface pressure at various areas per molecule is determined (64). The interaction of polyoxyethylene alkyl ethers with cholesterol monolayers has been investigated (61). Surfactants based on lauryl (C_{12}) and stearyl (C_{18}) alkyl chains with varying degrees of ethoxylation were used. The data suggested that, at very low surfactant concentration and a large area per molecule, cholesterol films were fluidized, resulting in a change from the gaseous to the liquid expanded state. As the area per molecule was reduced by compression, the surfactants were ejected from the film. As the surfactant concentration in the subphase was increased, however, a concentration-dependent biphasic response was observed (Fig. 10). An increase in surface pressure, with no ejection at high compression, was followed, at high surfactant concentration, by a reduction in surface pressure. This latter observation suggested that the surfactants were removing the cholesterol from the surface, perhaps by mixed micelle formation. Those surfactants with a lauryl alkyl chain appeared to be capable of removing cholesterol from the surface at a concentration of one of two orders of magnitude less than those based on a stearyl alkyl chain. This has interesting implications for the effect of these surfactants on the permeability characteristics of skin for which polyoxyethylene lauryl ethers appear to enhance permeability to a much greater extent than the polyoxyethylene stearyl ethers (11). More data are required, however, before any positive correlations can be drawn.

V. EFFECTS OF NONIONIC SURFACTANT ON PERCUTANEOUS ABSORPTION

To exert an effect in the skin, the surfactant must first itself penetrate into the stratum corneum. The rate of penetration of polyoxyethylene surfactants into the skin is generally quite low, although some possess a greater intrinsic rate of permeation than their anionic counterparts (65). For a series of lauryl ether ethoxylates, the molecules of low HLB ($C_{12}E_1$, $C_{12}E_2$) penetrated the skin at a higher rate than more hydrophilic surfactants with longer ethoxy chain lengths, $C_{12}E_6$ and $C_{12}E_{10}$ (66). There are many variables that will affect the extent of permeation of the surfactant and, hence, its potency as an enhancer. The vehicle used to deliver the drug and enhancer to the skin surface will affect the partitioning behavior of the enhancer and possibly the physical characteristics of the skin. The degree of enhancing activity is also strongly dependent on the surfactant structure and concentration (2,67). Therefore, attempts to correlate data from

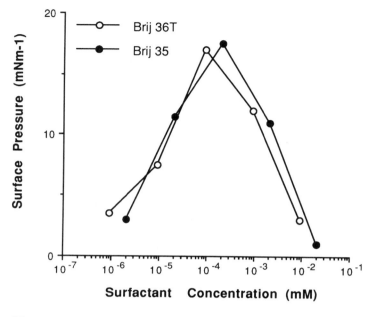

Figure 10 Surface pressure vs. surfactant concentration plots using, as an example, surfactants of the Brij 30 series.

different sources becomes very difficult, with each investigator using different systems and a variety of different animal species and anatomical application sites (68,69); also, as noted earlier, batch-to-batch variation among the polydisperse surfactants will add to the complexity of the situation. As with other membranes (discussed in Section III), surfactants enhance or retard the rate of absorption through the skin. This is dependent on how they are used and in what concentration (67).

The polysorbates have increased percutaneous absorption in several studies. Polysorbates 20, 40, 60, and 80, when present in low concentrations <0.5% v/v caused increased flux of both hydrocortisone and lidocaine through hairless mouse skin from a propan-2-ol/H_2O vehicle (8,9,70). When used in conjugation with propylene glycol (PG) the extent of enhancement was increased significantly, suggesting some synergism between the PG and the surfactants. Polysorbates have been shown to increase the permeation of salicylic acid, sodium salicylate, and flufenamic acid through rabbit skin in vivo from white petroleum bases containing 5 or 10% dimethyl sulfoxide (DMSO) (4,6); as with PG, some synergism was observed between DMSO and the surfactant. Polysorbate 80 increased the permeation of chloramphenicol through hairless mouse skin (71), whereas Mezei and Ryan (10) observed that polysorbate 85 increased the transepidermal water loss from excised rabbit skin. All these studies show that polysorbates can affect the barrier properties of the skin; however, polysorbate 20 had no effect on the absorption of naloxone through human skin (5), and similarly, polysorbate 60 had little effect on the permeation of naproxen through rat, rabbit, or human skin (7). From these studies, it is not possible to form any definite quantitative structure–activity relation for the polysorbates as permeation enhancers.

Polyoxyethylene aryl ethers are known to have potent membrane-disrupting activity and are widely used as solubilizing agents for membrane-bound enzymes (29). Despite this, there is little evidence to show that these surfactants will act as enhancers of percutaneous absorption. Walters et al. (11) found that the rate of skin permeation of methyl nicotinate across mouse skin was unaltered by both octyl and nonyl phenol decaethoxylates. The aryl ethers can also retard the percutaneous absorption of compounds. Dalvi and Zatz (72) observed that micellar concentrations of nonyl phenol pentadecaethoxylate considerably reduced the permeation of benzocaine through hairless mouse skin. It has been reported elsewhere that the damage potential on the skin from anionic surfactants is reduced by the presence of long ethoxy chain acyl ethers (73). The nonionic surfactant presumably retards the penetration of the ionic surfactant.

As with the other classes of surfactants, there are conflicting reports about the effects of poloxamers. Members of the poloxamer series had little effect on the flux of naloxone through human cadaver skin in vitro (5). However, poloaxamers 231 and 182 significantly increased the flux of salicylic acid and sodium salicylate through rabbit skin (4).

Polyoxyethylene alkyl ethers and esters enhance the percutaneous absorption of many compounds and appear to be the most potent enhancers among the nonionic surfactant classes. The efficacy of these surfactants appears to be very structure-dependent, and several structure–activity studies have been carried out. Walters et al. (11,12) studied the effect of a wide range of alkyl ether ethoxylates, which varied in both alkyl and ethylene oxide chain lengths, upon the permeation of methyl nicotinate through hairless mouse skin in two-chambered diffusion cells. They found that the surfactants with a linear alkyl chain length greater than C_8 and ethoxy chain length of less than E_{14} significantly increased the permeation of methyl nicotinate (Fig. 11). Maximum enhancement was obtained with Brij 36T ($C_{12}E_{10}$) followed by Brij 96 ($C_{18}=E_{10}$), Brij 56 ($C_{16}E_{10}$) and Brij 52 ($C_{16}E_6$). The effectiveness of Brij 36T as an enhancer upon the permeation of both hexyl and methyl nicotinate has been noted by other investigators (34,74). In a study of the effects of 15 nonionic agents on the permeation of sodium salicylate and salicylic acid through rabbit skin in vitro, significant enhancement was obtained

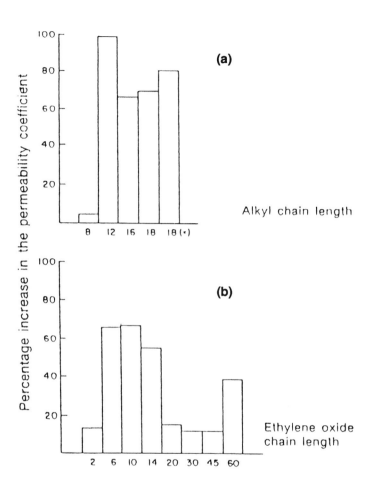

Figure 11 Enhancement of methyl nicotinate permeation as a function of surfactant structure: (a) with a constant ethylene oxide chain length of 10; (b) with a constant alkyl chain length of 16. (From Ref. 11.)

with Brij 30 ($C_{12}E_4$) and Brij 92 ($C_{18}=E_2$) when the surfactants were delivered to the skin in a simple white paraffin base containing 10% DMSO (4). Brij 92 ($C_{18}=E_2$) was also shown to be a good enhancer for flufenamic acid under the same test conditions (6). The flux of naloxone was enhanced by lauryl alcohol ($C_{12}E_0$) and $C_{12}E_4$, but $C_{12}E_{20}$ had little effect (5). Also, in this latter study, it was observed that the dodecyl (C_{12}) chain was often the optimum alkyl chain length for enhancement with both nonionic and ionic surfactants. Other work has shown that $C_{18}=E_5$ enhanced the permeation of nitroglycerin (13) and that $C_{12}E_2$ enhanced the flux of both theophylline and adenosine in vitro (75).

In a recent study, the effect of a homologous series of pure dodecyl ether ethoxylates ($C_{12}E_0$–$C_{12}E_8$) on the permeation of steroids through porcine skin in vitro was investigated (41). Application of surfactant to the skin greatly increased the mass penetrating the skin of the polar steroid hydrocortisone (HC) and the more lipophilic steroid estradiol (OE). The extent of penetration enhancement was highly dependent on the ethoxy chain length of the surfactant. Figure 12 shows the mean calculated enhancement ratios (mass that permeated surfactant treated skin at time t/mass that permeated untreated skin at time t) for OE permeation after 24, 48, 60, and 72 hr, plotted against the ethoxy chain length of the surfactant. As ethoxy chain length of surfactant increased from $C_{12}E_0$ to $C_{12}E_3$, the ER increased to a maximum with $C_{12}E_3$-treated skin. With enhancers of ethoxy chain length longer than three ($C_{12}E_3$–$C_{12}E_8$), the ER reduced with increasing surfactant ethoxy chain length. Figure 13 shows the mean ER ($n=6$) for HC after 24, 48, 60, and 72 hr, plotted against surfactant ethoxy chain length. For OE, the maximum effect was obtained with $C_{12}E_3$. However, as time of permeation increased, the effects of longer ethoxy chain surfactants became more pronounced, and the relative effect of the more hydrophobic molecules decreased. After 72 hr, there was little difference between the ER with $C_{12}E_3$, $C_{12}E_4$, and $C_{12}E_5$, the values with $C_{12}E_6$–$C_{12}E_8$ being only slightly lower. This differed from the study of OE permeation, for which the hydrophilic surfactants had far less effect. This suggests that there may be different mechanisms of action operative when surfactants enhance the permeation of polar and nonpolar compounds. The latter permeability data was well correlated with information obtained from the studies of model membranes using the same series of surfactants (described in Sect. IV).

Estradiol is a comparatively nonpolar compound and, as such, would be expected to pass freely across the lipid bilayers. All the surfactants caused some increase in fluidization of the lipid bilayers, and this was reflected in the permeation studies, as all the surfactants produced some degree of permeation enhancement. The maximum enhancement for estradiol was observed with $C_{12}E_3$ at all time points. In the related DSC study, this surfactant was the best fluidizer of the lipid bilayers. The corresponding FPS analysis suggested $C_{12}E_3$ was acting by fluidizing the acyl chains in the core of the bilayer, shown by its effect on DPH, but relative lack of efficacy with ANS. The increase in OE permeation through the skin, therefore, showed good correlation with the physicochemical studies of bilayer fluidization. This data suggests that OE penetrates the stratum corneum by the fluidized lipid bilayer core.

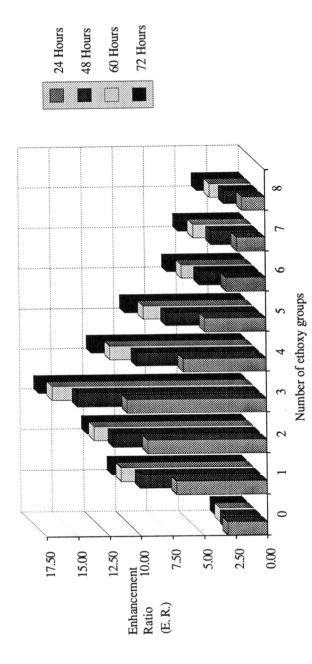

Figure 12 The enhancement ratios (ER) of the surfactants, $C_{12}E_0–C_{12}E_8$, for estradiol permeation through porcine ear skin measured at 24, 48, 60, and 72 hr. The bars shown are the mean values of six skin samples. (From Ref. 41.)

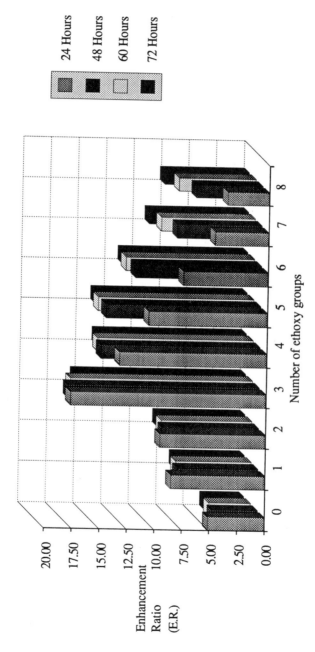

Figure 13 The enhancement ratios (ER) of the surfactants, $C_{12}E_0$–$C_{12}E_8$, for hydrocortisone permeation through porcine ear skin measured at 24, 48, 60, and 72 hr. The bars shown are the mean values of six skin samples. (From Ref. 41.)

Hydrocortisone can be regarded as a relatively polar molecule. However, as with estradiol, $C_{12}E_3$ was the most potent permeation enhancer, especially during the first 24 hr of the experiment. Later the enhancement ratio for $C_{12}E_3$ decreased, this was explained by depletion of the surfactant. It is unlikely that HC would permeate freely across the lipid bilayers. Therefore, $C_{12}E_3$ may have exerted its bilayer perturbing effects by allowing the polar molecule to partition across these potential barriers more easily. A similar mechanism was suggested for the enhancement of polar molecules by laurocapram (Azone) (28). For HC, the longer ethoxy chain length molecules $C_{12}E_5$–$C_{12}E_7$ were more effective enhancers than they were for OE permeation. In the corresponding FPS studies, $C_{12}E_5$–$C_{12}E_7$ were active in the headgroup region of the bilayer, as shown by their effect upon ANS. Disruption of the lipid headgroups by the long ethoxy chains would reduce the structure of the bound water surrounding them and tend to swell the aqueous regions of lipid lamellae, thereby providing a suitable solvent for hydrocortisone. Because of the increased solvent capacity of these regions of the lipid lamellae for HC, one would expect a faster net rate of permeation of this compound. The effect of the longer ethoxy chains would not be expected to be important for the enhancement of permeation of nonpolar molecules such as OE, which would be expected to penetrate more rapidly across the lipid bilayers.

VI. DISCUSSION

From the data presented in this chapter, it can be seen that nonionic surfactants can have a considerable effect on membrane permeability and, as such, have a potential use as skin penetration enhancers. The data presented was drawn from a variety of sources and encompasses many different model systems and membranes. In this section, an attempt will be made to draw together various aspects of this information, with the aim of rationalizing the use of nonionic surfactants as skin penetration enhancers.

To obtain the optimum effect in terms of permeation enhancement and drug delivery, careful selection of the surfactant and the formulation of the product is required. In this chapter, much emphasis has been placed on determination of structure–activity relation to identify potent permeation enhancers among the nonionic surfactants. This includes studies on model membranes, natural biological membranes, and the skin. The data in the previous sections have concentrated on alterations induced in the packing of membrane lipid bilayers and the lipid lamellae of the stratum corneum. There appears to be a remarkable correlation between fluidization of simple model membranes and the ability to enhance penetration of drugs through the skin. To affect these lipid regions, the surfactant would first have to penetrate into them. Therefore, the overall potency of particular surfactant is likely to be a combination of the molecules ability to penetrate into the lipid region and its ability to fluidize the lipid bilayers. Consideration of the data presented in Sections III, IV, and V for alkyl ether ethoxylate surfactants highlights these effects.

In many of the studies concerning the membrane activity of the alkyl ether ethoxylates, the optimum alkyl chain length for biological activity was C_{12}, molecules of longer or shorter alkyl chain length were less active. The potency of the C_{12} has been noted and discussed elsewhere (2,5,67). It is thought that this chain length may be optimal to penetrate and disrupt the lipid bilayer structure. Brij 36T ($C_{12}E_{10}$) was able to fluidize simple membranes in several studies (see Sect. IV). However, among a series of pure monodisperse C_{12} surfactants, the shorter ethoxy chain length molecules, $C_{12}E_2$–$C_{12}E_5$, were far more potent fluidizers of membrane lipids than surfactants with longer hydrophilic chains. The industrial polymeric surfactants may contain small amounts of lower HLB components of high membrane activity in a surfactant mixture stated as being of longer ethoxy chain length. The overall mode of action of the surfactants may also be greatly affected by the vehicle. Longer ethoxy chain molecules in aqueous solution will be able to form large micelles that have the potential to extract both lipids and proteins from membranes. This phenomenon would be highly dependent on the presence of water at the skin surface and would be less likely to occur with lipophilic surfactants, which form far smaller micelles.

Surfactants are known to both interact with and affect the keratin of the stratum corneum (34,76,77). Little attention has been paid to this possible mechanism of action of surfactants in this chapter. The involvement of surfactant–protein interaction in many of the studies described cannot be ruled out. However, the close relation observed between permeation enhancement and lipid bilayer fluidization observed in several studies would suggest that the lipid lamellae of the stratum corneum and not the keratin of the corneocytes is the major site of action of nonionic surfactants.

The penetration of the surfactant molecule into the lipid lamellae of the stratum corneum is strongly dependent on the partitioning behavior and solubilities of the surfactant. This would initially suggest that the more lipophilic the surfactant, the greater its ability to penetrate into the lipid membrane. This will, however, depend on the vehicle in which the enhancer and the drug are applied to the skin. In most of the studies described, the surfactants were present in aqueous solution. Optimum enhancement was observed with molecules containing an average of six to ten ethylene oxide groups condensed to a C_{10-18} alkyl group (11,23). However, when the surfactant was deposited directly onto the skin surface from a volatile solvent, the more lipophilic the surfactant, the higher its rate of penetration into the skin (66). Also, when the surfactant and drug were deposited by this method, optimum enhancement was observed with more lipophilic surfactants than for those found in the aqueous solution studies (41). The higher rate of penetration into the skin and possible higher intrinsic membrane activity of the lower HLB molecules may be restricted in aqueous solution by their low solubility in water, although this should favor partitioning of these surfactants into the lipids if they can achieve intimate contact with the skin. In an oil-based vehicle, the solubility and delivery to the skin surface of lipophilic surfactants would be improved; however, the vehicle/skin partition coefficient for the low HLB surfactants will be raised, reducing their penetration into the skin. This may explain the relatively low effect of $C_{12}E_3$ and $C_{12}E_6$ relative to $C_{12}E_9$ on the absorption of insulin from corn oil-based suppositories (24). The composition of the formulation, therefore, will have a great effect on the membrane activity of surfactants. Similarly the presence of water at the skin surface, caused by occlusion of the skin, may affect the efficacy and mode of action of surfactant penetration enhancers.

From the foregoing discussion, it can be seen that there are many factors that can affect and can complicate the use of surfactants as penetration enhancers. To achieve the maximum effect of the surfactant on percutaneous absorption, the delivery of both surfactant and drug to the skin should be optimized. The simplest formulation, but probably one of the most effective, would be to produce a saturated solution or dispersion of the drug to be administered in a pure monodisperse surfactant that has high membrane-fluidizing activity. Small lipophilic surfactant molecules, such as pure $C_{12}E_3$, are liquid at normal skin and room temperature, have a good solvent capacity, and are very effective fluidizers of lipid membranes. It is unlikely that a single surfactant would be the optimum enhancer for all drug molecules, the choice of enhancer would have to be tailored to the specific drug. However, simple mixtures such as this, incorporated into a therapeutic device, with a synthetic membrane to control the rate of delivery to the skin, may prove effective for enhanced transdermal drug delivery.

VII. CONCLUSIONS

To determine the potency of a compound as a skin penetration enhancer, it is ultimately necessary to study its effect on the permeation rates of drug compounds through skin, preferably human in origin. However, by studying the effect of the enhancer on model membrane systems, such as liposomes and monolayers, and by the extrapolation of data from other biological membranes, it is possible to gain insight into both the mechanism of enhancement and the efficacy of the particular compound as an enhancer. In light of this, it may be possible to use some of the techniques described with model membranes as quick, simple screens for potential penetration enhancers.

REFERENCES

1. Attwood, D. and Florence, A. T. *Surfactant Systems; Their Chemistry, Pharmacy and Biology.* Chapman & Hall, London (1983).
2. Florence, A. T., Tucker, I. G., and Walters, K. A. Interactions of nonionic alkyl and aryl ethers with membranes and other biological systems. In *Structure/Performance Relationships in Surfactants*, M. J. Rosen (ed.). *ACS Symp. Ser. 253*:189–207 (1984).
3. Walters, K. A. Surfactants and percutaneous absorption. In *Prediction of Percutaneous Penetration.* Scott, R. C., Guy, R. H., and Hadgraft, J. (eds.). IBC Technical Services, London, pp. 148–162 (1990).
4. Shen, W.-W., Danti, A. G., and Bruscato, F. N. Effect of nonionic surfactants on percutaneous absorption of salicylic acid and sodium salicylate in the presence of dimethyl sulphoxide. *J. Pharm. Sci. 65*:1780–1783 (1976).
5. Aungst, B. J., Rogers, N. J., and Shefter, E. Enhancement of naloxone penetration through human skin in vitro using fatty acids, fatty alcohols, surfactants, sulfoxides and amides. *Int. J. Pharm. 33*:225–234 (1986).
6. Hwang, C.-C. and Danti, A. G. Percutaneous absorption of flufenamic acid in rabbits: Effect of dimethyl sulphoxide and various nonionic surfactants. *J. Pharm. Sci. 72*: 857–860 (1983).
7. Chowhan, Z. T. and Pritchard, R. Effect of surfactants on percutaneous absorption of naproxen I. Comparisons of rabbit, rat and human excised skin. *J. Pharm. Sci. 67*: 1272–1274 (1978).
8. Sarpotdar, P. P. and Zatz, J. L. Evaluation of penetration enhancement of lidocaine by nonionic surfactants through hairless mouse skin in vitro. *J. Pharm. Sci. 75*:176–181 (1986).
9. Shahi, V. and Zatz, J. L. Effect of formulation factors on penetration of hydrocortisone through mouse skin. *J. Pharm. Sci. 67*:789–792 (1978).
10. Mezei, M. and Ryan, K. J. Effects of surfactants on epidermal permeability in rabbits. *J. Pharm. Sci. 61*:1329–1331 (1972).
11. Walters, K. A., Walker, M., and Olejink, O. Nonionic surfactant effects on skin permeability characteristics. *J. Pharm. Pharmacol. 40*:525–529 (1988).
12. Walters, K. A. and Olejink, O. Effects of nonionic surfactants on the hairless mouse skin penetration of methyl nicotinate. *J. Pharm. Pharmacol. 35*(Suppl):81P (1983).
13. Tiemessen, H. L. G. M. Nonionic surfactant systems for transdermal drug delivery. PhD Thesis, Leiden (1989).
14. Elias, P. M. Lipids and the epidermal permeability barrier. *Arch. Dermatol. Res. 270*:95–117 (1981).
15. Elias, P. M., Cooper, E. R., Korc, A., and Brown, B. E. Percutaneous transport in relation to stratum corneum structure and lipid composition. *J. Invest. Dermatol. 76*:297–301 (1981).
16. Wertz, P. W., Swartzendruber, D. C., and Downing, D. T. The role of the corneocyte lipid envelope in the structure and function of the barrier layer. In *Prediction of Percutaneous Penetration*, R. C. Scott, R. H. Guy, and J. Hadgraft (eds.). IBC Technical Services, London, 1990, pp. 405–411.
17. Walters, K. A., Dugard, P. H., and Florence, A. T. Nonionic surfactants and gastric mucosal transport of paraquat. *J. Pharm. Pharmacol. 33*:207–213 (1981).

18. Wilson, C. G. and Thomas, N. E. Interaction of tissues with polyethylene glycol vehicles. *Pharm. Int. 5*:94–97 (1984).

19. Whitmore, D. A., Brookes, L. G., and Wheeler, W. P. Relative effects of different surfactants on intestinal absorption and the release of proteins and phospholipids from the tissues. *J. Pharm. Pharmacol. 31*:277–283 (1979).

20. Zaslavsky, B. Y., Ossipov, N. N., Krivich, V. S., Baholdina, L. P., and Rogozhin, S. V. Action of surface-active agents on biological membranes II. Hemolytic activity of nonionic surfactants. *Biochim. Biophys. Acta 507*:1–7 (1978).

21. Levy, G., Miller, K. E., and Reuning, R. H. Effect of complex formation on drug absorption III: Concentration- and drug-dependent effect of a nonionic surfactant. *J. Pharm. Sci. 55*:394 (1966).

22. Florence, A. T. and Gillan, J. M. N. Non-ionic surfactants and membrane transport of thioridazine in goldfish. *J. Pharm. Pharmacol. 27*:152–159 (1975).

23. Walters, K. A., Florence, A. T., and Dugard, P. H. Nonionic surfactants and the membrane transport of barbiturates in goldfish. *Int. J. Pharm. 10*:153–163 (1982).

24. Ichikawa, K., Ohata, I., Mitomi, M., Kawamura, S., Maeno, H., and Kawata, H. Rectal absorption of insulin suppositories in rabbits. *J. Pharm. Pharmacol. 32*:314–318 (1980).

25. Baillie, A. J., Assadi, A., and Florence, A. T. Influence of nonionic surfactant structure on motility inhibition of *Tetrahymena elliotti* as a model for surfactant–membrane interactions. *Int. J. Pharm. 53*:241–248 (1989).

26. Gadd, A. L. and Curtis-Prior, P. B. A modified transmembrane migration method for evaluating spermicidal potency of some nonoxynol compounds. *J. Pharm. Pharmacol. 40*:215–216 (1988).

27. Levin, R. J. Structure/activity relationships of a homologous series of surfactants (nonylphenoxypolyethoxyethanols) on the rat vaginal bioelectric activity over the oetrous cycle. *Pharmacol. Toxicol. 62*:131–134 (1988).

28. Cserharti, T., Szogyi, M., and Bordas, B. QSAR study on the biological activity of nonyl-phenyl-ethylene-oxide polymers. *Gen. Physiol. Biophys. 1*:225–231 (1982).

29. Helenius, A. and Simons, K. Solubilisation of membranes by detergents. *Biochim. Biophys. Acta 415*:29–79 (1975).

30. Knutson, K., Potts, R. O., Guzak, D. B., Golden, G. M., McKie, J. E., Lambert, W. J., and Higuchi, W. I. Macro- and molecular physical chemical considerations in understanding drug transport in the stratum corneum. In *Advances in Drug Delivery Systems*. Anderson, J. W. and Kim, S. W. (eds.). Elsevier Scientific, New York, pp. 67–87 (1986).

31. Golden, G. M., McKie, J. E., and Potts, R. O. The role of stratum corneum lipid fluidity in transdermal drug flux. *J. Pharm. Sci. 76*:25–28 (1987).

32. Barry, B. W. Mode of action of penetration enhancers in human skin. *J. Controlled Release 6*:85–97 (1987).

33. Beastall, J. C., Hadgraft, J., and Washington, C. Mechanism of action of Azone as a penetration enhancer: Lipid bilayer fluidity and transition temperature effects. *Int. J. Pharm. 43*:207–213 (1988).

34. Ashton, P. Surfactant effects in percutaneous absorption. PhD Thesis, University of Wales (1988).

35. Gay, C. L., Murphy, T. M., Hadgraft, J., Kellaway, I. W., Evans, J. C., and Rowlands, C. C. An electron skin resonance study of skin penetration enhancers. *Int. J. Pharm.* 49:39–45 (1989).

36. Chapman, D. Phase transitions and fluidity characteristics of lipids and cell membranes. *Q. Rev. Biophys.* 8:185–235 (1975).

37. Jain, M. J. and Wu, N. M. Effect of small molecules on the dipalmitoyl lecithin liposomal bilayer III. Phase transition in lipid bilayer. *J. Membr. Biol.* 34:157–201 (1977).

38. French, E. J., Pouton, C. W., and Steele, G. Fluidisation of distearoylphosphatidyl-choline bilayers by nonionic surfactants of single ethoxy chain length. *J. Pharm. Pharmacol.* 40(Suppl):38P (1988).

39. Small, D. M. Lateral chain packing in lipids and membranes. *J. Lipid Res.* 25:1490–1500 (1984).

40. French, E. J., Pouton, C. W., and Steele, G. Fluidisation of lipid bilayers by nonionic surfactants: Structure–activity studies using a fluorescent probe. In *Prediction of Percutaneous Penetration*. Scott, R. C., Guy, R. H., and Hadgraft, J. (eds.). IBC Technical Services, London, pp. 308–315 (1990).

41. French, E. J. The enhancement of percutaneous absorption by nonionic surfactants. PhD Thesis, University of Bath (1991).

42. Weber, G. Rotational brownian motion and polarisation of the fluorescence of solutions. *Adv. Protein Chem.* 8:415–459 (1953).

43. Klein, R. A. Thermodynamics and membrane processes. *Q. Rev. Biophys.* 15:667–757 (1982).

44. Shinitzky, M., Dianoux, A. C., Gitler, C., and Weber, G. Microviscosity and order in the hydrocarbon region of micelles and membranes determined with fluorescence probes. I. Synthetic membranes. *Biochemistry* 10:2106–2113 (1971).

45. Sklar, L. A., Hudson, B. S., and Simoni, R. D. Conjugated polyene fatty acids as fluorescent probes: Synthetic phospholipid membrane studies. *Biochemistry* 16:819–828 (1977).

46. Azzi, A. The application of fluorescent probes in membrane studies. *Q. Rev. Biophys.* 8:237–316 (1975).

47. Hubbell, W. L. and McConnell, H. M. Molecular motion in spin labelled phospholipids and membranes. *J. Am. Chem. Soc.* 93:314–326 (1971).

48. Jost, P., Libertini, L. J., Herbert, V. C., and Griffith, O. H. Lipid skin labels in lecithin multibilayers. A study of motion along fatty acid chains. *J. Mol. Biol.* 59:77–98 (1971).

49. Gay, G. L., Hadgraft, J., Kellaway, I. W., Evans, J. C., and Rowlands, C. C. The effect of skin penetration enhancers on human stratum corneum lipids: An electron spin resonance study. In *Prediction of Percutaneous Penetration*. Scott, R. C., Guy, R. H., and Hadgraft, J. (eds.). IBC Technical Services, London, pp. 322–332 (1990).

50. Goodman, M. and Barry, B. W. Action of penetration enhancers on human stratum corneum as assessed by differential scanning calorimetry. In *Percutaneous Absorption*, Vol. 2. Bronaugh, R. and Maibach, H. I. (eds.). Marcel Dekker, New York, pp. 567–593 (1987).

51. Boustra, J. A., Peschier, L. J. C., Brusse, J., and Boddé, H. E. Effect of *N*-alkyl-azocycloheptan-2-ones including Azone on the thermal behaviour of stratum corneum. *Int. J. Pharm.* 52:47–54 (1989).

52. Attwood, D. and Udeala, O. K. The interaction of antihistamines with lecithin monolayers. *J. Pharm. Pharmacol. 27*:806–810 (1975).
53. Huidoboro-Toro, J. P., Caressa, M., and Fischer, S. Interaction of morphine with cholesterol monolayers. *Biochim. Biophys. Acta 436*:237–241 (1976).
54. Snart, R. S. and Sanyal, N. N. Interaction of polypeptide hormones with lipid monolayers. *Biochem. J. 108*:369–373 (1968).
55. Nakagaki, M. and Okamura, E. Penetration of leucine and norleucine into lecithin monolayers from underlying aqueous solutions. *Bull. Chem. Soc. Jpn. 55*:3381–3385 (1982).
56. Vilallonga, F. A. and Phillips, E. W. Surface activities of barbital, phenobarbital and pentobarbital and their interaction energies with phospholipid monolayers. *J. Pharm. Sci. 69*:102–104 (1980).
57. Jacobson, K., Wenner, C. E., Kemp, G., and Papahadjopoulis, D. Surface properties of phorbol esters and their interaction with lipid monolayers and bilayers. *Cancer Res. 35*:2991–2995 (1975).
58. Demel, R. A., Cromberg, F. J. L., VanDeenan, L. L. M., and Kinsky, S. C. Interaction of polyene antibiotics with single and mixed lipid monomolecular layers. *Biochim. Biophys. Acta 150*:1–14 (1968).
59. Vilallonga, F. A. and Garrett, E. R. Kinetics and mechanisms of monolayer interactions. II: Effect of chain length of alkyl ionic surfactants on their interaction with dipalmitoyl glycerol, dipalmitoylphosphatidylethanolamine and dipalmitoyllecithin. *J. Pharm. Sci. 62*:1605–1609 (1973).
60. McGregor, M. A. and Barnes, G. T. Equilibrium penetration of monolayers VI: Cholesterol cetrimonium bromide systems. *J. Pharm. Sci. 67*:1054–1056 (1978).
61. Walters, K. A., Florence, A. T., and Dugard, P. H. Interaction of polyoxethylene alkyl ethers with cholesterol monolayers. *J. Colloid Interface Sci. 89*:584–587 (1982).
62. Lewis, D. and Hadgraft, J. Mixed monolayers of dipalmitoylphosphatidylcholine with Azone or oleic acid at the air–water interface. *Int. J. Pharm. 65*:211–218 (1990).
63. Adamson, A. W. *Physical Chemistry of Surfaces*. John Wiley & Sons, London (1976).
64. Barnes, G. T. On the kinetics of monolayer penetration. *J. Colloid Interface Sci. 27*:806–810 (1975).
65. Black, J. G. and Howes, D. Skin penetration of chemically related detergents. *J. Soc. Cosmet. Chem. 30*:157–165 (1979).
66. Nishiyama, T., Iwata, Y., Nakajima, K., and Mitsui, T. In vivo percutaneous absorption of polyoxyethylene lauryl ether surfactants in hairless mice. *J. Soc. Cosmet. Chem. 34*:263–271 (1983).
67. Walters, K. A. Penetration enhancers and their use in transdermal therapeutic systems. In *Transdermal Drug Delivery*. Guy, R. H. and Hadgraft, J. (eds.). Marcel Dekker, New York, pp. 197–246 (1989).
68. Lampe, M. A., Burlingame, A. L., Whitney, J. A., Williams, M. L., Brown, B. E., Roitman, E., and Elias, P. M. Human stratum corneum lipids: Characterization and regional variations. *J. Lipid Res. 24*:120–130 (1983).
69. Wester, R. C. and Maibach, H. I. In vivo animal models for percutaneous absorption. In *Percutaneous Absorption*. Bronaugh, R. L. and Maibach, H. I. (eds.). Marcel Dekker, New York, pp. 251–266 (1985).

70. Sarpotdar, P. P. and Zatz, J. L. Percutaneous absorption; enhancement by nonionic surfactants. *Drug. Dev. Ind. Pharm. 12*:1625–1647 (1986).
71. Aguiar, A. J. and Weiner, M. A. Percutaneous absorption studies of chloramphenicol solutions. *J. Pharm. Sci. 58*:210–215 (1969).
72. Dalvi, U. G. and Zatz, J. L. Effect of nonionic surfactants on penetration of dissolved benzocaine through hairless mouse skin. *J. Soc. Cosmet. Chem. 32*:87–94 (1981).
73. Eagle, S. C., Barry, B. W., and Scott, R. C. Inhibition of the damaging activity of divalent anionic surfactants on human skin. In *Prediction of Percutaneous Penetration.* Scott, R. C., Guy, R. H., and Hadgraft, J. (eds.). IBC Technical Services, London, pp. 417–425 (1990).
74. Ashton, P., Hadgraft, J., Brain, K. R., Millar, A., and Walters, K. A. Surfactant effects in topical drug availability. *Int. J. Pharm. 41*:189–195 (1988).
75. Kadir, R., Stemper, D., Liron, Z., and Cohen, S. Penetration of theophylline and adenosine into excised human skin from binary and tertiary vehicles: Effect of a nonionic surfactant. *J. Pharm. Sci. 78*:149–153 (1989).
76. Dominguez, J. G., Parra, J. L., Infante, M. R., Peljero, C. M., Balaguer, F., and Sastre, T. A new approach to the theory of adsorption and permeability of surfactants on keratinic proteins: The specific behaviour of certain hydrophobic chains. *J. Soc. Cosmet. Chem. 28*:165–182 (1977).
77. Breuer, M. M. The interactions between surfactants and keratinous tissues. *J. Soc. Cosmet. Chem. 30*:41–64 (1979).

6

Interaction Between Anionic Surfactants and Skin

J. Gordon Black

Unilever Research, Sharnbrook, Bedford, United Kingdom

I. INTRODUCTION

The skin is the largest organ of the body, and one of its main functions is to provide humans with an almost completely impermeable barrier to the external environment. The external surface of the skin, the stratum corneum, or horny layer, normally is soft, smooth, and flexible, but this condition can be radically altered in certain disease states and also, to an extent, by the vagaries of the weather and by contact with chemicals. The stratum corneum is constantly being renewed as cells divide in the basal layer of the epidermis and move upward, differentiating into the stratum corneum which, on morphological grounds, is termed "dead," but still retains certain biochemical activities.

Historically, soap has been around for centuries, but after World War II, other synthetic detergents (e.g., alcohol sulfate) were introduced when soaps (or its raw materials) were in short supply. Since that time many other synthetic detergents have been introduced for specialist applications or in the search for better mildness in products deliberately applied to the skin.

Contact of the skin with detergents can, under appropriate conditions, result in a superficial dryness, roughness, and scaling, often exaggerated by ambient condition of low relative humidity or temperature. In addition, erythema and swelling can occur as an indication of the involvement of the viable layers of the skin.

This chapter will describe some of the skin's response to contact with the anionic detergents, particularly some of the changes taking place in the stratum

145

corneum, penetration of the detergent molecules themselves through the corneum (and skin) into the body, and the ability of other molecules to penetrate the skin to a greater extent in the presence of or after pretreatment of the skin with anionic detergents. Kastner (1) has reported on local tolerance of animal skin to anionic surfactants, and Philp (2) has reviewed the dermatological response of human skin.

II. SOME SURFACTANT INTERACTIONS

A. Protein Denaturation

A study of Emery and Edwards (3) had shown that solutions of soaps (sodium salts of saturated fatty acids) of different chain lengths caused skin irritation, those soaps with 12 and 14 carbon residues being the most irritant, whereas the shorter (C_8) and longer (C_{18}) chains had less of an effect. The authors repeated these studies with detergents (sodium alkyl sulfates) using the same carbon chain range (C_8–C_{18}) and included tests with these detergents after the addition of some inorganic salts usually found in soap powders (4). They were able to show that a type of response was obtained with the alkyl sulfates similar to that with the salts of the saturated fatty acids, although the maximum irritability was less with the corresponding detergent compound. The addition of sodium sulfate or sodium chloride (both neutral salts) enhanced the irritant action of all the substituted fatty acids, and this was most marked by the inclusion of sodium carbonate (an alkaline salt), which they attributed to an increase in alkalinity, in addition to the common ion effect.

The work of Emery and Edwards (4) and McMeekin (5), who showed that the alkyl sulfates with more than eight-carbon (C_8) residues were excellent protein precipitants, suggested that protein denaturation might be involved in the skin's response to detergents. Van Scott and Lyon (6) performed experiments in which dried and dry defatted plantar keratin was incubated with 1% solutions of several soap powders and synthetic detergent products. Their parameter of denaturation was an increase in the number of titratable sulfydryl (-SH) groups (7), and they concluded that protein denaturation was an important mechanism in the production of dermatitis. This alteration of the keratin molecule was believed to be caused by the rupture of certain interpolypeptide linkages, *not* the disulfide bridges (8), so that internal -SH groups became more accessible to the chemical reagents used in their detection.

Blohm (9), showed how the results of Emery and Edwards (4) are closely paralleled by the denaturing (-SH group exposing) action of sodium dodecyl sulfate (SDS) on a purified protein (ovalbumin) system. This, he claimed, demonstrated a relation between the skin-irritating and protein-denaturing effects of sodium dodecyl sulfate.

Blohm also showed (9) that the binding of the dye indigo tetrasulfonate to human skin was prevented after pretreatment of the skin with sodium lauryl sulfate, because of competition for the binding sites on the stratum corneum. Choman (10) using dermal collagen prepared from calf skin, treated with a homologous series of sodium soaps (C_8–C_{18}) at or below the critical micelle concentrations (CMCs), observed partial or complete inhibition of uptake of the dye indigo carmine for the C_{10}, C_{12}, and C_{14} soaps at concentrations above the critical micelle concentration, and no inhibition with the C_8, C_{16}, and C_{18} members of the series. Imokawa and Mishima (11) also used the acidic dye indigo carmine on human forearm skin pretreated with the anionic surfactants sodium lauryl sulfate, alkylbenzene sulfonate, alpha-olefin sulfonate, and dodecyl-polyoxyethylene sulfate. The horny layer was stripped off using cyanoacrylate resin, the adherent indigo carmine extracted, and the dye intensity measured spectrophotometrically. The data showed that lauryl sulfate and alkylbenzene sulfonate were adsorbed to a greater extent than the olefin sulfonate and ethoxysulfate.

In a series of publications, Imokawa et al. reported an apparent correlation between adsorption of surfactants on to isolated callus and the roughening effect of skin, for which they showed (12) that the anionic surfactants alkyl sulfates, alpha-olefin sulfonates, alkylbenzene sulfonates, paraffin sulfonates, alkylether sulfonates, and soaps with an alkyl chain length of the C_{12} caused a greater effect than shorter or longer chain lengths. They further showed (13), that the denaturing ability of these compounds as measured by changes in the optical rotation of bovine serum albumin also gave a good correlation with the intensity of skin roughness caused by these detergents.

However, investigations into the skin compatibility of monoalkyl phosphates by Imokawa and Tsutsumi (14) showed that they caused only minimal skin roughening. The ability of these alkyl phosphates to denature protein, as measured by the release of sulfhydryl groups from bovine skin powder, is anomalous with their mildness to skin, and the role of protein denaturation as a mechanism in skin irritation is thus questioned.

Miyazawa et al. (15) used ovalbumin and human serum albumin to investigate the protein-denaturing ability of commercially available surfactants, as measured by the reduction in peak height of the elution curves of the proteins from aqueous gel-permeation chromatography. Of the anionic surfactants studied, sodium lauryl sulfate and alkylbenzene sulfonate were equally potent, and both were more so than lauryl ether sulfate. Moreover, the reduction in peak height correlated with the irritancy of the surfactant. For sodium lauryl sulfate, the percentage denaturation increased rapidly with increasing sodium lauryl sulfate concentration and became 100% at concentrations of sodium lauryl sulfate greater than 1 mM, the critical micelle concentration of sodium lauryl sulfate in the buffer solution. Thus the monomer concentration of sodium lauryl sulfate is a critical feature in protein denaturation. The authors further showed that the effect of sodium lauryl sulfate could be reduced to varying degrees by the addition of various amphoteric surfactants, possibly owing to a reduction of the total monomer concentration by the formation of hydrophobic complexes.

B. Enzyme Inactivation

Wilmsmann (16) was the first to use the inherent enzymic ability of some proteins to assess the physiological compatibility of anionic surfactants. The inhibition of saccharase (invertase) by different surfactants corresponded to the same ranking of the irritation values in skin patch tests and rabbit eye tests. Such was the correlation that Wilmsmann recommended that only a few preparations must be tested on animals or humans.

Rutherford and Pawlowski (17) combined the techniques of superficial biopsies from the upper arm of human volunteers treated for 3 hr with two different concentrations of dodecylbenzene sulfonate, known to differ in their irritancy to skin, with the histochemical staining for acid phosphatase, a marker enzyme present in the stratum corneum. Although macroscopically there was no visual inflammatory reaction, the more concentrated test solution caused a consistent loss of staining for acid phosphatase, which the authors interpreted as being caused by the loss of the enzyme from the corneum cells as a result of membrane damage by the anionic surfactant.

Prottey et al. (18) quantified the effects of surfactants on the acid phosphatase activity in the corneum obtained by tape stripping, as measured fluorimetrically. Panelists dipped one hand into distilled water and the other into a 0.2% solution of a mixture of alkylbenzene sulfonate and lauryl ether sulfate at 41°C for 10 min. Measurements of acid phosphatase were made before and at 30 min after dipping. The surfactant solution produced consistently greater reduction of acid phosphatase activity than did water, presumably by the denaturation of the enzyme protein by the detergent. With use of a wider range of anionics, at 0.10% for 10 min at 41°C, these investigators (18) showed a good inverse relation of reduction in acid phosphatase with the assessed hand dryness score.

The effect of anionic surfactants on a variety of other enzymes has been reviewed by Schwuger and Bartnik (19).

C. Binding

Faucher and Goddard (20) used lauryl [^{35}S]sulfate to determine its adsorption to the stratum corneum of neonatal rats, which had well-developed barrier properties relative to loss of water vapor. Appreciable quantities were adsorbed after a short lag time of 15–30 min, which was linearly dependent on the square root of time, thereby indicating a diffusion process. A diffusion mechanism of adsorption implies that it is the monomer of sodium lauryl sulfate and not the micelle that binds to the substrate. Adsorption was increased markedly in the presence of NaCl, which lowers the critical micelle concentration of sodium lauryl sulfate. Therefore, the salt must act on the substrate to promote the uptake of sodium lauryl sulfate. Binding was considerably reduced by the addition of a nonionic surfactant owing to formation of mixed micelles and not to competition for binding sites. As a consequence, the critical micelle concentration of sodium lauryl sulfate was lowered, reducing the monomer concentration of sodium lauryl sulfate and, thereby, lowering the binding of this agent to the corneum.

The binding of a homologous series of alkyl sulfates at 0.075 M to human callus was repeated by Dominguez et al. (21), who showed that maximum adsorption occurred at C_{12}, with slightly less binding by C_{14} and C_{16} alkyl sulfates and considerably less binding by the C_{10} homologue. To explain the special behavior of the C_{12} chain length, it was proposed (21) that the hydrophobic chain could adapt its structure to a coiled shape when the concentration of the surfactant was below the critical micelle concentration, either in the solid support or in the aqueous phase. Cooper and Berner pointed out that the absence of maxima in other solution properties make this explanation questionable (22).

Conrads and Zahn, investigating the interaction of sodium lauryl sulfate with human heel callus, showed that maximum binding occurred at low pH (23). At concentrations of sodium lauryl sulfate below the critical micelle concentration, about 80% of surfactant was bound at pH 2, decreasing as the pH was raised to pH 10. At higher concentrations, above the critical micelle concentration, the shape of the adsorption curve was similar, indicating the same type of binding mechanism. The greater solubilization of protein was claimed to be due to the denaturing–solubilization properties of sodium lauryl sulfate and was accompanied by loss of amino acids and protein. The mean value of the amino acids extracted by sodium lauryl sulfate was significantly greater than that of the blank controls. With more specific techniques of protein analyses, such as gel electrophoresis and immunoblotting, the authors demonstrated the extraction of a range of proteins, depending on the experimental conditions.

D. Swelling

It has been reported by several workers that anionic surfactants cause the stratum corneum to swell, after the observations of Goette (24) that the sodium salts of fatty acids and of alkyl sulfates of chain lengths C_8–C_{16} caused isolated epidermis to swell, and that such a response could be correlated with skin irritation. For example, Putterman et al. (25) tested several anionic surfactants at concentrations above their critical micelle concentration for their ability to produce swelling by measuring the surface area of squares of isolated guinea pig stratum corneum. The greatest swelling was found with sodium laurate and sodium lauryl sulfate. Replacing the sodium cation with ammonium and tri-ethanolammonium cation did not significantly affect the swelling. Both sodium dodecylbenzene sulfonate and sodium oleate gave an increase in swelling comparable with the alcohol sulfates. Protein denaturants, such as 8 M urea and 5 M guanidine hydrochloride, and lipid solvents were without effect, and the authors concluded that, because of the reversibility of laurate-induced swelling and the loss of most of the birefringence in corneum treated with laurate, swelling was due to a reversible conformation change as a result of cooperative binding of the detergent.

Earlier Scheuplein and Ross reported (26) a visible expansion of a disk of isolated stratum corneum by as much as 50–80% of the area and proposed that the laurate anion caused the uncoiling and extension of α-keratin filaments, producing β-keratin and an expanded membrane. The birefringence of the corneum was greatly diminished by the treatment with sodium laurate at 5% for 24 hr, but was restored after soaking in water, when the original dimensions of the disk were restored. A reversible α-to-β conversion of the protein was proposed as being consistent with these experimental observations.

Robbins and Fernee observed an increase of about 30% in the crosswise length of the epidermal membrane preparation after 24 hr in 0.068 M sodium lauryl sulfate (27). They showed that for the even-numbered homologous series of alkyl sulfate C_8–C_{16}, the classic optimum swelling for the C_{12} chain length, and, as all the chain lengths were at constant molarity and with the same counterion, the importance of hydrophobic interaction to swelling was demonstrated. They also found that least swelling of the membrane occurred with sodium lauryl sulfate at acidic pH, so that ionic binding, which they claimed was maximal at acidic pHs and would present more hydrophobic tails that would associate and repel water, did not increase the water uptake of the membrane as much as did the hydrophobic binding at neutral pH.

Rhein et al. examined the relation between swelling of the stratum corneum and the structure of various surfactants (28). They found that the swelling response was concentration-dependent and appeared to level off at approximately 8 mM sodium lauryl sulfate, the critical micelle concentration, which implies that swelling is primarily due to the monomer of sodium lauryl sulfate. Swelling also increased with extended exposure times, which the authors interpreted as a disruption of the secondary and tertiary structure of proteins. However, above a given concentration, about 80 mM, swelling increased for the anionics sodium lauryl sulfate, alkylbenzene sulfonate, and alkyltriethoxy sulfate. Increasing the degree of ethoxylation at constant alkyl chain length gave significantly less swelling, which might have been due to reduced penetration of the larger surfactant molecule into the protein, or to a reduced critical micelle concentration, hence, lower monomer concentration, which would result in less binding to protein. For the homologous series of alkylbenzene sulfonates, alpha-olefin sulfonates, and paraffin sulfonates, maximal swelling always occurred with the C_{12} and C_{14} isomers. A higher hydrophobic bond energy, modulated by a less effective penetration of the longer-chained homologues, and a lower hydrophobic bond energy for the shorter-chained homologues, together with a higher monomer concentration, probably explains the maximum swelling for C_{12} and C_{14} chain lengths.

The swelling of a collagen film, as measured by the uptake of tritiated water (29) was used to predict the irritancy of a homologous series of two anionic surfactants. The swelling response was concentration-dependent for linear alkyl-benzene sulfonate (LAS) and sodium lauryl sulfate, but there was no change in swelling with concentration for ammonium triethoxysulfate after incubation with the test surfactant in 0.1 mM phosphate buffer, pH 7.0, at 50°C for 24 hr. Collagen swelling was also determined for the homologous series of alkyl sulfates with chain lengths C_8–C_{16} and for concentration of 2–30 mM. At 10 mM and above, maximum swelling of the collagen film occurred at C_{12}. At 8 mM and below maximum swelling occurred at C_{14} or C_{16}.

The effect of increasing the degree of ethoxylation of the parent homologue ammonium lauryl sulfate was to decrease the swelling of the collagen film inversely with the ethylene oxide content. The swelling caused by sodium lauryl sulfate increased as the pH was raised from 5 to 7 to 9 in agreement with Choman (30) and Robbins and Fernee (27).

Blake-Haskins et al. (29) concluded that the swelling of collagen began with the adsorption of the anionic surfactants, primarily by hydrophobic interactions of the alkyl chain with the hydrophobic regions of the protein, at near neutral pH and, to a lesser extent, ionically between the head group of the surfactant and charged sites on the protein.

Tavss et al. (31) showed a rise in pH when anionic detergents were mixed with bovine serum albumin solutions of the same pH. They found that the anionics that caused the greatest rise in pH also caused the greatest degree of skin irritation. The reason for the increase in pH is probably due to the complex formation between the positively charged groups on the protein by the negatively charged groups of the detergent. The remaining "basic" groups absorb protons from the solvent, thereby increasing the hydroxide ion concentration.

III. SURFACTANTS AND THE INTEGRITY OF
THE SKIN BARRIER

As the stratum corneum is the barrier to the penetration of chemicals into the skin, damage to this structure, whether by solvents, surfactants, abrasion, or irradiation, for example, can be expected to reduce the protection offered by the skin. As well as permitting easier access into the body, damage to the corneum also manifests itself in an increase in the loss of water out of the body, the so-called transepidermal water loss (TEWL), as measured by electrolytic hygrometry (32) or by vapor pressure gradient (33). These techniques have been used to assess changes in the barrier properties of skin found when stripping off the stratum corneum (34), or in patients with dermatitis (35), or after application of detergents. For example, Van der Valk et al. (36) applied 2% sodium lauryl sulfate and sodium laurate, in a chamber, to the volar forearm of 27 healthy volunteers for 24 hr and after 1 hr graded the skin's response and measured the water loss using a Servo Med Evaporimeter (33) in a temperature- and relative humidity-controlled room. Sodium lauryl sulfate caused a marked increase in water loss, whereas sodium laurate had less effect, not much greater, in fact, than that of the various controls. The results of the visual-scoring system corresponded with the results of the measurement of skin water vapor loss. Hassing et al. (37) placed a 1% solution of proprietary toilet soap bars in plastic cups on the forearm skin of nine volunteers for 24 hr and, after a further 24 hr, measured skin water vapor loss. Their results suggested that the effect of the pH of the soap solution on the skin's surface was less important that previously reported.

Murahata et al. (38) used a modified chamber irritation test, with an 8% solution of an all-purpose bar soap, of a complexion bar, and of 11 other unspecified products on the forearm of 74 subjects daily for 5 days. The TEWL was measured directly with a Servo Med Evaporimeter in a controlled atmosphere. They demonstrated a correlation between the clinical evaluation of irritation and TEWL readings, taken on day 1 and day 5, and suggested that the TEWL technique may be a more sensitive indicator of skin damage than visual assessment.

Dugard and Scheuplein investigated the mechanism whereby solutions of ionic surfactants increased the permeability of skin (39). They measured the changes in electrical conductance of isolated epidermal membranes from human skin after contact with solutions of soaps and alkyl sulfates from C_8 to C_{16} in chain length and all at concentrations less than the critical micelle concentration. They found that the C_8 compounds showed no effect, the C_{10} a slow, but distinct, increase in conductance, with maximal effects at C_{12} and C_{14}, and less at C_{16}. These changes were reversible, by as much as 90%, and the two series of anionic detergents were similar in effect. The authors concluded that the reversibility of the permeability changes ruled out extraction of lipids and other molecules as the sole explanation of the action, and they favored an interaction of the surfactants with the protein of the stratum corneum.

Increases in electrical properties of the forearm skin of human volunteers exposed to 30% aqueous sodium lauryl sulfate at 45°C for 3 min daily, with rinsing and drying, were reported by Serban et al. (40). These changes in conductance and capacitance occurred well in advance of the visible signs of irritation, and the authors suggested that these parameters might be used as a sensitive indicator of the gradual loss of barrier properties of the stratum corneum from treatment with various types of skin irritants.

Bahl (41) reported on the use of electron spectroscopy for chemical analysis (ESCA) of separated stratum corneum to estimate the relative amounts of lipid removal after treatment with certain solvents and the anionic surfactants sodium lauryl sulfate and sodium lauryl ether sulfate. They showed that lipid removal was greater after treatment with sodium lauryl sulfate than with the ether sulfate and proposed a correlation with skin permeability, skin swelling, and skin irritation.

IV. SURFACTANTS AND WATER BINDING

The interaction of anionic surfactants with the skin can result in a loss of corneum flexibility. Various authors—Blank (42), Singer and Vinson (43), Middleton (44)—investigating skin dryness, all showed that the amount of water bound by isolated intact stratum corneum was directly related to the relative humidity (RH) of the air. Blank and Shappirio (45), Singer and Vinson (43), and Middleton (46) further showed that exposure of human, rat, or guinea pig callus to soaps or anionic surfactants reduced the ability of the corneum to hold water. It was noted that these surfactant solutions extracted much more water-soluble substances than did water, and that the loss of these materials might be responsible for the increased brittleness of the treated corneum membranes. Earlier Blank (42) had shown how water, and not lipid, was important in preventing the dry skin condition.

Middleton (46) proposed that normally the cells of the stratum corneum contained water-soluble substances within a semipermeable membrane and that the action of surfactants was to extract lipid from the cell membrane, thereby allowing the water-soluble compounds to be washed out. Accordingly, the corneum was unable to retain water under conditions of high relative humidity.

V. SURFACTANT AND EXTRACTION OF LIPID
COMPOUNDS

Middleton (46) presented data to show that sodium lauryl sulfate extracted a phospholipidlike substance from guinea pig footpad, which by definition, contained no sebaceous glands and, hence, avoided the complication of contaminating sebaceous lipids. Under the same conditions, sodium isethionate extracted no measurable quantities of this substance. After pretreatment of the corneum with these anionic surfactants, water extracted more water-soluble substances, as measured by their absorbance at 275 nm, from the sodium lauryl sulfate- than from the isethionate-treated corneum. Thus, the relatively harsh detergent sodium lauryl sulfate had a significant effect on the water-binding properties of isolated stratum corneum and extracted significantly more water-soluble compounds than the relatively mild detergent sodium isethionate which, in turn, had no significant effect on water binding.

Singer and Vinson (43) also showed that surfactants reduced the water-binding capacity of corneum membranes. They showed that bar soap containing sodium isethionate had less of an effect than various other soaps and claimed that the ranking of effect on water binding corresponded with the mildness of the soaps, as measured by in vivo tests, although no data were given.

The earlier investigations into the mechanism of water binding by the stratum corneum have emphasized the importance of lipids which, after extraction with solvents or detergents, have allowed easier removal of water-soluble compounds and subsequent lowering of the water-holding capacity.

The discovery of the ceramides and the absence of phospholipids (47) in the lipids of the stratum corneum and the review by Elias (48) of lamellar lipids in the intercellular spaces have stimulated investigations into the structure–function of such lipids and their possible role in controlling percutaneous absorption. Elias illustrated how the effects of solvents and surfactants might disrupt the stratum corneum and allow substances to percolate between cells (48). Previously, the intercellular spaces were thought to be of insufficient volume to explain the rapid flux of certain compounds (49). However, Elias and Leventhal (50) had reported on how the intercellular volume fraction increased from 1 to 5–30% following secretion of lamellar bodies, making the suggestion that such an increase could allow a more significant penetration by the intercellular route than previously expected (48). Pretreatment of isolated stratum corneum with lipid solvents or sodium lauryl sulfate permitted the markers ferritin or horseradish peroxidase to penetrate into the depths of the corneum only by the intercellular route and not by traversing the cells (51). Barry (52) reported that sodium lauryl sulfate disrupted the entire corneum membranes, affecting both protein and lipid components. The swelling of the corneum by water uptake allows easier chemical permeation. The increase in the volume of the intercellular spaces facilitates entry of the sodium lauryl sulfate molecules into the intercellular laminar lipids, causing further disruption of the molecular structure of the horny layer.

In a series of papers Imokawa and collaborators have reemphasized the importance of lipids in maintaining the state of hydration of the corneum in relation to chapping and scaling (53) and how the reduced water-holding properties of the corneum could be improved by topical application of isolated intercellular lipids, particularly the sphingolipid fractions (54).

Treatment of healthy forearm skin of volunteers with 5% sodium lauryl sulfate for up to 30 min caused drying and scaling of the stratum corneum without erythema. There was a decrease in hydration, and electron microscopy of biopsies taken at 24 hr after detergent treatment showed a selective depletion of the intercellular lipids, with disruption of the lamellar structures. Skin lipids were collected by extraction for a limited time with acetone/ether, fractionated by thin-layer chromatography (TLC), and the bands corresponding to squalene, wax ester, triglyceride, and free fatty acids collected and combined to obtain a sebaceous-rich lipid fraction.

An additional extraction of the same area of skin gave a fraction containing cholesterol ester, free fatty acid, cholesterol, ceramide, and glycolipid. This latter group, as a 10% emulsion in a water-in-oil cream, increased conductance and decreased skin scaling after two daily topical applications to the detergent-treated skin, whereas application of the former group of lipids had no effect.

A chromatographic separation into cholesterol ester, free fatty acid, cholesterol, and sphingolipid, and their application to detergent-treated skin as a 1% water-in-oil cream, showed that only the cholesterol ester or sphingolipid fractions caused an increase in conductance, although both these lipid fractions and the free fatty acid fraction had a tendency to reduce skin scaling. From these data, the authors claim that the sphingolipids, possibly in combination with other neutral lipids, are important in establishing or maintaining the water-holding capacity of the corneum.

Fulmer and Kramer also reported (55) on the changes in the lipid composition of the stratum corneum after sodium dodecyl sulfate was used to induce a dry skin condition in human subjects, who were treated daily for 4 weeks with 4% sodium dodecyl sulfate on the lower leg. An independent dermatologist assessed the increase of surface roughness and scaliness, which was accompanied by a decrease in the corneum hydration, as measured by electrical impedance. From shave biopsies, lipid analyses revealed significant changes in specific lipid classes, although the total quantity of lipids per unit weight of stratum corneum protein was unaltered. The free cholesterol increased at the expense of the cholesterol ester, as well as the destruction of certain ceramides, and a reduction in the amounts of longer-chained free fatty acids (C_{22}–C_{28}). The authors interpreted their findings as a consequence of sodium dodecyl sulfate perturbing the formation of the stratum corneum, rather than a gross extraction of lipids by the anionic surfactant.

VI. SURFACTANT PENETRATION, IN VITRO

Many factors combined to encourage investigators to use isolated tissue for studies of skin absorption. Chemical methods with good sensitivity for the analysis of detergents were lacking, and the supply of pure detergents was limited. The increasing availability of radioactively labeled detergents and a supply of human skin from autopsies made this combination a popular one for studies of the penetration of detergents into skin.

With isolated human abdominal skin, Blank and Gould (56) compared the penetration of sodium 1-[^{14}C]dodecanoate with that of sodium 1-[^{14}C]dodecyl sulfate. The concentration of the test solutions was 0.005 M, which is below the critical micelle concentration of each, and the exposure time was 18–24 hr at room temperature (20°–23°C). Tape strippings were taken and their radioactive content was measured. Chemical analysis of surfactants was also used, but was limited by a low sensitivity of the method and by the strong binding of the anionic agent to protein. The route of absorption into the excised skin was also examined by autoradiography.

The counting of radioactivity in tape strippings showed that most of the anionic surfactants in the skin were recovered in the first two strippings of the corneum. The data for sodium dodecanoate showed appreciable radioactivity in the epidermis and dermis, whereas with sodium dodecyl sulfate, little or none was recovered from the dermis.

Autoradiography of skin, from which the stratum corneum had been removed by tape stripping, after exposure to sodium 1-[^{14}C]dodecanoate and to sodium 1-[^{14}C]dodecyl sulfate supported the ability of sodium dodecanoate and sodium dodecyl sulfate to penetrate into the epidermis and dermis. Fogging of the emulsion occurred in the epidermis and dermis of the skin exposed to sodium 1-[^{14}C]dodecanoate, less so in the sebaceous glands, and to a still smaller extent in the sweat glands. Blood vessels also showed fogging of the emulsion. The authors cautiously pointed out that the presence of shadows in the emulsion associated with the glands of the skin did not necessarily indicate a route of entry of the sodium 1-[^{14}C]dodecanoate by the respective ducts, but might indicate only an accumulation of the soap, as the autoradiograms were prepared after a single prolonged exposure of the skin to the soap. In contrast, autoradiograms prepared from skin treated with sodium 1-[^{14}C]dodecyl sulfate showed very little fogging of the emulsion over the epidermis or dermis, and none associated with the sebaceous and sweat glands or hair follicles.

Aqueous solutions of sodium dodecanoate and sodium dodecyl sulfate have different pH values; to control this variable, Blank and Gould investigated the penetration into skin of these radioactively labeled anionic detergents from buffered solutions (56). The pH values of the buffered solutions varied within the range 9.3–12.7 and the duration of contact with skin was 18 or 21 hr, respectively. With both solutions, the epidermis appeared damaged when the pH was 11 or higher, making it impossible to use the stripping method. Quite small amounts of each surfactant were present in the dermis of skins exposed to solutions buffered to pH 11 or below, but above this pH much greater amounts of both were found in the dermis. Differences in the ability of sodium dodecanoate to penetrate more easily than sodium dodecyl sulfate, as found with unbuffered solutions, were not consistent, nor was the penetration of sodium dodecanoate consistent from unbuffered and buffered solutions.

In a later paper, Blank and Gould (57) investigated the amount of penetration into excised human skin of sodium dodecanoate from dilute, buffered solutions of pH 7.5–12 and compared these data with the degree of erythema that developed in human skin in situ. They showed first that the pH of unbuffered 0.005 M sodium dodecanoate decreased by 1.5 pH units during the 5 hr contact with isolated skin, but buffered sodium dodecanoate decreased by less than 0.2 pH units during the 20 to 24 hr contact with excised skin. Moreover, they found that penetration into the dermis was minimal between pH 8.5 and 10.5, but increased below pH 8.5 and above pH 10.5. When excised skin was pretreated overnight with a dilute solution of sodium phosphate (pH 12.1), then exposed to a buffered solution of sodium dodecanoate (pH 10.0) that had previously showed virtually no penetration into excised skin, readily measured amounts of sodium dodecanoate, based on radio-activity measurement, were found in the dermis. Furthermore, pretreatment with buffer of pH 7.5, without sodium dodecanoate, followed by exposure to sodium dodecanoate buffered at pH 9.5, gave minimal values of sodium dodecanoate in the dermis. The authors concluded that the high alkalinity damaged the skin barrier to penetration.

The reason for the high penetration of sodium dodecanoate into excised skin from solutions buffered in the range pH 7.5–8.5 was explained by a study of the relation between penetration and the diethyl ether–water penetration coefficients. The partition coefficient was high at pH 8.1 and decreased linearly to a low value at pH 9.0 and above. Thus, the observed high penetration in the pH range of 7.5–8.5 was believed to be due to an increased lipid solubility.

Application of 0.005 M buffered solutions of sodium dodecanoate to human skin in situ showed that, during 6 hr contact, erythema and pruritus developed with solutions of pH 7.5, in agreement with the high penetration observed in vitro, but no erythema or pruritus was recorded when the pH of the applied solution was 9.5, at which pH virtually no penetration had been found in vitro.

In a further study, Blank and Gould (58) compared the absorption into the dermis of isolated human abdominal skin of a homologous series of pure alkyl sulfates, ranging from octyl to octadecyl sulfate, and of a series of pure alkylben-zene sulfonates. Two radioactive sulfur-containing detergents, sodium dodecyl sulfate and alkylbenzene sulfate, of underfined mixed homologues, were also examined. The concentration of the nonradioactive surfactants was measured spectrophotometrically after extraction from the separated dermis. Following extended contact (18–20 hr) of the isolated skin with 0.005 M aqueous solutions [or 60% (v/v) aqueous acetone solutions to solubilize the hexadecyl and octadecyl sulfates], less than 15 nmol·cm^{-2}—the sensitivity limit of the method—of the various surfactants, had penetrated into the dermis (i.e., a penetrations of less than approximately 5 µg·cm^{-2}). Various methods of decreasing the binding of surfactants failed to show that penetration then occurred. Removal of the upper layers of the stratum corneum did not increase the penetration of dodecyl sulfate into the dermis, but complete tape stripping of the corneum or exhaustive extraction of skin lipids with organic solvents did increase the penetration of dodecyl sulfate into the dermis. The authors concluded that the barrier to penetration seemed to be in the lower stratum corneum.

In a study of radioactively labeled potassium octadecanoate through isolated human abdominal skin, Bettley (59) found that for both 0.4 M (1.3% w/v) and 0.2 M (6.4% w/v) potassium ^{131}I-octadecanoate, penetration was 0.42–1.83% on day 4 and, thereafter, increased considerably over 24–26 days, indicating progressive damage by the pure soap to the epidermis.

Later, Bettley (60) used the potassium salts of octanoic, dodecanoic, and hexadecanoic acids labeled with ^{14}C. Human abdominal skin was obtained postmortem, and the epidermis separated by heating and mounted in a diffusion cell to which the soap solution at 0.04 M was added, while the dermal side of the skin was in contact with distilled water. The radioactivity of samples taken from each chamber daily for 7 days was determined. A total of 24.4% of the original quantity of potassium dodecanoate penetrated through the isolated human epidermis, whereas only 5.3% of potassium octanoate, and only 0.15% of potassium hexadecanoate penetrated. The irritancy of the potassium soaps was assessed after a 48 hr patch test on the upper back of 28 human volunteers, of whom 18 reacted to potassium dodecanoate, whereas only 2 responded to potassium hexadecanoate and 2 to potassium octanoate. Bettley concluded that the ability of potassium dodecanoate to penetrate skin most easily was compatible with its greater powers of irritancy.

With use of whole guinea pig skin mounted in a continuous-flow diffusion cell with a collecting chamber of small volume, to reduce dilution of the perfusate, Scala et al. (61) studied the percutaneous absorption of 0.03 M (or 1%) sodium tetrapropylenebenzene sulfonate at pH 7. Initially, penetration was low, until about 4 hr, when small amounts of radioactivity were just detectable in the perfusate. Over a 20 hr period, the diffusion curve was nonlinear, showing that the barrier properties of the skin were decreasing during contact with the detergent. When separated guinea pig dermis was placed in the diffusion cell, penetration was observed earlier and to much greater extent. Here, the diffusion was linear after 6 hr contact, showing that a steady state had been reached. It was not possible to use separated guinea pig epidermis in this system, but a comparison of the perfusion through whole skin with that through separated dermis showed that the epidermis provided the main barrier to absorption through skin. The authors concluded that, because of the time lag before radioactivity from sodium tetrapropylenebenzene [^{35}S]sulfonate appeared in the perfusate of isolated skin, little surfactant would be absorbed through skin under normal-use conditions. They also pointed out the importance of the duration of contact of the surfactant with skin and of the concentration of the penetrant in diffusion through skin.

Absorption of potassium dodecyl [^{35}S]sulfate from aqueous 0.0016 M solutions through excised human abdominal skin, mounted in diffusion cells, was studied by Emery and Dugard (62). No detergent appeared in the diffusate when whole skin or the isolated horny layer were used, but appreciable amounts were present when stripped skin was tested, again confirming that the barrier properties of skin reside in the stratum corneum. Interestingly, the absorption of the potassium dodecyl [^{35}S]sulfate in dimethyl sulfoxide was reduced, in contrast with the usual effect of promotion of absorption assigned to this aprotic solvent (63).

Fiker et al. (64) investigated the extent of retention and absorption by human and mouse skin in vitro of sodium dodecyl sulfate, using the methylene blue method of determination. Interestingly, they found that cellophane appeared to be a good model of human skin. At 1 g·L^{-1} sodium dodecyl sulfate, at a pH of 6, 9, or 12, the authors recorded a maximum absorption of 13 μ·cm^{-2} and a retention of 166 μg·cm^{-2} for human skin at pH 12. Most of the absorption occurred within the first 2 hr, and extending the duration of contact to 24 hr did not increase the absorption significantly. Human skin and depilated mouse skin were very similar in their behavior.

Howes (65) investigated the penetration through isolated rat skin and human epidermis of five homologous pure soaps and three pure synthetic detergents, all of which were radioactive. The dermal side of the skin was bathed with saline, which was stirred magnetically. At 24 hr, for rat skin, and at 48 hr for human epidermis, the epidermal surface was rinsed and the rinse water kept for measurements of radioactivity. An autopsy of the skin and human epidermis was taken for determination of radioactivity.

In rat skin, sodium octadecanoate did not penetrate during the 24 hr of the experiment, and sodium hexadecanoate was detectable only at 24 hr. The sodium decanoate, dodecanoate, and tetradecanoate all showed the same low penetration at 2 hr, a moderate penetration at 6 hr, and a larger penetration at 24 hr. None of the three pure synthetic detergents, sodium dodecyl sulfate, sodium dodecanoyl isethionate, and sodium dodecyl-1-benzene-*p*-sulfonate, gave measurable penetration during 24 hr. At the end of the experiment, rinsing of the rat skin removed 60–70% of the applied soaps and isethionate and 30–40% was retained by the skin. For dodecyl sulfate and dodecylbenzene sulfate, the rinse water contained only 30% of the applied radioactivity, and 70% was retained by the skin.

In human epidermis, a similar response to the soaps was recorded, except that the sodium dodecanoate gave greater penetration at 6 and 24 hr than in rat skin and sodium decanoate gave a greater penetration at 24 hr than in rat skin. With the synthetic detergents, no dodecylbenzene sulfonate penetrated during 48 hr, but both dodecyl sulfate and dodecanoyl isethionate showed progressively increased penetration over 48 hr, which indicated a loss of barrier properties. All samples of human epidermis showed a degree of swelling at 48 hr that was most notable with the dodecyl sulfate treatment. Retention of radioactivity of human epidermis was greatest with dodecyl sulfate treatment, after which approximately 75% was not removed by rinsing. Some 30–50% of dodecanoyl isethionate and dodecyl-benzene sulfonate was retained by human epidermis after rinsing.

Faucher and Goddard (66) used neonatal rat stratum corneum as a model membrane to study the penetration of sodium lauryl [^{35}S]sulfate through skin. The sodium lauryl sulfate was bound to the stratum corneum in large amounts, up to 50% by weight at high (10%) concentrations. Penetration occurred, even at low concentrations, after a lag period of some hours. The authors calculated a diffusion constant of about 10^{-10} cm^2·sec^{-1}, which they compared with the diffusion constant of sodium lauryl sulfate in water of 10^6 cm^2·sec^{-1}. At higher concentrations the flux through the corneum did not level off, despite these concentrations exceeding the critical micelle concentration. As the micelles are not believed to penetrate, and only the monomer is capable of penetrating, the authors suggested that the increased penetration might be due to alterations to the corneum by the surfactant, as previously proposed by Scala et al. (61) and Scheuplein and Ross (26).

Gibson and Teall (67), who used an in vitro penetration cell, reported on the treatment of rat skin slices with sodium laurate, sodium lauryl sulfate, or sodium lauroyl isethionate on the release of the enzymes, acid phosphates (AP), lactate dehydrogenase (LDH), and N-acetylglucosaminidase (NAG). They found that adsorption and penetration of the detergents were both concentration-dependent, with sodium laurate penetrating more than sodium lauryl sulfate. A time lag before enzyme release was measurable, reflecting the slow rate of penetration of C$_{12}$ surfactants and the time for the enzyme to diffuse out of the tissue. Generally, release of LDH was greater than that of AP or NAG from treatment with sodium laurate or sodium lauryl sulfate, whereas sodium lauroyl isethionate caused no release of any enzyme over a comparable concentration range.

VII. SURFACTANT PENETRATION, IN VIVO

Interest in measuring absorption through skin in vivo arose as it became obvious that, despite the attractions of an isolated skin system, in vitro measurements of absorption of substances such as anionic detergents, which bind strongly to skin, did have some shortcomings. A comparison of the penetration of sodium dodecyl [35S]sulfate into living and excised guinea pig skin was made by Choman (68). Clipped guinea pig skin was treated with sodium dodecyl [35S]sulfate for 60 min without rinsing, and the treated area was excised. Sections of the frozen skin were cut parallel to the surface of the skin from the dermal side to avoid the transfer of radioactivity from an area of high deposition to one of low deposition, which would occur in the traditional method of obtaining transverse sections of skin. Four hours after sacrifice, other areas of the dorsal skin were excised and considered to be nonliving. Two were placed in a static stainless steel diffusion chamber and sodium dodecyl [35S]sulfate placed on the epidermal surface. The distilled water in contact with the dermal side was monitored for radioactivity by evaporating samples on a glass plate, taken at various times, and exposing the residue to x-ray film. Other areas of the nonliving skin were treated with sodium dodecyl [35S]sulfate and, after 60 min, autoradiograms were prepared from skin sections.

The results showed that in vivo skin absorption occurred to a depth of some 800 μm, whereas, in the nonliving skin, absorption was recorded to only some 250 μm. The position of radioactivity on the autoradiograms of the living skin coincided with the position of the pilosebaceous appendages. No detectable radioactivity was recorded at any time up to 24 hr from the dermal perfusate in the diffusion cell. The author concluded that skin in vivo was more permeable to sodium dodecyl sulfate than skin in vitro, but, by the nature of this technique, he was unable to quantify his data.

The first direct study of percutaneous absorption of alkyl sulfates in vivo was reported by Sprott (69). Anesthetized rats were prewashed with a 1% (w/v) aqueous solution of sodium dodecyl sulfate or sodium hexadecyl sulfate, rinsed, and dried. Immediately, a solution of the appropriate sodium n-alkyl [35S]sulfate was applied to the pretreated skin for 10 min, after which the skin was rinsed and dried, but not protected with a patch, and the rats placed in individual metabolism cages. The excretion of radioactivity in the separated urine was measured daily for 9 days. The results showed that approximately 40% of the applied radioactivity was recovered from the rats treated with sodium dodecyl sulfate, whereas some 20% was recovered in the urine from the rats treated with sodium hexadecyl sulfate. In both cases, the rate of excretion was rapid, with approximately half of the total recovery being excreted in the first day. When the duration of contact of sodium hexadecyl sulfate was increased from 15 to 30 min, the excretion of radioactivity in the urine was doubled and, significantly, absorption could be demonstrated in the short time of 15 min by the presence of radioactivity in the blood. Other types of surfactants were able to be absorbed through skin. The α-sulfonated fatty acids and alkyl carboxylic acid esters of isethionic acid were stated to be absorbed through skin, although experimental data were not provided.

Penetration into rat skin of sodium hexadecyl sulfate was also reported following exposure of the skin for 10, 30, and 60 min to hexadecyl $[^{35}S]$sulfate. After application and without rinsing, the treated skin was excised and separated by heat into the epidermis and dermis. The frozen dermis was then cut into 25 μm sections in the plane parallel to the skin surface. Radioactivity of the separated epidermis and individual sections of the dermis was measured. The amount of hexadecyl sulfate in the epidermis was constant during 60 min. The dermis contained small, but significant, amounts of radioactivity (approximately 0.01% of the amount in the epidermis) which decreased with depth into the skin, although the total radioactivity in the 150 μm of dermis seemed to remain constant for the various exposure times.

Studies in rats of percutaneous absorption of a series of homologous soaps from saturated chain lengths C_{10}–C_{18} were reported by Howes (65). A model soap system (30 mM, approximately 1% w/v) in which the five pure Na soaps were soluble at 37° was used. Separate solutions were prepared containing, in turn, each of the 1-$[^{14}C]$soaps (6 mM), which was applied to a defined area of the dorsal skin of anesthetized rats. After 15 min contact, the skin was rinsed and dried and a protective, nonocclusive patch was fitted to the rats to prevent ingestion of the radioactive soap by grooming of the treated area. Other rats were fitted with restraining collar to allow prewashing with a non-radioactive model soap solution before applications of the various radioactive soap solutions. The extent of percutaneous absorption was calculated from the recovery of radioactivity in the expired breath, urine, feces, and carcass after excision of the treated area of skin, at 6 hr after application. For the sodium salts of the five n-1-$[^{14}C]$fatty acids, the order of absorption through rat skin was $C_{12} > C_{10} = C_{14} > C_{16} = C_{18}$ when there was no pretreatment of the skin. The absorption for C_{12} soap at 6 mM (0.13% w/v) was 0.675 μg·cm^{-2} during the 6 hr of the experiment, and the absorption for the C_{16} soap was approximately ten times less, emphasizing the importance of chain length in absorption. After three prewashes, the order of penetration was $C_{12} = C_{10} > C_{14} > C_{16} > C_{18}$, for which only the quantities of both C_{12} and C_{10} soaps had increased significantly to approximately 1.2 μg·cm^{-2}.

Howes (65) also investigated the percutaneous absorption of three synthetic detergents by the rat. In this instance, aqueous solutions of the relatively insoluble sodium 1-$[^{14}C]$dodecyl-1-benzene-p-sulfonate (3 mM), sodium 1-$[^{14}C]$dodecyl sulfate (24 mM), or sodium 1-$[^{14}C]$dodecanoyl isethionate (25 mM) were applied and the localization by autoradiography of the detergents in skin, as well as quantities absorbed through skin, were studied. There was heavy deposition of all the synthetic detergents in the surface of the skin and in the upper hair follicles, but only sodium dodecyl sulfate was seen to penetrate into the lower hair follicles and into the dermis.

The absorption through skin of dodecylbenzene sulfonate at 3 mM was below the sensitivity of detection (<0.1 $\mu g \cdot cm^{-2}/ \cdot 24\ hr^{-1}$) as was the absorption of the dodecanoyl isethionate from a 25 mM solution (0.3 $\mu g \cdot cm^{-2} \cdot 24\ hr^{-1}$), whereas at 25 mM (0.7%), the penetration of sodium dodecyl sulfate was 0.26 $\mu g \cdot cm^{-2} \cdot 24\ hr^{-1}$. When dodecanoyl isethionate of higher specific activity, thereby conferring much greater sensitivity to the detection of radioactivity, was used, a low penetration, 0.09 $\mu g \cdot cm^{-2}$ in 24 hr, was recorded by application of a 20 mM aqueous solution (approximately 0.3% w/v). Thus, for a constant chain length of C_{12}, various headgroups strongly influenced the ability of the surfactant to be absorbed through skin.

A comparative study of the absorption of pure ^{14}C-labeled detergents through guinea pig skin was reported by Prottey and Ferguson (70). Different headgroups were substituted on the hydrophobe, which remained constant at 12-carbon atoms. Aqueous solutions of 5 mM were applied to a defined area of clipped guinea pig skin for 10 min, then the skin was rinsed, dried, and protected with a nonocclusive patch for 24 hr. Absorption through skin was calculated from the amount of radioactivity excreted in the expired breath, urine, and feces, together with that remaining in the carcass after removal of the treated area of skin, and corrected for the disposition of a dose of each surfactant given intraperitoneally. The nature of the headgroup was found to be very important in determining the extent of percutaneous absorption. Of the anionics examined, sodium laurate was the best penetrant. Sodium dodecyl triethoxysulfate and sodium dodecanoyl isethionate were intermediary, whereas sodium dodecyl sulfate and sodium dodecyl sulfonate gave the least absorption.

Another comparative study on the absorption of pure ^{14}C-labeled alcohol sulfates, alcohol ether sulfates, and alcohol ethoxylates of varying chain length and degree of ethoxylation, through rat skin was reported by Black and Howes (71). The data showed that penetration was low for the alcohol sulfates and alcohol ether sulfates, but greater for the alcohol ethoxylates. For each anionic agent, penetration was proportional to the applied concentration and the number of applications, but increased more gradually with extended duration of contact.

By comparing the amount of radioactivity excreted together with that remaining in the main organs after application of alpha-[14C]olefin sulfonate to the intact skin of rats, without wiping off, or after removal at 0.5 hr or 1.5 hr after application, Minegishi et al. (72) concluded that percutaneous absorption was almost finished by 1.5 hr after application. When the stratum corneum was removed, penetration of a 0.02% solution of the anionic surfactant increased to nearly 50%, compared with 0.63% from treatment to intact skin of a 0.2% detergent solution.

VIII. SURFACTANT-INDUCED PENETRATION

Bettley and Donoghue (73) used heat-separated human epidermis from abdominal skin in a Perspex cell and measured daily for 20–30 days the decrease in weight from loss of water through the epidermis under recorded conditions of temperature and humidity. A 1% solution of a standard hospital toilet soap bar increased the water loss to a maximum of 25–39 mg·day^{-1} at 5–7 days, compared with the water control rate of 5–10 mg daily. At 5% soap, the rate of water loss increased steadily to about 70 mg·day^{-1} at day 14, and replacement of the soap solution by water caused a return to the control level in 3–4 days. A similar increase in the rate of water loss was recorded with 5% solution of potassium hexadecanoate. The commercial detergent Teepol (secondary alkyl sulfates) caused an increase in the rate of water loss of the order of 15 mg·day^{-1}, an effect that is intermediary between the water (control) and soap response.

In describing a new improved brass cell for measurement of water diffusion through whole rat skin, Isherwood (74) recorded the effect of 1, 2, and 3% (w/v) potassium hexadecanoate. The results showed a linear increase in the mean rate per day, during 4 days, of the water diffusion rate, from 0.13 mg·cm^{-2}·hr^{-1}, the control rate, to 0.20, 0.41, and 0.64 mg·cm^{-2}·hr^{-1} for 1, 2, and 3% solutions, respectively.

In a diffusion cell with a continuously circulating fixed volume of physiological saline in which the accumulation of radioactivity was recorded, Sprott (69) investigated the effect of chain length (C_8–C_{18}) of the sodium salts of fatty acids and sodium n-alkyl sulfates upon the permeability to tritiated water of isolated rat whole skin. In this study, the skin was exposed to solutions of the detergent and tritiated water. At 0.50 mM and pH 10.8, to ensure solubilization of C_{16} and C_{18} soaps, the C_8, C_{10}, C_{12}, and C_{14} soaps increased the penetration of tritiated water. Of the alkyl sulfates at 0.50 mM, C_{12}, C_{14}, and C_{16} increased the penetration of tritiated water, whereas the effects of C_8, C_{10}, and C_{18} were of doubtful significance. The C_{12} and C_{14} soaps and alkyl sulfates gave similar increases in the absolute penetration rate. It is interesting that the lower members of the soap series had a greater effect on the penetration rate than the intermediary ones, whereas the higher members were without effect. The more moderate effect on the penetration rate of tritiated water of the alkyl sulfates appeared to be greater at longer chain lengths. When the pH of the solutions of the alkyl sulfates was raised by buffers from 6.1 to 9.1 and 10.8, the effect on the permeability of tritiated water was reduced because of an increase in the control value caused by the more alkaline pH itself.

Scheuplein and Ross investigated the effect of soap and detergent on the permeability of tritiated water through isolated human abdominal epidermis (26). Sodium dodecanoate at 1% (w/v) caused a large increase in the permeability to tritiated water after an initial lag period of approximately 5 hr. The permeability curve increased exponentially, indicating that damage by the soap to the epidermis was continuous. When the concentration of sodium dodecanoate was increased to 5% (w/v), the permeability of the isolated epidermis to tritiated water rose more quickly after a reduced lag phase. These investigators also observed that the epidermis regained some of its barrier properties when the soap solutions were removed, but that use of the more concentrated solutions caused permanent damage. At 5% (w/v), Scheuplein and Ross (26) found that sodium dodecanoate had a greater and earlier effect on the permeability of isolated human epidermis to tritiated water than had sodium dodecyl sulfate. Raising of the pH of the sodium dodecyl sulfate to that of sodium dodecanoate (pH 10) had little effect on increasing the permeability of tritiated water by sodium dodecyl sulfate. These authors concluded from additional studies with sodium sulfate and acetic acid that the dodecanoate and dodecyl sulfate were the effective anions of soap and alkyl sulfate, respectively. Scheuplein and Ross believed that the mechanism of the effect of sodium dodecanoate on the stratum corneum was due to a reversible α- to β-conversion of keratin resulting from a denaturation by the soap, which facilitated the diffusion of water through the more porous membranes.

Sprott (69) used tritiated water to assess the effect of toilet soap bars on the permeability of rat skin. Groups of rats were clipped and washed for 5 min with 4% (w/v) solutions of the toilet soaps, one of which was a conventional bar containing the sodium salts of the fatty acids from saponified tallow and palm kernel oil. The other toilet bar contained a high proportion of sulfonated fatty acids and fatty acid esters of isethionic acid. After rinsing, one group of rats from each treatment had tritiated water applied to the skin. The rats were killed at 5 min after application of tritiated water, and samples of heart blood were withdrawn, weighed, and freeze-dried. The water from the cold traps of the lyophylizer was counted to determine its content of tritium. Both groups of rats washed with solutions of the toilet bars showed significantly increased tritium content in the blood, but the difference between the conventional soap bar and the toilet bar containing synthetic detergents was not statistically significant.

Other groups were rinsed after application of the tritiated water, placed in metabolism cages, and separate urine was collected for 72 hr. There was a tendency for the urine of the rats washed with solutions of the toilet bars to contain greater amounts of radioactivity than the control group, but only the effect of the conventional soap was statistically greater.

With use of the diffusion chamber, Bettley (75) investigated the effect of various surface-active agents, including soaps of different chain lengths, sodium dodecyl sulfate, alkyl benzene sulfonate, all at 0.04 M, on the penetration of sodium ions through isolated human epidermis after 1- and 2-weeks contact. Compared with sodium tetradecanoate and sodium hexadecanoate, both of which were similar to the control, sodium dodecanoate exerted a striking effect on the penetration of sodium ions. Sodium dodecyl sulfate and sodium dodecylbenzene sulfonate were approximately equal in their effect and only about half as potent as sodium dodecanoate. Neither pH nor surface tension appeared to be directly related to the increase in permeability.

Sodium lauroyl sarcosinate had no effect, sodium sulfosuccinate lauric mono-isopropanolamine polyglycol had a slight effect on the permeability to potassium ions, whereas sodium sulfosuccinate lauric monoethanolamine had marked effects. The effect of sodium sulfosuccinate lauryl polyglycol on potassium ions was approximately equal to that of sodium dodecyl sulfate and sodium dodecyl-benzene sulfonate on sodium ions, whereas sodium sulfosuccinate lauric mono-ethanolamide had a relatively greater effect on potassium ions than had sodium lauroyl sarcosinate and sodium dodecylbenzene sulfonate on sodium ions. The effects of these various anionic detergents would be only partly related to their ability to denature protein of isolated human epidermal stratum corneum (76).

There have been many reports on the way in which surface-active agents enhance the absorption of electrolytes, particularly those known to elicit a contact dermatitis or delayed hypersensitization, such as nickel and chromate salts. Nilzen and Wikstrom (77) showed that, although neither nickel sulfate nor sodium dodecyl sulfate alone would cause an eczematous response, the combination did produce a contact dermatitis. Similarly, Kvornung and Svendsen (78) reported that secondary alkyl sulfate (Teepol) facilitated the sensitization response to nickel chloride and potassium dichromate in susceptible patients. In human patch tests, these authors were able to show a skin response to the allergen in a more dilute solution when the challenge solution contained Teepol. Vinson and Choman (79) showed that sodium dodecyl sulfate and sodium dodecylbenzene sulfonate applied to the skin of guinea pigs in a two-stage multiple-application test produced an eczematous response to nickel sulfate, and they observed the deep penetration of nickel into the skin. The application of soap or the other test anionic detergents, Igepon A and Igepon T, did not elicit a nickel response under the conditions of the test.

Friberg et al. (80) investigated the effect of soap and alkylaryl sulfonate on the penetration of mercuric chloride and methyl mercury dicyandiamide, both radio-actively labeled, through guinea pig abdominal skin by disappearance measure-ments. Pretreatment of the skin by painting with a soft brush for 2 min twice daily with 1% aqueous solution of soap did not affect the absorption of either of the two mercury compounds. However, a 1% aqueous solution of the aklylaryl sulfonate did show a tendency to increase the absorption of the methyl mercury dicyan-diamide. Radioactive mercury was present in the kidneys, liver, and blood of the guinea pigs. When the mercuric chloride or methyl mercury dicyandiamide was dissolved in the soap or alkylaryl sulfonate solution and applied to the dorsal skin of the guinea pigs, Skog and Wahlberg (81) showed that, as Friberg et al. (80) had reported, only the alkylaryl sulfonate affected the absorption of the methyl mercury dicyandiamide. There was no difference between the absorption through guinea pig dorsal or abdominal skin. However, the disappearance technique is not sufficiently sensitive to quantify the degree of absorption.

In comparison of the absorption of sodium chloride and mercuric chloride in soap or alkylaryl sulfonate through normal or stripped guinea pig skin, Wahlberg reported (82) that absolute absorption was related to concentration of the applied salt solution and was greater through stripped skin. In similar disappearance measurements with sodium ^{51}C-chromate in solutions of 0.1, 1.0, and 10% sodium dodecyl sulfate, Wahlberg (83) showed that at 0.239 M sodium chromate in 10% sodium dodecyl sulfate, there was a significantly increased absorption, compared with the salt in distilled water.

The effect of surfactants upon the absorption of radioactively labeled sodium [^{131}I]iodide, chosen to represent a highly polar, water-soluble substance, and also because of the ease with which its rapid localization can be measured by the scanning in vitro of the thyroid, was reported by Sprott (69). Rats were washed with solutions of two toilet bars of different composition, followed by application of [^{131}I]iodide. Autoradiography of sections of the thyroid from rats killed 15 min after application of radioactive marker showed that the silver grain density in the rat washed with the toilet bar containing the sodium salts of the fatty acid esters of isethionic acid and sodium dodecylbenzene sulfonate. In a second identically washed group of rats, the thyroid [^{131}I]iodine radioactivity rose rapidly to a level that was greater in animals washed with the nonsoap toilet bar, compared with animals washed with the soap bar. Water-washed rats showed a level of accumulation of ^{131}I in the thyroid. Although it was clear that both toilet bars increased the permeability of skin in this single experiment, the statistical significance of differences between soaps and synthetic detergents was unresolved.

Bettley (75) used sodium salicylate as a marker for soap damage to human epidermis. The penetration of sodium salicylate through isolated abdominal epidermis was measured chemically before and after addition of 0.034 M (1% w/v) potassium hexadecanoate. During the first week, the average penetration of sodium salicylate in the control cell was 82.5 µg or approximately 21 µg cm^{-2}·day^{-1} and at the end of the second week penetration was essentially the same. However, in the presence of the soap, penetration of sodium salicylate increased from the control level of 82.5 to 675 µg at the end of the first week, to 1200 µg after 2 weeks, and to 1430 µg after 3 weeks. Thus, the action of the soap was to increase progressively the penetration of the salicylate.

Bettley (75) showed that the permeability of the epidermis from human abdominal skin to glucose (200 mg% w/v) was rarely above the sensitivity of the method. In the presence of 1% (w/v) potassium hexadecanoate, the permeability of the epidermis to glucose increased during the test period of 3 weeks, although inspection of the data suggest that there is no statistical significance in penetration in the presence of soap at 1, 2, or 3 weeks, as Bettley (75) found with sodium salicylate.

Sprott (84) investigated the effects of four pure *n*-alkyl sulfates on the penetration of [^{35}S]thiourea and [^{14}C]urea through isolated whole rat skin. Only dodecyl sulfate gave an increase in the recorded absolute penetration rate of [^{35}S]thiourea.

Scala et al. (61) investigated the effect of sodium tetrapropylenebenzene sulfonate or soap on the absorption of [^{14}C]nicotinic acid and [^{14}C]thiourea through isolated guinea pig whole skin. In the absence of the detergent, the absorption of [^{14}C]nicotinic acid had a lag time of 5–6 hr, after which time absorption was low, but linear. Preexposure of the skin to 0.5% tetrapropylenebenzene sulfonate for 1 hr did not significantly increase the penetration of nicotinic acid, but preexposure for 3 hr did. In both instances of preexposure, the subsequent penetration of nicotinic acid was linear with time. However, when the nicotinic acid was placed in the solution of tetrapropylenebenzene sulfonate or soap, the penetration became nonlinear, with a quantitative change in rate similar to that observed for the penetration of tetrapropylenenbenzene sulfonate and soap themselves. Like nicotinic acid, thiourea showed a linear, but low, rate of penetration that became nonlinear in the presence of tetrapropylenebenzene sulfonate.

The effect of sodium dodecyl sulfate on the absorption of chloramphenicol through isolated hairless mouse skin was reported by Aguiar and Weiner (85). They showed that absorption through the skin of hairless mice was time-dependent and that there was no lag time in absorption, which the authors attributed to the thinness of the stratum corneum. Absorption was proportional to temperature, from which the authors calculated an apparent activation energy of 15,900 cal·mol^{-1}. Addition of 0.2% sodium dodecyl sulfate caused the permeability of the skin to chloramphenicol to double, whereas addition of 0.4% sodium dodecyl sulfate had only a slightly greater effect than the 0.2%. At a concentration of sodium dodecyl sulfate (0.02%) below the critical micelle concentration, the effect of the surfactant was to reduce the penetration of chloramphenicol through isolated hairless mouse skin. The authors suggest that, below the critical micelle concentration, the surfactant may complex with the drug and that, at the high concentrations, the surfactant may damage the stratum corneum.

Studies into the response of human, guinea pig, and rabbit skin to 2,4-dinitrochlorobenzene (DNCB), a known irritant and sensitizer, after preexposure of the skin with up to 2% (w/v) aqueous solutions of soap and alkylbenzene sulfonate were reported by Skog (86). In humans and guinea pigs, preexposure to the surfactants tended to increase the response to DNCB, particularly when the subjects had been sensitized to it. In rabbits no gross differences in the response to DNCB were observed between pretreated and nonpretreated skin.

The bacteriostatic compound 3,5,3′,4′-tetrachlorosalicylanilide (T4CS) in radioactive form was applied in 75% (v/v) aqueous 2-methoxyethanol to rats, the skin of which had been prewashed with water or 1% (w/v) sodium dodecyl sulfate (69). Excess of the T4CS was removed after 5 min contact with the skin, and the radioactivity remaining on the skin and excreted in the urine on 5 consecutive days was measured. Washing of the rats with detergent seemed to increase the capacity of the stratum corneum and epidermis to bind T4CS and to promote its absorption through skin, compared with the water-washed (control) rats, although the differences were small.

The treatment of guinea pigs with aqueous solutions of soap (5% w/v) or alkyl ether sulfate (0.045 N) for 1 min had little effect on the permeability to sarin, an organophosphorus cholinesterase inhibitor (87). A significantly greater effect on permeability was recorded when the duration of contact was increased to 5 and 30 min. The progressive damage to skin with time was not altered by rinsing off the surface-active agents with water, indicating that their effect was not reversible. A slow recovery of the barrier properties was observed (88), which might be related to the regeneration of nondenatured proteins by the epidermis. It would have been interesting to use this well-defined system (89) to study the effect of surfactants on the skin barrier properties in relation to concentration of surfactant and to compare the differences between various chemical structures of detergents of the anionic class.

That anionic surfactants have different effects on the skin barrier properties was shown in the studies of Black et al. (90) with pyridine-2-thione-N-oxide, also called zinc pyrithione (ZnPT). The absorption of Zn[^{3}H]PT through rat skin washed with shampoos containing different detergent actives was greatest when the active was sodium dodecyl sulfate, and least when triethanolamine lauryl sulfate was used. Sodium lauryl ether sulfate gave an intermediary absorption of Zn[^{3}H]PT.

The effect of sodium lauryl sulfate on the percutaneous absorption of butanol, as a microemulsion, through guinea skin was studied by Boman et al. (91) by sampling arterial blood at regular intervals through a catheter. For different concentrations of SDS and water, there were marked increases in the blood concentration of butanol, compared with the levels after application of neat solvent, which the authors believed might be due to denaturation of keratin and hydration of the stratum corneum by SDS, thereby facilitating skin absorption of butanol.

Lindberg et al. (92) used the technique of energy dispersive x-ray microanalysis to investigate the effect of sodium lauryl sulfate on the penetration of nickel through guinea pig stratum corneum. The authors found in the sodium dodecyl sulfate-treated skin a greater nickel penetration, which they believed might be due to an increase in the "water channel" volume of the stratum corneum.

Enhancing the penetration of the drug naloxone through isolated human skin by using a variety of compounds, including sodium lauryl sulfate, sodium laurate, or sodium oleate, at 10% in polyethylene glycol (PEG) 400 was studied by Aungst et al. (93). They found a flux of 3.8 ± 0.5 for sodium oleate and 4.6 ± 0.9 for sodium lauryl sulfate, whereas sodium laurate gave a flux of 7.3 ± 0.8, all of which were much less than found for fatty acids of various chain lengths. Vehicles other than PEG 400 were also examined. In propylene glycol and isopropanol, sodium lauryl sulfate approximately doubled naloxone flux, compared with the vehicles alone, whereas there was no effect when in PEG 400. In a mineral oil vehicle, however, the naloxone flux increased some 30 times. The authors noted that maximum penetration was observed with C_{12}-saturated hydrophobic groups, and that molecules with unsaturated groups were more effective than were saturated ones.

They further point out that the majority of the most abundant skin lipids are of C_{16} chain length or longer and consider that shorter fatty acid chains could disrupt the crystalline lipid packing, causing a more fluid and permeable membrane.

All studies have shown that absorption of anionic detergents through skin is low and that determinations by in vitro and in vivo methods yield results that are not directly comparable, probably mainly because of the strong binding of detergents to protein. The effects on the skin barrier are also progressive, so that increased duration of exposure will increase the absorption of the detergent. Higher concentrations will also promote absorption. Although synthetic anionic detergents in aqueous solution have a pH near neutrality, the alkalinity per se of aqueous soap solutions may reduce the barrier properties of skin. The effect of detergents on the skin barrier also allows better absorption of other compounds, but their ability to induce an irritation of the skin, in common with other popular penetration enhancers, may limit their application in delivery systems.

REFERENCES

1. Kastner, W. In *Anionic Surfactants: Biochemistry Toxicology, Dermatology*, Gloxhuber, Ch. (ed.). Marcel Dekker, New York, p. 139 (1980).
2. Philp, J. McL. In *Anionic Surfactants: Biochemistry, Toxicology, Dermatology*. Gloxhuber, Ch. (ed.). Marcel Dekker, New York, p. 309 (1980).
3. Emery, B. E. and Edwards, L. D. *J. Am. Pharm. Assoc. 29*:251–254 (1940).
4. Emery, B. E. and Edwards, L. D. *J. Am. Pharm. Assoc. 29*:254–255 (1940).
5. McMeekin, T. L. *Fed. Proc. 1*:125 (1942).
6. Van Scott, E. J. and Lyon, J. B. *J. Invest. Dermatol. 21*:199–203 (1953).
7. Anson, M. L. *Adv. Protein Chem. 2*:361–386 (1945).
8. Van Scott, E. J. and Flesch, P. *Arch. Dermatol. Syphilol. 70*:141–154 (1954).
9. Blohm, S. F. *Acta Derm. Venereol. 37*:269–275 (1957).
10. Choman, B. R. *J. Invest. Dermatol. 40*:177–182 (1963).

11. Imokawa, G. and Mishima, Y. *Contact Dermatitis* 5:357–366 (1979).
12. Imokawa, G., Sumura, K., and Katsumi, M. *J. Am. Oil Chem. Soc.* 52:479–483 (1975).
13. Imokawa, G., Sumura, K., and Katsumi, M. *J. Am. Oil Chem. Assoc.* 52:484–489 (1975).
14. Imokawa, G. and Tsutsumi, H. *J. Am. Oil Chem. Soc.* 55:839–843 (1978).
15. Miyazawa, K., Ogawa, M., and Mitsui, T. *Int. J. Cosmet. Sci.* 6:33–46 (1984).
16. Wilmsmann, H. *Am. Perf. Cosmet.* 78:21–26 (1963).
17. Rutherford, T. and Pawlowski, A. *Br. J. Dermatol.* 91:503–506 (1974).
18. Prottey, C. and Coxon, A. *Int. J. Cosmet. Sci.* 6:263–273 (1984).
19. Schwuger, M. J. and Bartnik, F. G. In *Anionic Surfactants, Biochemistry, Toxicology, Dermatology.* Gloxuber, Ch. (ed.). Marcel Dekker, New York, p. 1 (1980).
20. Faucher, J. A. and Goddard, E. D. *J. Soc. Cosmet. Sci.* 29:323–337 (1978).
21. Dominguez, J. G., Parra, J. L., Infante, M. R., Pelejero, C. M., Balaguer, F., and Sastre, T. *J. Soc. Cosmet. Chem.* 28:165–182 (1977).
22. Cooper, E. R. and Berner, B. In *Surfactants in Cosmetics.* Rieger, M. M. (ed.). Marcel Dekker, New York, pp. 195–210 (1985).
23. Conrads, A. and Zahn, H. *Int. J. Cosmet. Sci.* 9:29–46 (1987).
24. Goette, E. K. *Kolloid Z.* 117:42–47 (1950).
25. Putterman, G. J., Wolejsza, N. F., Wolfram, M. A., and Laden, K. *J. Soc. Cosmet. Chem.* 28:521–532 (1977).
26. Scheuplein, R. J. and Ross, L. *J. Soc. Cosmet. Chem.* 21:853–873 (1970).
27. Robbins, C. R. and Fernee, K. M. *J. Soc. Cosmet. Chem.* 34:21–34 (1983).
28. Rhein, L. D., Robbins, C. R., Fernee, K., and Cantore, R. *J. Soc. Cosmet. Chem.* 37:125–139 (1986).
29. Blake-Haskins, J. C., Scala, D., Rhein, L. D., and Robbins, C. R. *J. Soc. Cosmet. Chem.* 37:199–210 (1986).
30. Choman, B. R. *J. Invest. Dermatol.* 37:263–271 (1961).
31. Tavss, E. A., Eigen, E., and Kligman, A. M. *J. Soc. Cosmet. Sci.* 39:267–272 (1988).
32. Baker, H. and Kligman, A. *Arch. Dermatol.* 94:441–452 (1967).
33. Nilsson, G. E. *Med. Biol. Eng. Comput.* 16:209–218 (1977).
34. Frodin, T. and Skogh, M. *Arch. Dermatol. Venereol.* 64:537–540 (1984).
35. Werner, Y. and Lindberg, M. *Arch. Dermatol. Venereol.* 65:102–105 (1985).
36. Van der Valk, P. G. M., Nater, J. P., and Bleumink, E. *J. Invest. Dermatol.* 82:291–293 (1984).
37. Hassing, J. H., Nater, J. P., and Bleumink, E. *Dermatologica* 164:314–321 (1982).
38. Murahata, R. I., Crowe, D. M., and Roheim, J. R. *Int. J. Cosmet. Sci.* 8:225–231 (1986).
39. Dugard, P. H. and Scheuplein, R. J. *J. Invest. Dermatol.* 60:263–269 (1973).
40. Serban, G. P., Henry, S. M., Cotty, V. F., and Marcus, A. D. *J. Soc. Cosmet. Chem.* 32:407–419 (1981).
41. Bahl, M. K. *J. Soc. Cosmet. Sci.* 36:287–296 (1985).
42. Blank, I. H. *J. Invest. Dermatol.* 18:433–441 (1952).
43. Singer, E. G. and Vinson, L. J. *Proc. Sci. Sect. Toilet Goods Assoc.* 46:29–33 (1966).
44. Middleton, J. D. *Br. J. Dermatol.* 80:437–450 (1968).
45. Blank, I. H. and Shappirio, E. B. *J. Invest. Dermatol.* 25:391–401 (1955).
46. Middleton, J. D. *J. Soc. Cosmet. Chem.* 20:399–412 (1969).
47. Gray, G. M, and White, R. J. *J. Invest. Dermatol.* 70:336–341 (1978).

48. Elias, P. M. *Int. J. Dermatol.* *20*:1–19 (1981).
49. Scheuplein, R. J. and Blank, I. H. *Physiol. Rev.* *51*:702–747 (1971).
50. Elias, P. M. and Leventhal, M. E. *Clin. Res.* *27*:525a (1979).
51. Elias, P. M. and Friend, D. S. *J. Cell Biol.* *63*:93a (1974).
52. Barry, B. W. *Int. J. Cosmet. Sci.* *10*:281–293 (1988).
53. Imokawa, G. and Hattori, M. *J. Invest. Dermatol.* *84*:282–284 (1985).
54. Imokawa, G., Akasaki, S., Minematsu, Y., and Kawai, M. *Arch. Dermatol. Res.* *281*:45–51 (1989).
55. Fulmer, A. W. and Kramer, G. J. *J. Invest. Dermatol.* *81*:598–602 (1986).
56. Blank, I. H. and Gould, E. *J. Invest. Dermatol.* *33*:327–336 (1959).
57. Blank, I. H. and Gould, E. *J. Invest. Dermatol.* *37*:485–488 (1961).
58. Blank, I. H. and Gould, E. *J. Invest. Dermatol.* *37*:311–315 (1961).
59. Bettley, F. R. *Br. J. Dermatol.* *73*:448–454 (1961).
60. Bettley, F. R. *Br. J. Dermatol.* *75*:113–116 (1963).
61. Scala, J., McOsker, D. E., and Reller, H. H. *J. Invest. Dermatol.* *50*:372–379 (1968).
62. Emery, G. and Dugard, P. H. *Br. J. Dermatol.* *81*(Suppl. 4):63–68 (1969).
63. Staughton, R. B. and Fritsch, W. *Arch. Dermatol.* *90*:512–517 (1964).
64. Fiker, S., Janeckova, V., and Kacovska, V. *Acta Fac. Med. Univ. Brun 41*:177–180 (1972).
65. Howes, D. *J. Soc. Cosmet. Chem.* *26*:47–63 (1975).
66. Faucher, J. A. and Goddard, E. D. *J. Soc. Cosmet. Chem.* *29*:339–352 (1978).
67. Gibson, W. T. and Teall, M. R. *Food Chem. Toxicol.* *21*:581–586 (1983).
68. Choman, B. R. *J. Soc. Cosmet. Chem.* *11*:138–145 (1960).
69. Sprott, W. E. *Trans. St. John's Hosp. Dermatol. Soc.* *51*(2):56–71 (1965).
70. Prottey, C. and Ferguson, T. *J. Soc. Cosmet. Chem.* *26*:29–46 (1975).
71. Black, J. G. and Howes, D. *J. Soc. Cosmet. Chem.* *80*:157–165 (1979).
72. Minegishi, K. I., Osawa, M., and Yamaha, T. *Chem. Pharm. Bull. (Tokyo) 25*:821–825 (1977).
73. Bettley, F. R. and Donoghue, E. *Nature 185*:17–20 (1960).
74. Isherwood, P. A. *J. Invest. Dermatol.* *40*:143–145 (1963).
75. Bettley, F. R. *Br. J. Dermatol.* *77*:98–100 (1965).
76. Wood, D. C. F. and Bettley, F. R. *Br. J. Dermatol.* *84*:320–325 (1971).
77. Nilzen, A. and Wikstrom, K. *Acta Derm. Venereol.* *35*:292–299 (1955).
78. Kvornung, S. A. and Svendsen, I. B. *J. Invest. Dermatol.* *26*:421–426 (1956).
79. Vinson, L. J. and Choman, B. R. *J. Soc. Cosmet. Chem.* *11*:127–137 (1960).
80. Friberg, L., Skog, E., and Wahlberg, J. E. *Acta Derm. Venereol.* *41*:40–52 (1961).
81. Skog, E. and Wahlberg, J. E. *Acta Derm. Venereol.* *42*:17–20 (1962).
82. Wahlberg, J. E. *Acta Derm. Venereol.* *45*:335–343 (1965).
83. Wahlberg, J. E. *Acta Derm. Venereol.* *48*:549–555 (1968).
84. Sprott, W. E. In *De Structura et Functione Stratorum Epidermidis*. Barrierae, S. D., Lejhanee, G., and Hybasek, P. (eds.). Publ. Facultas Medica Universitatis Brunensis, pp. 219–232 (1965).
85. Aguiar, A. J. and Weiner, M. A. *J. Pharm. Sci.* *58*:210–215 (1969).
86. Skog, E. *Acta Derm. Venereol.* *38*:1–14 (1958).
87. Fredricksson, T. *Acta Derm. Venereol.* *49*:55–58 (1969).

88. Fredricksson, T. *Acta Derm. Venereol. 49*:481–483 (1969).
89. Fredricksson, T. *Acta Derm. Venereol. 43*:91–101 (1963).
90. Black, J. G., Howes, D., and Rutherford, T. *Actualites de Dermocosmetologie VII.* Centre European de Dermocosmetologie, Lyon, pp. 127–142 (1975).
91. Boman, A., Blute, I., Fernstrom, P., Carlfors, J., and Rydhag, L. *Contact Dermatitis 21*:92–104 (1989).
92. Lindberg, M., Sagstroan, S., Roomans, G. M., and Forslind, B. *Scan. Microsc. 3*: 221–224 (1989).
93. Aungst, B. J., Rogers, N. J., and Shefter, E. *Int. J. Pharm. 33*:225–234 (1986).

7

Azone

Mechanisms of Action and Clinical Effect

Jonathan Hadgraft and Dafydd G. Williams

*The Welsh School of Pharmacy, University of Wales,
Cardiff, Wales*

Geoffrey Allan

Whitby Research, Inc., Richmond, Virginia

I. INTRODUCTION

Azone (known generically as laurocapram) is a material that was developed specifically as a skin penetration enhancer that could be used for both improving the absorption of topical agents and for use in optimizing the design of transdermal devices. Additionally, it can be incorporated into transdermal systems such that their design can be optimized. Drugs that are poorly absorbed through the skin cannot be used transdermally, but the addition of an appropriate enhancer may increase the flux through the skin sufficiently that therapeutic levels can be achieved in the plasma. The ideal properties of an enhancer have been quoted in several recent publications and include the following factors

1. It should be pharmacologically inert.
2. It should be nontoxic, nonirritant, and nonallergenic.
3. Its action should be rapid and for a predictable duration of time.
4. Its action should be reversible.
5. It should be specific in its action.
6. It should be chemically and physically stable.
7. It should be colorless, odorless, and tasteless.

In any assessment of an enhancer, the foregoing criteria have to be addressed in depth, and it is important to be able to identify the mechanisms by which it acts.

The mechanism of action of chemical enhancers has been the subject of many investigations over the past decade. Recent advances in the identification of the route of drug penetration through the skin and the application of biophysical techniques to study the structure of skin has facilitated the understanding. The techniques include spectroscopic (Fourier transform Infrared [FTIR], nuclear magnetic resonance [NMR], electron spin resonance [ESR], x-ray diffraction, fluorescence) and thermal analyses of skin. Additionally, it is possible to obtain useful information from the interactions of enhancers with some structured model lipids representative of those found in the skin.

This chapter will provide a brief account of the route of penetration and describe the ways in which Azone can modify the structure of the skin to enhance permeability. Spectroscopic and thermal methods have been used to probe these. With the advent of sophisticated molecular modeling it is possible to speculate on the interactions that may be occurring between Azone and skin components. In many instances synergistic effects can be found between an enhancer and other formulation additives. These effects will be considered from a physicochemical standpoint. The degree of enhancement will be related to the physicochemical characteristics of the permeant. Finally, the clinical work that has been conducted on the effectiveness of Azone will be reviewed.

II. PHYSICOCHEMICAL PROPERTIES OF AZONE

The chemical structure of Azone (laurocapram; 1-dodecylazacycloheptan-2-one) is shown in Figure 1. It is a clear, colorless, liquid, with a relative molecular mass (M_r) of 281.49 Da, a melting point of $-7°C$, and a boiling point of $160°C$ at 0.05 mmHg. The octanol–water partition coefficient can be estimated from Hansch analysis and the log P of 6.21 shows that it is an extremely lipophilic material. It is likely to associate itself with the lipids contained in the stratum corneum and is unlikely to partition significantly into the underlying viable tissue. It is also possible to calculate the solubility parameter by using a fragmental approach. The number obtained is 9.06 H, which can be compared with that estimated by Liron and Cohen (1) for the stratum corneum as being between 9.7 and 10.0 H. Since the numbers are very similar, Azone would be expected to dissolve readily in the skin lipids, but be poorly absorbed into the systemic circulation. This has been verified by Wiechers et al. (2), who used radiolabeled Azone and determined its distribution and accumulation within the skin by a tape-stripping technique. The amount absorbed through the skin, as assessed by urinary excretion, was small. Most of the Azone that penetrated into the skin resided in the upper layers of the stratum corneum.

For formulation considerations, it is compatible with most organic solvents. In the development of topical formulations containing water-soluble drugs, it can be incorporated into emulsions, gels, and other biphasic systems. However, the efficacy of action can be reduced by the presence of some agents (e.g.,

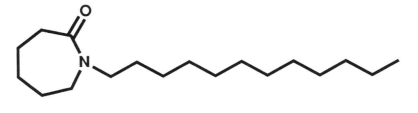

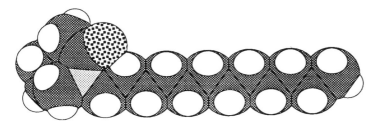

Figure 1   The chemical structure of Azone and a three-dimensional representation of the molecule.

petrolatum). The reduction in effect is probably a result of the petrolatum preventing the Azone from entering the stratum corneum caused by a decrease in its thermodynamic activity.

III. THE ROUTE OF PENETRATION OF DRUGS THROUGH THE SKIN

Katz and Poulsen (3) published an excellent review that detailed the different possible routes of drug penetration through the skin. At that time, it was not possible to differentiate between the pathways, and the subject was a matter for conjecture. Two years later, Michaels et al. (4) considered the stratum corneum as having a "bricks and mortar structure," with transfer occurring either through the dead cells or by a more tortuous intercellular route. From that publication, it was not possible to determine the precise route of penetration of the drugs under investigation, but the concepts were subsequently employed to distinguish the possible mechanisms involved in percutaneous penetration. Albery and Hadgraft (5) examined the absorption of some esters of nicotinic acid and, as a result of a kinetic analysis of the data, showed that these molecules penetrate through the intercellular channels. The approximate diffusional path length of these is 330 μm. Following this, several research groups have identified the intercellular route as being dominant. Therefore, it is of importance to determine the nature and composition of the intercellular channels.

The lipid structure has been reviewed by Wertz and Downing (6). The lipids of the stratum corneum are a complex mixture that structure themselves into multiple lamellae. The thickness of a double bilayer appears to lie in the range 9.7–12.8 nm. The main constituents are cholesteryl esters, free cholesterol, fatty acids, and various ceramides (sphingosines and phytosphingosines). Unlike other biological membranes, there is no phospholipid present. The lipid sheets provide the skin's resistance to water loss and also control the ingress of materials through the epidermis and into the systemic circulation. Consideration of both the microscopic detail of the stratum corneum and results from thermal analysis of skin, provide evidence that a lipoprotein complex exists. This has been attributed to a corneocyte envelope, the precise structure of which is still under investigation. It has been postulated that the hydroxyceramides form an anchor between the corneocyte envelope and the intercellular lamellae.

A molecule diffusing through the stratum corneum, therefore, encounters a structured array of lipids. Consequently, its progress may be accelerated if the structuring is reduced and the lipids are disordered. This may be a result of its own interaction with the lipids or of another species codiffusing with it. It is useful to examine the ways in which molecules, such as Azone, can interact with a lamellar structure.

IV. THE INTERACTION OF AZONE WITH STRUCTURED LIPIDS

The chemical structure of Azone (see Fig. 1), shows that there is a long alkyl chain and a region that is more polar—the lactam grouping. A simple way to demonstrate the degree to which the lactam group influences the polarity of the molecule is to consider partitioning behavior. There are four orders of magnitude difference between the estimated log P (using fragmental constants) of Azone, compared with the all-carbon analogue. The lactam grouping, therefore, would be expected to interact with the polar regions of a structured lipid array. The carbon side chain would then insert itself into the alkyl chain regions of the lipids.

To examine the potential for interaction with lipids, experiments have been conducted using liposomes composed of dipalmitoyl phosphatidylcholine (DPPC). Although there are no phospholipids present in the skin, these vesicles were used as a reproducible model, with as few variables as possible, to simulate potential changes that may be induced by the presence of Azone in the lipids of the stratum corneum. To assess the changes, the phase transition temperature of the DPPC liposomes was determined, using a simple light-scattering technique.

Addition of increasing amounts of Azone to the DPPC liposomes resulted in a lowering of the phase transition temperature, as shown in Figure 2. In addition to simple determinations of the effect of Azone on the phase transition temperature, the effect on a fluorescent probe incorporated into the liposome was also investigated (7). The results indicate that Azone does interact with structured lipids making them more fluid, which will produce a concomitant reduction in the diffusional resistance experienced by the penetrating species.

It is possible to consider the interactions of Azone with structured lipids in more detail by using monolayers of DPPC spread at an air–water interface (8). Large surface expansions are found as a result of the interaction of Azone and the DPPC molecules, and the presence of increasing concentrations of the enhancer gradually reduced and finally abolished the liquid-expanded to liquid-condensed phase transitions. The surface expansion indicates, in conjunction with molecular graphics, that the Azone headgroup is in a bent conformation relative to the alkyl chain and that the ring structure lies in the plane of the polar headgroups of the phospholipid. Molecular energetic calculations show that the energy differences between the linear and bent conformation is less than 10 kcal·mol^{-1}, an amount that is easily accessible.

The use of monolayers has also been extended to the use of lipid mixtures, which are more representative of skin (9). Azone changed the solid film of cholesterol and the liquid-condensed film of ceramide to liquid-expanded films.

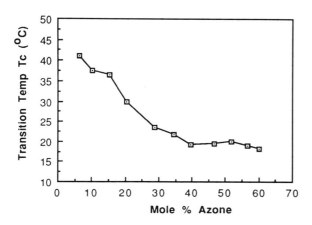

Figure 2 The influence of Azone on the phase transition temperature of DPPC liposomes.

Differential scanning calorimetry (DSC) studies have shown that Azone does not interact with the proteins within the stratum corneum, indicating that it does not enter the corneocytes in any significant amounts (10), therefore, suggesting partitioning into the intercellular lipid bilayer. The phase transitions that have been attributed to the melting of the lipids in the skin are lowered by the presence of Azone.

V. EFFECT ON SKIN PENETRATION

Azone has been an effective enhancer for a range of compounds. Both hydrophobic and hydrophilic molecules have their skin penetration enhanced, although greater enhancement with Azone has been seen with hydrophilic compounds. Ionized molecules do not readily penetrate the stratum corneum and, in this instance, Azone may be used as an ion-pairing agent with an anionic species to promote their partitioning into the lipid phase (11). This would then alter the thermodynamic activity of the anionic drug and, thereby, affect its bioavailability within the tissue.

Importantly, it seems that Azone is most effective when it is present at low concentrations in the formulation, usually between 1 and 10%. There appears to be a parabolic concentration dependence on its activity to enhance the penetration of other active molecules through the skin. The concentration of Azone needed to produce optimal penetration does, however, vary from drug to drug. Azone produces large enhancement when only a small amount of the active drug is present in the formulation (12). This can be advantageous when a potentially hazardous or particularly expensive compound may be applied to the skin in lower concentrations in the presence of Azone. In any assessment of penetration of drugs through the skin and the effect of enhancers, it is necessary to take into account the animal species that has been chosen for the work. Any enhancement of the percutaneous absorption of compounds using Azone will vary with biological species, as well as there being intraspecies variations.

The concentration-dependent–enhancing phenomenon of Azone with individual classes of pharmacologically active compounds will be examined further. Table 1 gives an overview of compounds that have been investigated in combination with Azone (13), together with the observed enhancement factors. Its enhancing property has been demonstrated predominantly in vitro in animal tissue.

The concentration of Azone that maximally enhances drug penetration varies both with different compounds and with the composition of topical vehicle. Enhanced penetration of both hydrophobic and hydrophilic molecules has been demonstrated, although greater enhancement has usually been reported with hydrophilic compounds (14).

A. Antibiotics

Transdermal enhancement of antibiotics may be helpful in the management of acne vulgaris and in the control of the resident microflora located on the skin surface. The microorganisms found in acne pustules and hair follicles [*Propionibacterium acnes* (*Corynebacterium acnes*), *Staphylococcus albus*, and *S. epidermidis*] all have lipolytic activity and increase the concentration of fatty acids in the sebum. The fatty acids are irritants and provoke an inflammatory response. Topical delivery of the antibiotics clindamycin, sodium fusidate, and erythromycin have been enhanced by incorporating Azone within the vehicle (15). Maximal enhancement of a 0.02% clindamycin formulation was seen with 8% Azone, which had the same activity in inhibiting the growth of *P. acnes* as a vehicle containing 0.1% clindamycin alone (12), thereby lowering the amount of the active drug required in the formulation.

Penetration of erythromycin was enhanced with Azone, with a 6% concentration of Azone giving half-maximal enhancement, reaching a maximal plateau level of erythromycin enhancement seen with 30–40% concentrations of Azone incorporated within the base (12).

With sodium fusidate, low concentrations of Azone in the vehicle gave a two- to threefold enhancement of drug flux; however, higher concentrations of the enhancer generally showed less drug enhancement. Concentrations of Azone in excess of 15% actually inhibited the activity of fusidic acid and, in formulations incorporating 50% or more, Azone abolished antibiotic activity altogether.

Metronidazole is a polar antibiotic that has been used in the treatment of trichomoniasis and amebiasis, and is of use in the prophylaxis of anaerobic infections. It has been used as a model drug for the investigation of the transdermal delivery of drugs in many situations, particularly with penetration enhancers (40). Azone at a concentration of 1% was equally as effective as 5 and 10% formulations in achieving enhanced transport of metronidazole. However, in the presence of propylene glycol, Azone increased the drug delivery 25-fold more than the control (56). Propylene glycol has been widely cited as an adjunct to dermatological formulations, acting as a cosolvent for other skin accelerants such as Azone (26,40,48). Some studies have suggested that propylene glycol alone can act as a skin penetration enhancer (40), or when operating as a synergist to other accelerants, by possibly solvating α-keratin and occupying hydrogen-bonding sites, thereby reducing drug–tissue binding. Repeated doses of metronidazole after a single dose of Azone gave further enhancement of the antibiotic, showing that the effect of Azone on the skin could remain after several days (40). However it should be noted that these experiments were conducted in vitro in a design in which there was no sink for the Azone.

Table 1 Overview of Compounds Investigated in Combination With Azone

Compound	% Azone in formulation	Study type	Skin type	Enhancement factor	Refs.
Amcinonide	2	In vivo	H	>2[a]	12, 15
Anthracene	3	In vivo	HM	Yes[b]	16
Betamethasone	2[c]	In vivo	H	2.2[a]	17
benzoate	2.5	In vivo	H	0.9[a]	17
8-Bromo cAMP	1	In vitro	HM	12	12, 16
6-Carboxyfluorescein	3	In vivo	R	2–3	18
Clindamycinphosphate	8	Ex vivo	HM	Yes[b]	12, 15
Desonide	2	In vivo	H	>2[a]	12, 15
Desoximetasone	1	In vivo	H	3–4[a]	12, 16
Dexamethasone					
acetate	5	In vivo	R	Yes[b,d]	19
palmitate	5	In vivo	R	Small[b,d]	19
Difluoromethyl-					
ornithine	10	In vitro	P	1.3	20
Erythromycin	5[c]	In vivo	HM	15	21
	50[c]	Ex vivo	HM	Yes[b]	15
Estradiol	2[c]	In vitro	H	1.4	22
	3	In vitro	H	1.3	22
Ethanol	5	In vitro	HR	2	23
Fluocinolone acetonide	2	In vivo	H	4–5[a]	12, 16
Fluorouracil	1.8	In vitro	HM	>80	15
	2[c]	In vitro	HM	>130	24
	2[c]	In vitro	H	~20	24
	2[c]	In vitro	H	100	24
	3	In vitro	HR	Yes[b]	25
	3	In vitro	HR	10–100	26
	3	In vitro	HR	~100	21
	3	In vitro	HM	>10	24
	3	In vitro	H	8	22
	3	In vitro	H	7	24
	5	In vitro	HM	50	27
	10	In vitro	HR	~10	28
Fusidate sodium	3[c]	Ex vivo	HM	2–3	12, 15
Griseofulvin	3	In vivo	H	yes[b]	16
	5[c]	In vitro	HM	>36	21
Hematoporphyrin-	2	In vitro	HM	8	29
derivative	10	In vitro	H	~9	30
Hydrocortisone	5[c]	In vitro	HM	45	21
	5[c]	Ex vivo	HM	~65	21
Hydroquinone	0.5	In vivo	H	1.2[e]	31
	2	In vitro	HM	>3	32
Ibuprofen	5	In vitro	HR	3	23
Idoxuridine	5[c]	In vitro	HM	>3000	33
Indomethacin	3	In vitro	HR	9	34
	5	In vitro	HR	4	23
	6[c]	In vitro	R	5	35
	6[c]	In vivo	R	3	35
	8	In vitro	HM	>7	32

Table 1 (Continued)

Compound	% Azone in formulation	Study type	Skin type	Enhancement factor	Refs.
Indomethacin Ca	6	In vitro	R	2	35
	6	In vivo	R	1.3	35
Insulin	0.1[c]	In vitro	R	7	36
	0.1[c]	In vitro	P	14	37
Isoproterenol	1[c]	In vitro	H	8	38
6-Mercaptopurine	3	In vitro	GP	30	39
Metronidazole	1	In vitro	H	25	40
Mitomycin	3.3	In vitro	R	Yes[b]	41
	3.3	In vitro	R	60	42
	3.3	In vitro	HM	40	42
Nifedipine	5[c]	In vivo	R	8[d]	43
Propranolol	2	In vivo	Ra	30[d]	44
	3[c]	In vivo	Ra	1.8[d]	44
Sulfanilamide	5	In vitro	HR	~70	23
Thymidine	2	In vitro	HM	>3	45
	2	In vivo	HM	Yes[b]	45
Triamcinolone	1.6[c]	In vivo	H	>3[e]	13
acetonide	1.6[c]	In vivo	H	4–9[a]	32
	2	In vitro	HM	>120	46
	3	In vivo	H	>2[a]	12, 15
	10	In vitro	HM	>5	12
Trifluorothymidine	5	In vitro	GP	224	47
	5[c]	In vitro	GP	287	47
	5[c]	In vivo	GP	Yes[b]	48
	10[c]	In vitro	GP	Large[b]	48
	10[c]	In vitro	H	Large[b]	48
Vasopressin	5	In vitro	HM	65	49
	5	In vitro	R	15	49, 50
Verapamil HCl	2[c]	In vivo	R	6[d]	51
	3	In vitro	R	~5	52
	3	In vitro	HM	44–130[f]	52
	3	In vitro	H	3	52
	12	In vitro	R	>20	52
	3	In vitro	HM	170	53
	Pretreat.[g]	In vitro	HM	360	54
Ara-A-2′,3′-di-O-acetate	15	In vitro	HM	100–1000	55
	Pretreat.[g]	In vitro	HM	100	54
Ara-A-5′-O-valerate	15	In vitro	HM	100–1000	55

Type of skin: H, human skin; HM, hairless mouse; R, rat; HR, hairless rat; GP, guinea pig; Ra, rabbit; P, pig.
[a]Based on vasoconstriction assay.
[b]Not quantitated or not quantifiable.
[c]Propylene glycol was coadministrated.
[d]Based on plasma concentrations.
[e]Based on amounts retrieved in the urine and feces.
[f]Spreading owing to biphasic pattern in control.
[g]Pretreated with 50 mg of Azone for 24 hr.

Generally for antibiotics, Azone enhancement of the active drug is concentration-dependent, with a maximal effect seen with 2–3% Azone concentrations within the topical vehicle; plateau effects are seen at 4–10% azone, and attenuation of response at higher Azone strengths (15).

B. Topical Sunscreens

An effective topical sunscreening agent should have the attributes of being able to stay on, or in, the outer skin layers over a long period, even if the individual perspires or is immersed in water. Selective absorption of the ultraviolet component of sunlight is provided by preparations containing benzophenone derivatives: these absorb radiation in the range 250–350 nm and prevent tanning as well as an erythematous response. *para*-Aminobenzoic acid (PABA) protects the skin from the damaging effects of ultraviolet light; therefore, there is a requirement for an effective vehicle for PABA that carries it into the skin quickly, forming a reservoir. Azone enhances the absorption of PABA through the skin, allowing formation of a reservoir, and also decreases its desorption rate within the stratum corneum (57). With a 3% Azone formulation, penetration of PABA into the skin was four times greater than treatment with PABA alone, with a maximum reservoir effect seen after 4 hr. Again, there is concentration-dependent enhancement, although no difference was seen between 1 and 3% Azone concentrations.

C. Glucocorticoids

Triamcinolone acetonide, a corticosteroid that has potent local anti-inflammatory action, is used topically in the treatment of various skin disorders, such as keloids, lichens, and sarcoidosis of the skin. It exerts its pharmacological effects after penetration of the skin barrier and reaching the target cells within the epidermis and dermis. The risk of systemic toxicity from the topical treatment of most acute dermatoses with steroids is slight, but is appreciable in chronic conditions in which large areas of the skin are treated, particularly with occlusive dressings. The main local adverse effects of topical steroids are drying and thinning of the epidermis, along with weakening of the collagen fibers within the dermis. Ruption of these collagen bundles can produce characteristic purple markings, *striae*, which are permanent and unsightly.

Incorporation of Azone in a formulation does enhance the permeation of triamcinolone acetonide into the skin (46). Test concentrations of 0.1–10% Azone increased the transdermal flux of triamcinolone acetonide (15), with a tenfold increase in flux seen with a 10% Azone formulation. It appears that the penetration enhancement of the steroid is dependent on the concentration of enhancer and reached a maximum flux with 10% Azone, however, higher concentrations of 40% of enhancer led to a decrease in the amount of active drug penetrating the tissue. There was a gradual decrease in efficacy of the corticosteroid as enhancer concentrations approached 100%, with a 2% Azone base seen to be as effective as the higher concentrations. Incorporating Azone with an active corticosteroid can decrease the amount of active drug required in the topical formulation required to exert a pharmacological effect, consequently, leading to a decrease in side effects and the chance of systemic absorption.

Skin blanching experiments with other steroids have shown that at Azone concentrations of 1–3% there is a two- to fourfold enhancement of the steroids desonide, fluocinolone acetonide, amcinonide, and desoxymetazone (12). Again, there was a gradual decrease in efficacy of enhancement as the concentration of Azone rose toward 100%.

D. Photochemotherapy

Psoriasis is a common skin disorder that affects 1–2% of the general population. It is characterized by patches of erythematous scaly skin, with the lesions being slightly raised with clearly defined margins to the surrounding unaffected skin. The psoriatic lesion itself has no effect on general physical well-being; however, there is often much mental distress because of the disfigurement induced by these psoriatic lesions. The erythema seen is due to proliferation of dermal blood vessels and the accumulation of lymphocytes and histocytes within the dermal papillae. These effects are secondary to the changes seen in the epidermis, where mitotic activity is greatly increased in the prickle cells as well as the basal layer. The higher cellular turnover rate leads to a condition known as *parakeratosis*, in which the keratin within the stratum corneum is poorly developed, the cells contain fragments of nuclei, the granular layer disappears, the prickle layer is thicker, but the corneum is thinner and weaker.

Two main classes of drugs are used to treat psoriasis: the tars and the corticosteroids. The tars are thought to act by depressing the rate of mitosis of the epidermal cells, whereas corticosteroids are said to act by inhibiting mitosis and by dermal vasoconstriction. Anthracene is a keratoplastic agent obtained from the distillation of coal tar and has been used alone in ointments at concentrations of 1–5% for the treatment of psoriasis. At these concentrations, it was often an irritant and has caused acne-type eruptions on the area applied. However, incorporation of 3% Azone into bases containing lower anthracene concentrations (0.02–0.05%) enhanced the penetration so that DNA synthesis in the psoriatic lesion was inhibited (16).

Another approach to treating psoriasis and other hyperproliferative cutaneous disorders is to use photochemotherapy. This is an ideal method that localizes the effects of a drug that is inactive in the body, but can be made photoactive within the skin, to exert a pharmacological effect. Hematoporphyrins, especially hematoporphyrin derivative (HPD), are localized in malignant tissues. The HPD, upon photoactivation, can cause single-strand breaks in the cellular DNA; HPD can be used in combination with UVA or red light to destroy selectively malignant tissues, leaving normal skin relatively undamaged. Incorporating Azone into the vehicle enhances HPD penetration (29,58). Penetration of HPDS with Azone increased in a concentration-dependent manner with 0.5–2% formulations, with a maximal enhancement seen with 2% Azone. Topical HPD in 2% Azone produces complete inhibition of epidermal synthesis, compared with the controls, thus giving a more effective vehicle delivery system for HPD.

Psoriasis and similar cutaneous disorders are characterized by increased cellular polyamine levels, which are synthesized in the cells by the biosynthetic pathway seen in the schematic representation (Fig. 3). The polyamines, spermidine and spermine, are powerful growth stimulators of biological cells, and exert several actions on the control of nucleic acid metabolism, which probably underlies their effects on growth. X-ray analysis indicated that the polyamines bind to the double-helix of DNA in three ways: across the minor groove, across the major groove, and aligned parallel to the individual DNA strands. By neutralizing the negative charges on DNA, the polyamines make the molecule more flexible; they also increase the stability of the double-helical form.

The polyamines also have a marked stimulatory effect on the activity of RNA polymerase, transcription is accelerated and, likewise, they stimulate the activity of DNA polymerase, so that the replication of DNA is facilitated. The

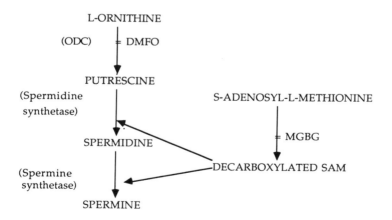

Figure 3 Polyamine biosynthetic pathway. DFMO, 2-difluoromethylornithine; MGBG, methylglyoxal bis-(guanylhydrazone); ODC, ornithine decarboxylase; SAMDC, S-adenosylmethionine decarboxylase.

cloverleaf-like structure of tRNA molecules is stabilized by polyamines, which form cross links between adjacent phosphate groups, and polyamines are involved in the joining of two ribosomal units (60S and 40S in mammals) forming the functional ribosome, probably by bridging the rRNA molecules in the two components, thereby stimulating protein synthesis.

Mitoguazone [methylgloxal bis(guanylhydrazone) MGBG] is a competitive inhibitor of *s*-adenosylmethionine decarboxylase (SAMDC), and is of limited use alone in the treatment of cutaneous malignancies because of its toxic effects; eflornithine (2-difluoromethylonithine; DFMO) is an irreversible inhibitor of ornithine decarboxylase (ODC) and has marginal activity in the treatment of psoriasis (20). Treatment with topical MGBG or DFMO alone does produce partial improvement in clinical psoriatic conditions, for which the proliferative skin multiplication needs to be inhibited. However, concurrent administration of both compounds in a 10% Azone vehicle produced a greater inhibition of DNA synthesis and depletion of polyamine levels than with either drug individually. This simultaneous topical delivery of DFMO and MGBG allows the use of smaller concentrations of MGBG in the presence of Azone, thereby reducing any dose-related side effects.

Severe intractable psoriasis may require treatment with more potent antimitotic compounds, since the object is the same as in the treatment of cancer, that is to prevent cellular proliferation. However, with the administration of such compounds there is the risk of inhibition of normal cellular synthesis, for example, within the bone marrow, leading to a decrease in effectiveness of the body's immune system. Incorporation of an effective penetration enhancer, such as Azone, may increase the topical bioavailability of such drugs, with lower concentrations required to produce a beneficial effect, thus reducing any normal cellular damage or damage to the immune system.

E. Antivirals

Fluorouracil (FU) is a cytotoxic agent used topically in the treatment of various epithelial neoplasms. The compound itself appears to have little direct inhibitory action, but competes for an active transport system for pyrimidines (59), is treated within the body like uracil, and converted to the active metabolite, 5-fluoro-deoxyuridine-5-phosphate by the corresponding nucleotide. This enzyme system, thymidylate synthetase, catalyzes the conversion of deoxyuridine-5-phosphate to deoxythymidine-5-phosphate for incorporation into cellular DNA. 5-Fluoro-deoxyuridine-5-phosphate acts as a false substrate for this enzyme and also has greater affinity for the enzyme than does the natural substrate. The false substrate is not incorporated into the DNA, but acts by inhibiting the enzyme so that DNA synthesis is blocked.

Azone has been shown to be useful in enhancing the permeability of FU across the stratum corneum (12,24–26) in treating herpes simplex virus lesions. Formulations including 1–5% Azone increased the permeability of FU in a concentration-dependent manner, with an 44-fold enhancement seen at lower concentrations of 1% Azone (27), increasing to an 80-fold increase with a 1.8% Azone formulation (15), compared with treatment with FU alone. Higher concentrations of Azone in the vehicle caused less enhancement, with a 50-fold enhancement seen with 5% Azone (27); however these values were still greater than with the control values obtained by treating the herpetic lesions with FU alone.

Incorporation of Azone increased the transport of the purine analogue and antiviral agent vidarabine (the 5'-valerate ester), 50- to 500-fold better than formulations without Azone (60). Vidarabine (9-β-arabinofuranosyladenine or ara-A), shows promising activity against herpes simplex and vaccinia viruses, and herpes keratitis (59). When incorporated into 10–20% formulations that contained Azone, higher steady-state epidermal vidarabine levels were obtained 50–200 times more frequently than with vidarabine by itself. Herpetic lesion scores, seen with hairless mice infected topically with herpes simplex virus (HSV), were improved with Azone-containing formulations of vidarabine, and the mortality rate was reduced significantly.

A series of experiments were designed to determine the optimal vehicle and minimum drug concentration that were required to achieve protective activity against herpetic skin lesions, paralysis, and mortality in hairless mice inoculated intracutaneously with HSV-1 and HSV-2 (61). Bromovinyldeoxyuridine (BVDU) has been found to be an effective antiviral compound, irrespective of the composition of its topical base; however, the amount of active constituent required for an inhibiting effect was greatly lowered when it was delivered at a 0.3% concentration in a base composed of 5% Azone in dimethyl sulfoxide (DMSO). This was found to be the optimal vehicle for the treatment of cutaneous HSV-1 with BVDU.

VI. CLINICAL STUDIES OF AZONE

A. Clinical Safety

1. Twenty-one Day Studies of Cumulative Irritation

Several clinical studies have been conducted in normal adult volunteers to investigate the irritative potential of different concentrations of Azone with various delivery systems. In one study (62), each of 11 subjects was treated with 2, 5, 25, 50, and 100% Azone in a Neutrogena vehicle and with three control preparations (i.e., Neutrogena, mineral oil, and Vaseline Intensive Care lotion). The materials were delivered by using a Webril patch with occlusion, applied to the same site, for 5 days a week over a 21 day period (63). Azone in concentrations through 50%

was not irritating; at a concentration of 100%, Azone was more irritating than a mineral oil control in 1 of the 11 subjects.

In another study (62), ten subjects received 100% Azone in a poroplastic patch, along with a control patch containing water only. Patches were applied in the foregoing, 5 days weekly for 21 days, to the same sites. None of the subjects reacted to either treatment.

In a third study (62), 26 subjects were exposed to 46% Azone incorporated into occluded Webril patches, applied 5 days weekly for 21 days. Estimates of skin irritation on a 5-point scale were made daily at the time of patch removal. Low irritancy potential was seen.

A study of 12 subjects was conducted to assess the correlation of two physiological measures of skin irritation, transepidermal water loss and cutaneous blood velocity, with traditional visual measures of irritation (62). Each subject had 12 test sites, 6 on each side of the back. One concentration of sodium lauryl sulfate (1%) and five concentrations of Azone (0, 1, 3, 10, and 30%) were used; each concentration was applied to duplicate sites, one on each side of the back. The six sites on one side of the back were covered with a Webril patch, and the six sites on the other side were left uncovered. Measurements of irritation were conducted at baseline, 7, 14, and 21 days.

The sites without patches were unaffected by all treatments, whereas the sites with patches containing sodium lauryl sulfate (1%) and 10 and 30% Azone were irritated. The physiological measures, transepidermal water loss, and cutaneous blood velocity, proved no better in detecting irritation than visual scoring.

2. Modified Draize Skin Sensitization Study

To evaluate the potential for Azone to induce irritation and sensitization, a repeat-insult patch test was performed on 200 subjects (62) by using the modified Draize method (64). Test patches with 50% Azone were applied with occlusion to the same site, three times, for a 3 week induction period. Two weeks later, the same kind of patch was applied to a site not previously exposed to Azone. After 2–3 days, the challenge patch was removed, and the degree of inflammation was evaluated. There was no evidence of allergic contact sensitization. During the induction phase, mild irritation of the stratum corneum was observed.

3. Photoirritative (Phototoxic) Study

The photoirritative (phototoxic) potential of 100% Azone was investigated in ten normal subjects (62) by using a modification of the Marzulli procedure (65). Test sites were prepared by tape stripping and then were moistened with 100% Azone; 1 hr later, the sites were irradiated by using the Woods Light Inspectolamp for 45 min at 23 cm. After 24 hr the test sites were evaluated. No evidence of photoirritation was observed.

4. Modified Photo Draize Skin Sensitization Study

The potential of 100% Azone for irritation and photosensitization was assessed by using a repeated-insult patch test on 25 normal subjects (62); the modified Draize procedure (as discussed earlier) was used. The test site was irradiated when each patch was removed. A challenge patch was applied for 24 hr to a new test site not previously exposed or irradiated, and then the new site was irradiated. Four days later the challenge site was evaluated. No evidence for allergic or photoallergic contact sensitization was observed.

In summary, clinical studies demonstrate that human skin can tolerate repeated applications of Azone over an extended period. Irritation tends to be associated with the use of high concentrations of Azone and with the use of occlusive patches on the application site.

B. Absorption, Metabolism, and Excretion Studies

Two studies were conducted to examine the absorption, metabolism, and excretion (ADME) of radioactively labeled Azone in the same three adult male volunteers. In the first study (2), 3.70 MBq of ^{14}C-labeled Azone was applied to 16 cm^2 of forearm skin, allowed to stand uncovered for 4 hr, and wiped off to recover any unabsorbed Azone. Blood samples, urine, and feces were collected for 5 days; and the stratum corneum was sampled by tape stripping 28 times at 5, 24, and 48 hr after application of the Azone.

Most of the applied radioactivity was recovered from the skin surface (92.5, 97.7, and 64.8% for the three subjects), and less than 1% was absorbed. Most of the radioactivity detected in the skin strippings was found in tape strips that sampled the outermost layers of the stratum corneum, 5 hr after application. By 24 and 48 hr, only a trace of radioactivity was detectable in skin strippings. These results indicate that most of the Azone remaining in the skin was restricted to the stratum corneum.

No radioactivity was detected in the blood, and very little was recovered from urine (0.132%) and feces (0.005%). Excretion in urine and feces was nearly complete after 5 days, with more than 94% of the excreted radioactivity found in the urine.

In the second study (14), 2.75 MBq of ^{14}C-labeled Azone was applied to 24 cm^2 of skin, and the area was occluded for 12 hr before wiping away the unabsorbed material. Use of a larger area of application, a longer application time, and a waterproof covering was expected to promote absorption of the Azone into the skin. Urine samples were extracted in methanol and analyzed by using high-performance liquid chromatography (HPLC) to detect metabolites of Azone. Recovery of radioactivity from the unabsorbed material was consistently high in this study (greater than 95% in all three subjects). Mean absorption appeared slightly higher than in the previous study, but was still minimal; 0.409% of the applied radioactivity was recovered in urine and 0.003% in feces. Urinary excretion again accounted for most (97%) of excreted radioactivity. Several metabolites of Azone were detected in urine that was collected within 24 hr of the application; only a trace of unchanged Azone was present.

The results of these two studies demonstrate that pure Azone is poorly absorbed into the body. Although Azone rapidly penetrates into the stratum corneum, it does not accumulate in the skin. The trace that is absorbed appears to be readily metabolized and excreted in the urine.

C. Examples of Clinical Applications

Azone has been used as a vehicle for both hydrophilic and lipophilic medications with topical or transdermal application (32). Classes of compounds that have been formulated with Azone include antibiotics, antihistamines, beta-blockers, bronchodilators, corticosteroids, neuroleptics, and nonsteroidal anti-inflammatory drugs. Two examples of clinical applications of Azone are summarized here: its use with methotrexate, a water-soluble antimetabolite; and its use with triamcinolone, a lipophilic corticosteroid.

1. Methotrexate

Methotrexate is an antimetabolite that is used in the systemic treatment of certain neoplastic diseases, adult rheumatoid arthritis, and severe psoriasis. Because of the extreme toxicity of this drug, its use in the treatment of psoriasis is restricted to patients for whom the condition is both severe and insufficiently responsive to less extreme forms of therapy. There would be obvious advantages in a method for administering methotrexate that could concentrate the drug at the site of action, the skin, while minimizing systemic exposure. As a water-soluble medication, however, methotrexate alone does not readily penetrate the stratum corneum; and initial efforts to treat psoriasis with local application of methotrexate were unsuccessful. The use of Azone as a vehicle for topically applied methotrexate was investigated in a pilot study of 42 adults with psoriasis vulgaris (66).

Four treatments were used: 3% Azone in a gel formulation with methotrexate at either 0.1, 0.5, or 1.0%; or the 3% Azone formulation alone. Each subject received two different, randomly assigned treatments on separate sites. Test medications were applied to 25 cm^2 sites of affected skin, twice daily, for 6 weeks. The test sites and untreated sites were scored weekly during therapy, and again 1 week after therapy was concluded. A 5-point scale for degree of erythema, scaling, and elevation was used. Scores for these measures were summed and compared with baseline values to assess the degree of improvement. Complete blood cell counts were performed weekly. Laboratory tests, including blood chemistry, urine analysis, and serum methotrexate levels, were performed at baseline, 3 and 7 weeks.

All treatments, including Azone alone, were associated with progressive improvement over the 6 week treatment period. Vehicle-only preparations for psoriasis commonly show short-term alleviation of symptoms, possibly owing to nonspecific moisturizing effects. In all groups, improvement reached a maximum at 6 weeks, and declined during the week after treatment ended. All treatment sites were significantly ($p < 0.001$) improved over untreated sites during all 6 weeks of therapy. At 6 weeks, improvement of the sites treated with 0.1% methotrexate was significantly greater ($p < 0.05$) than improvement of the sites treated with only Azone.

No systemic side effects were observed from the hematological and biochemical profiles; furthermore, methotrexate was not detected in the serum, suggesting that most or all of the applied drug remained at the site of treatment. The lack of improvement at untreated sites provides further evidence that the observed therapeutic effects occurred locally in the skin. These preliminary results suggest that Azone may facilitate the percutaneous penetration of methotrexate.

The pharmacokinetic characteristics of a topical 1% methotrexate–3% Azone gel were assessed in nine patients with moderately severe psoriasis (67). Methotrexate was applied every 12 hr for 3.5 days to psoriatic lesions, drug was discontinued, and after at least a 5 day washout period, patients received 5 mg orally every 12 hr for three doses. Methotrexate concentrations in serum and urine were measured by a kinetic enzyme assay based on the competitive inhibition of dihydrofolate reductase. The total area under the curve (AUC) was calculated using the trapezoidal rule. Percutaneous absorption was calculated from urinary excretion. Preliminary determinations for the AUC ranged from 35.1 to 101.6 ng/hr·mL^{-1} (mean 65.6 ng/hr·mL^{-1}) for day 4 of methotrexate topical application compared with 362.6–614.88 ng/hr·mL^{-1} (mean 491.8 ng/hr·mL^{-1}) for the first day of oral methotrexate. The AUC for oral methotrexate was 1.6–25.9 times that seen after treatment with topical methotrexate. The range for maximum methotrexate serum concentration with topical methotrexate on day 4 was 4.1–33.2 ng·mL^{-1} versus 60.4–160.8 ng·mL^{-1} with oral drug or 4–30 times lower on topical compared to oral drug. Percutaneous absorption of methotrexate ranged from 0.01 to 1.2% of the administered dose.

Adverse side effects of the topical preparation were primarily transient pruritus and burning and stinging in psoriatic lesions in six patients. Interestingly, after only 4 days of topical therapy, one patient showed no change, one patient had moderate improvement and seven patients had slight improvement of their psoriasis.

Increased penetration of methotrexate in the presence of Azone, has also been recently demonstrated in vitro, thereby confirming the in vivo findings (68).

2. Trimacinolone

Triamcinolone is a synthetic corticosteroid with a variety of systemic and topical applications. The efficacy of triamcinolone preparations with and without Azone was assessed in clinical studies of two dermatological disorders, psoriasis vulgaris and atopic dermatitis (62).

Psoriasis Adults with psoriasis vulgaris (n=160) were randomized into three treatment groups; triamcinolone acetonide 0.05% plus Azone 1.6%, triamcinolone 0.05% alone, and Azone 1.6% alone. Subjects applied test medication to all lesions twice daily for 6 weeks. Subjects were evaluated for severity of the disease at baseline; days 8, 15, 29, and 43 of treatment; and 2 weeks after treatment ended (day 57). Erythema, induration, and scaling were rated by using a 7-point scale, and global change in disease status was rated by using a 6-point scale.

All treatments, including Azone alone, were associated with improvement over baseline; there was, however, a slight decline after treatment ended. After 6 weeks of treatment, improvement did not differ significantly between triamcinolone plus Azone and triamcinolone alone. Patients treated with triamcinolone plus Azone showed significantly greater improvement after 6 weeks of treatment than those treated with Azone alone; treatment with triamcinolone alone and with Azone alone did not differ in effect after 6 weeks. No serious adverse events occurred, and reports of treatment-emergent adverse experiences did not differ among the three treatment groups.

Atopic Dermatitis Adults with atopic dermatitis (n=150) were randomized into three treatment groups; triamcinolone acetonide 0.05% plus Azone 1.6%, triamcinolone 0.05% alone, and Azone 1.6% alone. Subjects applied test medication to all lesions twice daily for 2 weeks. Subjects were evaluated for severity of the disease at baseline; hour 6; and days 3, 8, and 15. Erythema, induration, and pruritus were rated by using a 7-point scale, and a global evaluation of change in disease status was made by using a 6-point scale.

Triamcinolone plus Azone was generally associated with greater improvement than triamcinolone alone at day 3 and day 7. At day 15, patients treated with triamcinolone plus Azone showed greater improvement than those treated with triamcinolone alone, and the difference was statistically significant. Furthermore, triamcinolone plus Azone was associated with significantly greater improvement than Azone alone from day 3 through day 15. During the same period, patients treated with triamcinolone alone showed significantly greater in some, but not all, of the measures than patients treated with Azone alone.

No serious adverse events were reported; and the most common treatment-emergent adverse experience reported, exacerbation of symptoms, was believed by the investigators to represent disease progression, rather than an effect of treatment.

D. General Exposure of Patients to Azone

A total of 650 persons have been exposed to Azone; 328 were exposed to 1.6%
Azone, and 322 were exposed to higher concentrations. Within the group exposed
to 1.6% Azone, the overall incidence of adverse experiences was 17.7%; more
than half of these events were either "exacerbation of disease" (4.9% of total
subjects) or "itching/pruritus" (4.6% of subjects), both of which could reflect
treatment failure, rather than side effects. Symptoms of local irritation reported by
more than one subject were "burning/stinging" (1.5%) and "soreness/tenderness"
(1.5%); only one subject reported simple "irritation" (0.3%).

Of the subjects exposed to concentrations of Azone higher than 1.6%, 200
received 50% Azone as part of the modified Draize skin sensitization study, and
an additional 35 received 100% Azone in the studies of phototoxicity and photoallergic sensitization. A somewhat higher incidence of adverse experiences
(37.6%) was observed in this group; these reports were all in the category of
"irritation" and were due to a grade 1 erythema rating in the repeat-insult patch
test. Overall, the side effects observed in numerous volunteers or patients exposed
to Azone appear to be of limited clinical consequence.

E. Conclusions

The ADME and safety studies that have now been conducted with Azone show
that this compound is nonirritative and nonallergenic. Azone is readily absorbed
into the stratum corneum, but does not appear to accumulate in the body; metabolism is rapid, and metabolites are excreted in the urine. When combined with
topically applied medications indicated for the skin disorders of psoriasis vulgaris
and atopic dermatitis, Azone is generally associated with a greater pharmacological effect than the primary drug alone, which suggests that Azone does
promote skin penetration of the drug. The results of these clinical studies indicate
that Azone may prove useful in the transdermal delivery of systemic medications,
as well as in improving the absorption of specific dermatological agents.

REFERENCES

1. Liron, Z. and Cohen, S. *J. Pharm. Sci.* 73:538–542 (1984).
2. Wiechers, J. W., Jonkman, B. F. H., and de Zeeuw, R. A. *Pharm. Res.* 4:519–523 (1987).
3. Katz, M. and Poulsen, B. J. In *Handbook of Experimental Pharmacology*, Vol. 28. Brodie, B. B. and Gillette, J. (eds.). Springer Verlag, New York, pp. 103–174 (1971).
4. Michaels, A. S., Chandrasekaran, S. K., and Shaw, J. E. *AICHE J.* 21:985–996 (1975).
5. Albery, W. J. and Hadgraft, J. *J. Pharm. Pharmacol.* 31:140–147 (1979).

6. Wertz, P. W. and Downing, D. T. In *Transdermal Drug Delivery*. Hadgraft, J. and Guy, R. H. (eds.). Marcel Dekker, New York, pp. 1–17 (1989).
7. Beastall, J. C., Hadgraft, J., and Washington, C. *Int. J. Pharm. 43*:207–213 (1988).
8. Lewis, D., and Hadgraft, J. *Int. J. Pharm. 65*:211–218 (1990).
9. Schückler, F. and Lee, G. *Int. J. Pharm. 70*:173–186 (1991).
10. Goodman, M. and Barry, B. W. *J. Pharm. Pharmacol. 37*(suppl.):1–80 (1985).
11. Hadgraft, J., Walters, K. A., and Wotton, P. K. *J. Pharm. Pharmacol. 37*:725–727 (1985).
12. Stoughton, R. B. and McClure, W. O. *Drug Dev. Ind. Pharm. 9*:725–744 (1983).
13. Wiechers, J. W. "Absorption, Distribution, Metabolism And Excretion Of The Cutaneous Penetration Enhancer Azone." PhD Thesis, University of Leiden, pp. 42–66 (1989).
14. Wiechers, J. W., Drenth, B. F. H., Jonkman, J. H. G., and de Zeeuw, R. A. *Int. J. Pharm. 47*:43–49 (1988).
15. Stoughton, R. B. *Arch. Dermatol. 118*:474–477 (1982).
16. Stoughton, R. B. *Proc. Third Int. Symp. Psoriasis*, pp. 397–398 (1982).
17. Bennett, S. L., Barry, B. W., and Woodford, R. *J. Pharm. Pharmacol. 37*:298–304 (1985).
18. Oshima, T., Yoshikawa, H., Takada, K., and Muranishi, S. *J. Pharmacobiodyn. 8*: 900–905 (1985).
19. Ogiso, T., Ito, Y., Iwaki, M., Atago, H., Tanaka, C., Maniwa, N., and Ishada, S. *Chem. Pharm. Bull. 35*:4263–4270 (1987).
20. McCullough, J. L., Peckham, P., and Klein, J. *J. Invest. Dermatol. 85*:518–521 (1985).
21. Mirejovsky, D. and Takuri, H. *J. Pharm. Sci. 75*:1089–1093 (1986).
22. Goodman, M. and Barry, B. W. *J. Invest. Dermatol. 91*:323–327 (1988).
23. Ito, Y., Ogiso, T., and Iwaki, M. *J. Pharmacobiodyn. 11*:749–757 (1988).
24. Bond, J. R. and Barry, B. W. *J. Invest. Dermatol. 90*:810–813 (1988).
25. Adachi, Y., Hosoya, K., and Sugibayashi, K. *Chem. Pharm. Bull. 36*:3702–3705 (1988).
26. Sugibayashi, K., Hosoya, K.-I., Morimoto, Y., and Higuchi, W. I. *J. Pharm. Pharmacol. 37*:578–580 (1985).
27. Touitou, E. and Abed, L. *Int. J. Pharm. 27*:89–98 (1985).
28. Hosoya, K.-I., Shudo, N., Sugibayashi, K., and Morimoto, Y. *Chem. Pharm. Bull. 35*:726–733 (1987).
29. McCullough, J. L., Weinstein, G. D., and Lemus, L. L. *J. Invest. Dermatol. 81*:528–532 (1983).
30. McCullough, J. L., Weinstein, G. D., Douglas, J. L., and Berns, M. W. *Photochem. Photobiol. 46*:77–82 (1987).
31. Bucks, D. A. W., McMaster, J. R., Guy, R. H., and Maibach, H. I. *J. Toxicol. Environ. Health 24*:279–289 (1988).
32. Vaidyanathan, R., Rajadhyaksksha, V., Kim, B. K., and Anisko, J. J. In *Transdermal Delivery of Drugs*, Vol. 2. Kydonieus, A. F. and Berner, B. (eds.). CRC Press, Boca Raton, pp. 63–83 (1987).
33. Touitou, E. *Int. J. Pharm. 43*:1–7 (1988).

34. Sugibayashi, K., Nemoto, M., and Morimoto, Y. *Chem. Pharm. Bull. 36*:1519–1528 (1988).
35. Ogiso, T., Ito, Y., Iwaki, M., and Atago, H. *J. Pharmacobiodyn. 9*:517–525 (1986).
36. Priborsky, J., Takayama, K. and Nagai, T. *Pharm. Weekbl. Sci. Ed. 10*:189–192 (1988).
37. Priborsky, J., Takayama, K., Nagai, T., Waitzova, D., and Elis, J. *Drug Design Deliv. 2*:91–97 (1987).
38. Patel, R. A. and Vasavada, R. C. *Pharm. Res. 5*:116–119 (1988).
39. Okamoto, H., Hashida, M., and Sezaki, H. *J. Pharm. Sci. 77*:418–424 (1988).
40. Wotton, P. K., Mollgaard, B., Hadgraft, J., and Hoelgaard, A. *Int. J. Pharm. 1*:19–26 (1985).
41. Okamoto, H., Ohyabu, M., Hashida, M., and Sezaki, H. *J. Pharm. Pharmacol. 39*: 531–534 (1987).
42. Okamoto, H., Ohyabu, M., Hashida, M., and Sezaki, H. *J. Pharm. Pharmacol. 39*: 531–534 (1987).
43. Kondo, S., Mizuno, T., and Sugimoto, I. *J. Pharmacobiodyn. 11*:88–94 (1988).
44. Ogiso, T., Ito, Y., Iwaki, M., and Shintani, A. *J. Pharmacobiodyn. 11*:349–355 (1988).
45. Klein, J. A., McCullough, J. L., and Weinstein, G. D. *J. Invest. Dermatol. 86*:406–409 (1986).
46. Chow, D. S.-L., Kaka, I., and Wang, T. I. *J. Pharm. Sci. 73*:1794–1799 (1984).
47. Sheth, N. V., Freeman, D. J., Higuchi, W. I., and Spruance, S. L. *Int. J. Pharm. 28*:201–209 (1986).
48. Spruance, S. L., McKeough, M., and Sugibayashi, K. *Antimicrob. Agents Chemother. 26*:819–823 (1984).
49. Banerjee, P. S. and Ritschel, W. A. *Int. J. Pharm. 49*:199–204 (1989).
50. Banerjee, P. S. and Ritschel, W. A. *Int. J. Pharm. 49*:189–197 (1989).
51. Sekine, T., Machida, Y., and Nagai, T. *Drug Design Deliv. 1*:245–252 (1987).
52. Agrawala, P., et al. *J. Pharm. Sci. 77*:776–778 (1988).
53. Vaidyanathan, R., Flynn, G. L., and Higuchi, W. I. *Abstr. Pharm. Sci. 12*:126 (1982).
54. Okano, T., Miyajima, M., and Komadaet, F., et al. *J. Controlled Release 6*:99–106 (1987).
55. Shannon, W. M., Westbrook, L., Higuchi, W. I., et al. *J. Pharm. Sci. 74*:1157–1161 (1985).
56. Hoelgaard, A. *Second Int. Symp. Recent Adv. in Drug Deliv. Syst.* Salt Lake City, Utah (1985).
57. Liang, W. Q., Petersen, R. V., and Fang, S. M. *Proc. Int. Symp. Controlled Release Bioactive Materials* (13th) (1984).
58. Goldman, L., Gregory, R. O., and La Plant, M. *Lasers Surg. Med. 5*:453–456 (1985).
59. Bowman, W. C. and Rand, M. J. *Textbook of Pharmacology*, 2nd ed. Blackwell Scientific Publications, Oxford (1982).
60. Higuchi, W. I. *Abstr. Proc. Int. Symp. Recent Adv. Drug Deliv. Syst.* (1985).
61. De Clerq, E. *Antimicrob. Agents Chemother. 26*:155–159 (1984).
62. Whitby Research, Inc. Data on file.
63. Phillips, L., Steinberg, M., Maibach, H. I., and Akers, W. A. *Toxicol. Appl. Pharmacol. 21*:369 (1972).

64. Marzulli, F. and Maibach, H. *Adv. Mod. Toxicol. 4*:353 (1977).
65. Marzulli, F. and Maibach, H. *J. Soc. Cosmet. Chem. 21*:695 (1970).
66. Weinstein, G. D., McCullough, J. L., and Olsen, E. *Arch. Dermatol. 125*:227 (1989).
67. Olsen, E. A., Cato, A., Meyer, C., Baughman, S., and Allan, G. *Fifth Int. Psoriasis Symposium* (1991).
68. Brain, K. R., Hadgraft, J., Lewis, D., and Allan, G. *Int. J. Pharm. 71*:R9–11 (1991).

8

In Vitro Analysis of QSAR in Wanted and Unwanted Effects of Azacycloheptanones as Transdermal Penetration Enhancers

Harry E. Boddé, Maria Ponec, Ad P. IJzerman, A. Janet Hoogstraate, M. A. Ineke Salomons, and Joke A. Bouwstra

Leiden University, Leiden, The Netherlands

This study deals with the skin penetration enhancement and skin cell toxicity of Azacycloheptanones (Azones). The enhancement ratio for permeation across human stratum corneum in vitro increased sigmoidally with increasing azone alkyl chain length, for both nitroglycerin and the peptide DGAVP, with an inflection point at C_8 and C_{10}, respectively. Freeze-fracture electron microscopy, differential thermal analysis, and small angle x-ray diffraction all revealed increased disorder of the intercellular lipids with increasing azone alkyl chain length upon pretreatment of stratum corneum. In vitro inhibition of keratinocyte growth also became stronger with increasing azone alkyl chain length, hence there was parallelism between enhancement and cytotoxicity.

I. INTRODUCTION

Transdermal drug delivery systems and dermatological vehicles are greatly dependent for their efficacy on properly chosen skin penetration enhancers. In most cases, the rate limiting step for the inward penetration of the drug is in the stratum corneum. Consequently, the percutaneous or intracutaneous absorption of the drug may be slow and difficult to control. The use of skin penetration enhancers for decreasing the barrier capacity of the stratum corneum will not only increase the rate of drug absorption, but at the same time tend to convey a higher degree of rate control to the vehicle. An acceptable and applicable skin

199

penetration enhancer should ideally fulfill at least the following requirements
(1): its action should be specific, reversible, nontoxic, nonallergenic, and nonirritating. Hence, in a successful strategy for skin penetration enhancement, the
optimization of the unwanted effect (increased skin permeability) should go hand
in hand with minimization of the unwanted effects (irritant and allergic skin
responses.

An interesting class of potent enhancers are the N-alkylazacycloheptan-2-ones,
of which the dodecyl derivative (lauracapram, better known as Azone) (2) has
been shown to be very effective for both hydrophilic and hydrophobic drugs and
other agents (3). Although the mode of action of lauracapram and the other
azacycloheptanones is still under study, several papers which have appeared
in recent years have shed more light on this problem: strong indications exist
that azacycloheptanones directly interfere with the intercellular lipids in stratum
corneum, increasing the degree of order in their structure and hence rendering
them more permeable to a wide variety of agents (4–7).

Very little is known about the skin toxicity of laurocapram and other azacycloheptanones. In a recent study, Ponec et al. (8) have shown that a close correlation
exists between the in vitro skin cell toxicity of N-alkyl-azacycloheptanones on the
one hand, and their alkyl chain length on the other. It is the aim of this paper to
summarize the results of a set of structure-activity-relationship studies on wanted
and unwanted effects of azacycloheptanones on human skin, carried out in our
group. The studies deal with (a) effects on the skin barrier properties in vitro,
characterized by flux measurements, differential thermal analysis, small angle
x-ray diffraction, freeze-fracture electron microscopy and molecular modelling,
and (b) effects on in vitro cultured skin cells (keratinocytes and fibroblasts),
characterized by growth inhibition studies.

II. MATERIALS AND METHODS

A. Chemicals

9-Desglycinamide, 8-Arginine Vasopressin (DGAVP) citrate was a generous gift
of Dr. J. W. van Nispen (Organon international, Oss, The Netherlands). The
amino acid structure of this neuropeptide (Mw=1412) is:

H-Cys-Tyr-Phe-Gln-Asn-Cys-Pro-Arg-OH

The other permeant used was nitroglycerin p.a. (Merck, Darmstadt, Germany).

A number of N-alkyl-aza-Cycloheptanones (Azones) were synthesized by the
Department of Organic Chemistry (Leiden University, Leiden, The Netherlands),
including: ethyl-, hexyl-, octyl-, decyl-, dodecyl-, tetradecyl-, and hexadecyl-
Azone. The chemical structure of dodecyl-Azone is shown in Figure 5 (p. 211).

Propylene Glycol (PG) was obtained from J. T. Baker Chemicals B.V. (Deventer, The Netherlands). All chemicals used were of analytical grade and dissolved in freshly prepared bidistilled water. Purification and characterization of the azones has been described elsewhere (6).

B. Skin Preparation

The skin was prepared for the peptide permeation studies as follows.

Human inguinal skin was obtained from the Dutch Burn Society (Beverwijk, The Netherlands), from a 22 year old male donor. After removal of the sub-cutaneous fat, the skin was dermatomed at a thickness of about 200 μm and incubated on a filterpaper soaked in a 0.2% trypsin (Type III; from a bovine pancreas) solution in isotonic Phosphate Buffered Saline (PBS, pH=7.4) for 24 hours at 37°C. By this splitting technique the stratum corneum can be separated from the underlying epidermis. Because the remaining trypsin might effect the integrity of the stratum corneum and also interfere with peptide stability, the stratum corneum was subsequently treated with a 0.2% solution of trypsin inhibitor (Type II-S from soybean; Sigma Chemicals, The Netherlands) in PBS. Then the stratum corneum was dried and stored in a desiccator over sillicagel.

Before use the stratum corneum was punched into circular samples of 14 mm diameter and hydrated to a relative humidity of 50% at room temperature over a PBS solution of pH 7.4 (10). To this buffer penicillin and streptomycin were added to prevent bacterial growth, and amphotericin B to prevent fungal growth. Dialysis membrane disks (cut-off value: 5000 Da, Diachema Switzerland) with a diameter of 18 mm were placed on each side of the stratum corneum to avoid tissue damage. The dialysis membranes did not influence the peptide transport through the stratum corneum. When a penetration enhancer was used, the prehydration was followed by pretreatment with the enhancer. For that purpose the stratum corneum samples were submerged in the enhancer solution (PG, as a cosolvent, or a 0.15 M solution of the enhancer in PG) for 24 hours at room temperature. Thereafter the pretreated stratum corneum was sandwiched between two dialysis membrane disks.

For the nitroglycerin flux studies, SAXD, DTA, and FFEM studies, the stratum corneum samples were prepared likewise from full thickness human abdominal skin obtained from cosmetic surgical corrections.

For the SAXD and DTA studies, the stratum corneum samples were immersed in 0.15 M azone/PG mixtures for 24 hours.

For FFEM they were treated by applying about 200 μl of the 0.15 M solutions on the top surface for 24 hours under occlusion.

For the nitroglycerin flux studies, 200 µl of 10% azone solutions in PG were applied on the top surface of the stratum corneum samples for 24 hours in a closed chamber at 95% Relative Humidity.

C. Permeation Studies

Peptide flux studies were carried out as follows.

A sandwich of human stratum corneum and dialysis membranes was clamped horizontally in a diffusion cell made of poly-tetra-fluoro-ethylene (9), with a stirred donor compartment, initially containing 1 ml of a 5 mM solution of the peptide in PBS. The area of diffusion was 0.79 cm^2. The isotonic PBS solution (pH=7.4) was pumped through the acceptor compartment at a rate of 1 ml per hour and samples were collected at hourly intervals for 18 or 19 hours with a fraction collector. Experiments were performed at 33°C. Collected fractions were stored at −20°C until analysis.

For nitroglycerine permeation studies the pretreated/prehydrated stratum corneum samples were sandwiched between two (non-ratelimiting) silastic sheeting membranes (10), whereupon the sandwich was clamped in the diffusion cell. The aqueous nitroglycerin donor solution, prepared by a twenty-fold dilution of a 1% ethanolic solution of nitroglycerin, finally contained 0.05% nitroglycerin and 5% ethanol. Peptide- or nitroglycerine concentrations in the effluents collected from the acceptor chambers were determined, and the data analyzed as described in references (6) and (10).

D. Small Angle X-ray Diffraction (SAXD) and
Differential Thermal Analysis (DTA)

1.   Small Angle X-ray Diffraction

All measurements were carried out at the Synchrotron Radiation Source at Daresbury Laboratories using Station 8.2. This station has been built as part of an NWO/SERC agreement. A more detailed description of the equipment is given elsewhere (15). The diffraction patterns were normalized with respect to synchrotron beam decay and absorption of the sample using two ion chambers. The stratum corneum, approximately 5 mg in weight was put in a sample cell. The orientation with respect to the primary beam was approximately at random.

The scattering intensities are plotted as a function of Q defined as $Q = 4 \pi \sin \Theta/\lambda$, in which Θ is the scattering angle and $\lambda (= 0.15$ nm) the wavelength. At those Q-values at which a peak is located, Q is directly related to the repeat distance d, namely $Q = 2\pi/d$.

2. Differential Thermal Analysis

Approximately 20 mg of hydrated stratum corneum was used. All measurements were carried out in hermetically closed pans using a Maple Instruments differential thermal analyzer (Maastricht, The Netherlands). The scans were carried out in a temperature range from 0–130°C using a heating rate of 2°K/min. For further details see (7).

E. Freeze-Fracture Electron Microscopy

Small pieces of pretreated stratum corneum were cryo-fixed in liquid propane after having been folded in silver cylinders (12). The samples were fractured in a Balzers BAF 400. A thin layer of platinum (2.5 nm; 45°) and carbon (30 nm; 90°) were evaporated on the freshly broken surface of the samples in vacuo. The obtained replicas were cleaned with soluene (an 0.5 M solution of undecyl-dodecyl-dimethyl ammonium hydroxide in toluene) for at least one week. The soluene was removed by soaking the replicas in toluene for two days. The replicas were mounted on copper grids and examined in a Philips EM300 Electron Microscope operated at 80 kV.

F. Computations

Visualization and manipulation of Azone structures was performed with the molecular modelling program Chem-X (April 1989 update) running on a VAX 11/785 computer and employing a Pericom MX 7200 color display (Chem-X: Molecular Modelling System. Chemical Design Ltd., Oxford, U.K.). In order to save CPU time the hydrocarbon chain of the Azone molecule was shortened to yield N-propylazacycloheptan-2-one. The minimum energy conformation of this Azone analogue and subsequent conformational searches were computed on a Convex C-120 mini-super computer with the semi-empirical molecular orbital MOPAC program (Stewart, 1990). The AM1 Hamiltonian and Pulay's method of convergence were used.

The rotational flexibility between the ring system and the aliphatic side chain was studied as follows. The minimum energy conformation of 1-propylaza-cycloheptan-2-one calculated in MOPAC was used as a starting point for separate conformational searches also performed in MOPAC over two torsion angles (phi) with steps varying from 5 ($phi_{O6-C5-N4-C3}$) to 60 ($phi_{C1-C2-C3-N4}$), where C1, C2, and C3 are alkyl chain carbons, and C5 is the carbonyl C-atom next to the nitrogen in the ring, resp. The calculation of each step was started from the conformation found in the previous step. All other torsion angles in the molecule were allowed to relax fully.

G. In Vitro Cytotoxicity Assays

Three types of cytotoxicity assays have been carried out: (a) inhibition of pro-liferation of cultured human keratinocytes, (b) inhibition of proliferation of cul-tured human keratinocytes, and (c) inhibition of collagen contraction by human fibroblasts. An extensive description of these can be found in (8).

III. RESULTS AND DISCUSSION

A. Permeation Studies

The enhancement ratios obtained for nitroglycerin are given in Figure 1a, as a function of the pretreatments. The permeability coefficients of DGAVP are plotted similarly in Figure 1b. Enhancement factors obtained for the peptide are given in Table 1 for completeness.

By comparing the data obtained for the peptide and nitroglycerin, we notice that both give rise to a sigmoidal dependence of the enhancement effect on the chain length of the azone used, i.e., virtually no effect with short chain azones, and significant enhancement beyond a certain chainlength ('the inflection point'). The inflection point for nitroglycerine occurs at a shorter azone chain length than for the peptide. Beyond the inflection point the nitroglycerine enhancement factors yielded a plateau, those for DGAVP showed a maximum at C_{12} but remained significantly high for C_{14}.

Furthermore, the highest enhancement factor obtained for the peptide was higher than the one obtained for nitroglycerin (6,13). This is most likely not due to the difference in azone concentrations used (10% vs. 0.15 M), since 10% of the

Table 1 Permeabilities and Enhancement Factors of the Penetration of DGAVP through Human Stratum Corneum, Untreated or Pretreated with Enhancers

	Permeability ± S.D. (exp-11 cm/s)	Enhancement Factor ± S.D.
control	5.3 ± 2.1	1.00
PG	4.0 ± 0.8	0.75 ± 0.15
C_{14}-Azone	13.0 ± 0.9	2.45 ± 0.18
C_{12}-Azone	18.7 ± 1.9	3.53 ± 0.35
C_{10}-Azone	9.9 ± 0.6	1.86 ± 0.12
C_8-Azone	5.4 ± 0.6	1.03 ± 0.11
C_6-Azone	3.8 ± 0.2	0.71 ± 0.03

Data represent the mean S.D. of 3 experiments.

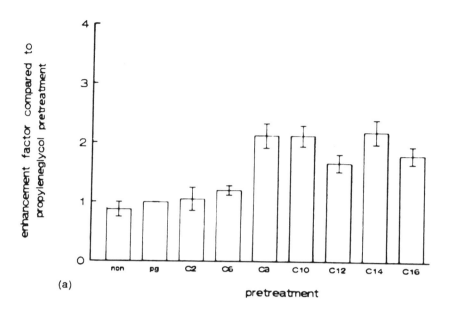

(a)

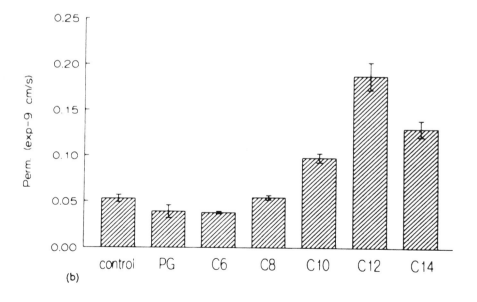

(b)

Figure 1 (a) Nitroglycerin flux enhancement ratios as a function of the azone pretreatments. (b) DGAVP permeabilities as a function of the azone pretreatments.

most potent one, dodecyl-azone, corresponds to about 0.35 M, so 0.15 M would (in a pretreatment) likely have produced an even smaller enhancement of the nitroglycerin flux.

In other words, the (much more polar) peptide 'requires' a more hydrophobic azacycloheptanone to enhance its flux, and 'profits' more from the improved skin permeability than does nitroglycerin.

B. Differential Thermal Analysis and Small Angle X-ray Diffraction

The essential results obtained with DTA have been compiled in Figure 2, which displays the gel-liquid transition enthalpies of the stratum corneum lipids as a function of the pretreatment with azones of increasing chain length. Interestingly, we observe a sigmoidal dependence of the enthalpy on the chain length, with an inflection point around C_8, probably indicating that only azones with chain lengths longer than C_6 interact strongly with the intercellular lipid bilayer structure, to the extent that the existing gel structure becomes disordered. It is important to note, that the PG pretreatment did not change the gel-liquid transition enthalpy of the stratum corneum lipids, hence it is likely that the effects obtained

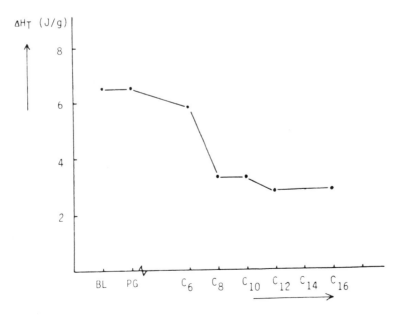

Figure 2 Lipid gel-liquid transition enthalpies vs. azone chain length.

with the PG/Azone mixtures should primarily be ascribed to the presence of the azones.

The SAXD observations (compiled in Figure 3) shed more light on the lipid structure perturbations induced by the pretreatments. Importantly, the PG pretreatment did not induce any significant change in the stratum corneum scattering curve in comparison to the control (Fig. 3a), not even in the position of the main diffraction peak, indicating that the lipid lamellae did not swell as a result of the treatment, and hence that the suggestion made in the literature (4) that PG would intercalate between the lamellae and thus facilitate the entrance of azone, is probably incorrect.

As a result of the Hexylazone/PG pretreatment the strong diffraction doublet (main peak, reflecting a 6.4 nm unit cell and the neighboring shoulder, reflecting a 13.4 nm unit cell, ref. 15) decreased in intensity, but maintained its position. This indicates that hexylazone interacted with the lipids in both unit cells without changing the interlamellar distances. Pretreatments with longer alkylazones resulted in stronger disordering and finally (with hexadecylazone) in complete disappearance of the doublet on the scattering curve. Thermal pretreatment studies (7) have indicated that the small shoulder observed in the scattering curve at the former main peak position upon treatments with octyl- or longer azones, most likely belongs to protein bound lipids, possibly those covalently bound to the cornified envelope (14). This would imply that the azones primarily perturb the intercellular, non-protein-bound lipids. Recently, Wide-angle X-ray diffraction (WAXD) studies confirmed the persistence of orthorhombic and/or hexagonal packing of the alkyl chains in the lipid bilayers upon dodecylazone/PG treatment, strongly suggesting that a lamellar structure, through perturbed, was still there (unpublished data).

Taken together, the DTA and SAXD observations suggest that PG does not, and PG/Hexylazone only moderately changes the stratum corneum lipid structure. They furthermore suggest that with increasing alkyl chain length (octyl, decyl, dodecyl and tetradecyl), alkyl-azones increasingly perturb the intercellular (non-protein-bound) lipid structure, by decreasing the order while maintaining lamellarity; with hexadecyl-azone the intercellular lamellar structure disappears. The disordering effect may be based on increased undulations and/or defects in the lamellar structure.

Four relevant FFEM micrographs are shown in Figure 4. The freeze-fracture procedure was designed such that almost perpendicular crossfractures through stratum corneum were obtained. Hence, the untreated control (Fig. 4a) displays crossfractured corneocytes, alternated by intercellular lipid domains, where the fracture plane runs partly along the lamellae (smooth surfaces), partly and step-wide across them (sharp cutting edges). The PG treatment alone does not change this pattern at all: only some of the PG tends to penetrate into the open spaces

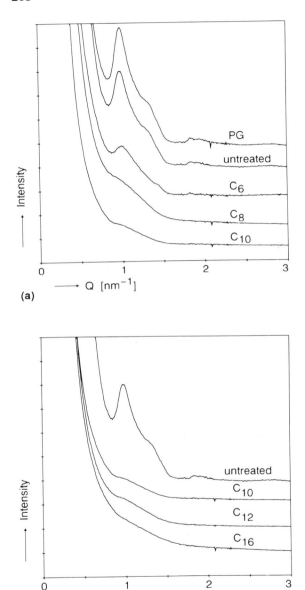

Figure 3 (a) Scattering curves of human stratum corneum after treatments with PG, C_6, C_8, or C_{10}. (b) After treatment with C_{10}, C_{12} and C_{16}.

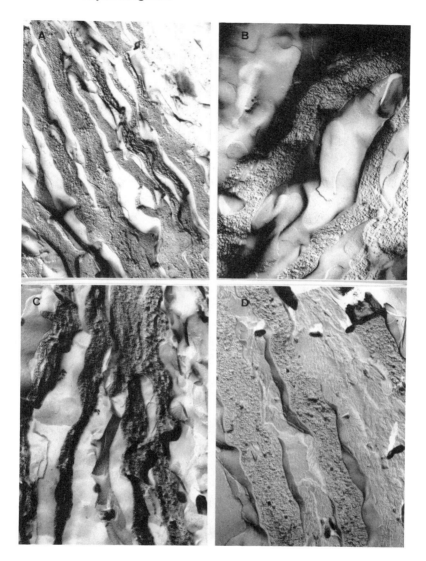

Figure 4 Electron micrographs of freeze-fracture replicas of (A) untreated (i.e., PBS treated), (B) PG treated, (C) PG/octylazone treated and (D) PG/dodecylazone treated human stratum corneum.

between the outer squames (compare Figs. 4a and b). Upon Hexyl-azone/PG treatment the intercellular lipids maintained their lamellar appearance, without defects. The fracturing behavior of the preparation on the surface was clearly different (not shown).

The Octyl-azone/PG treatment led to abnormal, disordered fracturing behavior in intercellular domains near the stratum corneum-preparation interface; further away from the interface, normal lamellar fracturing behavior could be observed (Fig. 4c).

Whereas the Decyl-azone treatment (not shown) looked like an aggravated version of the last treatment, the Dodecyl- (Fig. 4d) and Tetradecyl-azone (not shown) treatments both induced structural changes involving the entire inter-cellular domain except for border regions close to the cell envelopes. In all replicas the intercellular lipid material had a very disordered appearance, different from both the normal lipid structure and the topically applied preparation: fracture surfaces running parallel and close to the corneocyte surfaces were relatively smooth, but the crossfractures through the remaining intercellular material were very rough and revealed many notched, irregularly shaped edges. We interpret this intercellular material as a product of the interaction between the longchain azones and the intercellular lipids, having a disordered, irregular structure, which bears a vague resemblance to the original lamellar lipid phase but lacks regular lamellae. Such an appearance may well have been caused by crystal defects, induced by the azones.

C. Molecular Modelling

Recently, a spoon-shaped model of Azone has been proposed to account for its lipid disordering capability (6). This model was based on the crucial assumption, that the carbonyl moiety belonging to the amide group, being the strongest hydrogen bond former in the Azone molecule, would "try" to turn itself away from the lipid bilayer and into the polar region as much as possible. This would require a "twist" in the ring, almost inevitably pushing it upwards so as to create a "soup spoon" conformation. This conformation can be obtained by only imposing a torsion around the bond between the carbonyl-carbon and the adjacent nitrogen atom. We have included the corresponding energy calculations and the result shown in Figure 5 directly came forth from said assumption.

In fact the structure shown in Figure 5 was obtained by tilting the carbonyl group over 10 degrees from the minimum energy position.

The spoon conformation presented here should be easily attainable, since it is only 1 kcal/mol away from the minimum energy conformation; it would even become energetically favorable, when the carbonyl group would be able to form hydrogen bonds with polar groups facing it from an opposite head group region.

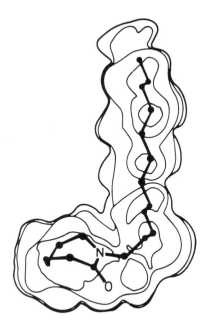

Figure 5 "Soup spoon" conformation with van der Waals contours of N-dodecylaza-cycloheptan-2-one, obtained by torsion of the peptide bond over 10 degrees, with phi(C_1-C_2-C_3-N_4) = 62 degrees.

The soup spoon conformation not only could provide a rationale for the flux enhancement by Azones, it might also explain why a minimal chain length would be needed: namely to ensure the required affinity of the Azone for the bilayer to make sure it inserts.

D.   Skin Cell Toxicity Assays

Figure 6 summarizes the results by showing the dependence of the observed IC_{50} values on the azone alkyl chain lengths. All three test methods used show a similar trend, i.e., a sharp decrease in IC_{50} from ethyl- to octyl-azone, followed by a plateau between octyl- and tetradecyl-azone, possibly indicating that the toxic effect of the azones is based on their interaction with the phospholipid membranes of the cells (keratinocytes or fibroblasts). With hexadecyl-azone, there seems to be a tendency for the IC_{50} to increase again, suggesting decreasing toxicity with increasing chainlength beyond C_{16}. Recently, DPPC/Azone mixed monolayer

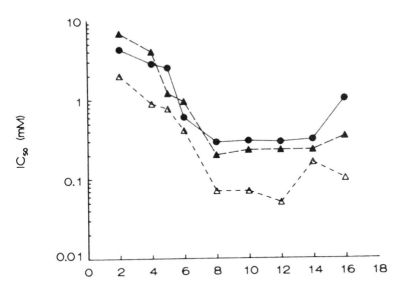

Figure 6 The IC_{50} values obtained from proliferation inhibition studies with keratinocytes (open triangles) and fibroblasts (dots) and from collagen contraction assays (closed triangles) upon administration of N-alkylazacycloheptan-2-one derivatives with increasing alkyl chain length.

studies using the dodecyl-, tetradecyl- and hexadecyl-azones, showed these to be capable of inducing expansion of the mixed monolayer over ideal mixing, dodecyl-azone being the most effective one. The expansive effect on phospholipid monolayers could be related to the 'soup spoon' conformation which might induce increased conformational freedom in the mixed monolayer; the same mechanism might be relevant for azone-mediated phospholipid membrane damage, and hence explain the toxic effect.

E. General Discussion

We have observed a sigmoidal chainlength dependence of the enhancement effects for DGAVP and nitroglycerine, as well as of the minimization of the lipid gel-liquid transition enthalpies, with inflections at C_{10}, C_8, and C_{10}, resp. This not only confirms the likelihood of the intercellular stratum corneum lipids constituting the major barrier component, but also strongly suggests that perturbation of the lipid structure by the azones is the common mechanism behind these observations.

The SAXD and freeze-fracture work has helped to clarify the nature of the lipid structure perturbations: the diffraction patterns clearly showed that the lamellar structure undergoes a disordering, which becomes more severe with increasing azone chainlength, while the interlamellar distances remain unchanged, up to the point where the entire lamellar structure disappears (C_{16}). The freeze-fracture electron micrographs generally confirmed this trend, suggesting that the lipid structure disordering effect most likely involved the induction of crystal defects and/or undulations in the lamellar lattice by strong interaction between the stratum corneum intercellular lipid and the azones. The 'soup spoon' conformation, which was shown to require relatively little energy, may provide a mechanism whereby the azones disrupt the ordering of the lipid lamellae: they would insert in the lipid bilayer (provided they have the critical chainlength required to do so) and subsequently disrupt the headgroup region with the bulky ring and hence induce extra conformational freedom in the lipid bilayer. The reason why DGAVP profits more from these structural changes in the intercellular lipid domain than does nitroglycerin is not clear: maybe Nitroglycerin partitions deeper into the lipid bilayer where the alkyl chain mobility is generally higher, while DGAVP tends to partition closer to the headgroup domain, where the bilayer is generally 'stiffer' and hence the insertion of an enhancer would have a relatively stronger effect.

Interestingly, the cytotoxicity studies showed a chainlength dependence of the IC_{50} values which generally follows the trend found with respect to the azone-stratum corneum interactions: the toxic effect increased with increasing chainlength, and showed a plateau beyond a certain inflection point (C_6–C_8). Hence the toxic effect (probably membrane-mediated) of the azones generally increases with increasing enhancement effect (most likely stratum corneum lipid mediated).

REFERENCES

1. Hadgraft, J., Penetration enhancers in percutaneous absorption, *Pharm. Int.* 5:252–254 (1984).
2. Stoughton, R. B., Enhanced percutaneous penetration with 1-dodecylazacycloheptan-2-one, *Arch. Dermatol.* 118:474–477 (1982).
3. Sheth, N. V., Freeman, D. J., Higuchi, W. I., and Spruance, S. L., The influence of Azone, propylene glycol and polyethylene glycol on in vitro skin penetration of trifluorothynidine, *Int. J. Pharm.* 28:201–209 (1986).
4. Barry, B. W., Mode of action of penetration enhancers in human skin, *J. Control. Rel.* 6:85–97 (1987).
5. Beastall, J. C., Hadgraft, J., and Washington, C., Mechanism of action of Azones as a percutaneous enhancer: lipid bilayer fluidity and transition temperature effects, *Int. J. Pharm.* 43:207–213 (1988).

6. Hoogstraate, A. J., Verhoef, J., Brussee, J., Ijzerman, A. P., Spies, F., and Boddé, H. E., Kinetics, ultrastructural aspects and molecular modelling of transdermal peptide flux enhancement by N-alkylazacycloheptanones, *Int. J. Pharm.* 76:37–47 (1991).

7. Bouwstra, J. A., Gooris, G. S., Brussee, J., Salomons-de Vries, M. A., and Bras, W., The influence of alkyl-azones on the ordering of the lamellae in human stratum corneum, *Int. J. Pharm.* 79:141–148 (1992).

8. Ponec, M., Haverkort, M., You Lan Soei, Kempenaar, J., Brussee, J., and Boddé, H. E. Toxicity screening of N-alkylazacycloheptan-2-one derivatives in cultured human skin cells: structure-toxicity relationships, *J. Pharm. Sci.* 78:738–741 (1989).

9. Tiemessen, H. L. G. M., Boddé, H. E., Van Koppen, M., Bauer, W. C., and Junginger, H. E., A two-chambered diffusion cell with improved flow through characteristics for studying the drug permeability of biological membranes, *Acta Pharm. Technol.* 34: 99–101 (1988).

10. Tiemessen, H. L. G. M., Boddé, H. E., Mollee, H., and Junginger, H. E. A human stratum corneum-silicone membrane sandwich to simulate drug transport under occlusion, *Int. J. Pharm.* 53:119–127 (1989).

11. Bouwstra, J. A., Peschier, L. J. C., Brussee, J., and Boddé, H. E., Effect of N-alkylaza-cycloheptan-2-ones including azone on the thermal behavior of human stratum corneum, *Int. J. Pharm.* 52:47–54 (1989).

12. Holman, B. P., Spies, F., and Boddé, H. E., An optimized freeze-fracture replication procedure for human skin, *J. Invest. Dermatol.* 9:332–335 (1990).

13. Boddé, H. E., Tiemessen, H. L. G. M., Mollee, H., and de Haan, F. H. N., Modelling percutaneous drug transport in vitro: the interplay between water, flux enhancers and skin lipids. In: *Prediction of Percutaneous Penetration*, R. C. Scott, R. H. Guy, and J. Hadgraft, eds.), IBC Technical Services Ltd., London, pp. 93–109 (1990).

14. Wertz, P. W., Swartzendruber, D. C., Kitko, D. J., Madison, K. C., and Downing, D. T., The role of corneocyte lipid envelopes in cohesion of stratum corneum, *J. Invest. Dermatol.* 93:169–172 (1989).

15. Bouwstra, J. A., Gooris, G. S., van der Spek, J., and Bras, W., Structural investigations of human stratum corneum by small-angle X-ray scattering, *J. Invest. Dermatol.* 97:1005–1012 (1991).

9

Oleyl Surfactants as Skin Penetration Enhancers

Effects on Human Stratum Corneum Permeability and In Vitro Toxicity to Cultured Human Skin Cells

Ron Kadir

Baselstreet, Tel Aviv, Israel

Harry L. G. M. Tiemessen

Sandoz AG Pharma Division, Basel, Switzerland

Maria Ponec, Hans E. Junginger, and Harry E. Boddé

Leiden University, Leiden, The Netherlands

Penetrant enhancer properties of oleyl surfactants with respect to drug transport through human stratum corneum in vitro were investigated under "occlusion simulation conditions," using nitroglycerin as a model penetrant. The permeation of nitroglycerin through stratum corneum, which was untreated or pretreated with solutions of the surfactants in propylene glycol (0.14 M) was enhanced the most by oleic acid (EF = enhancement factor = permeability ratio of the treated and untreated stratum corneum = 6). Among three oxyethylene oleyl ethers (EO-2⁻, EO-5, and EO-10 ether) the enhancement factor maximized at EO-5.

Epidermal keratinocytes growth inhibition studies using surfactants showed different surfactant chain length dependence. The toxicity of the oxyethylene oleyl ethers increased continuously with increasing oxyethylene chain length (i.e., their IC_{50} decreased). Furthermore, the toxicity of the EO-5 and EO-10 oleyl esters was an order of magnitude less than the toxicity of their ether analogues, probably due to enzymic degradation of the esters to the much less toxic oligo-oxyethylene and oleate moieties. Thus, this study leads to the interesting observation that a powerful skin penetration enhancer does not have to be strongly toxic for skin cells.

I. INTRODUCTION

Although the stratum corneum owes its barrier properties largely to its inter-cellular lipid it cannot be regarded as a simple lipid membrane due to its special composition and microstructure (1–4). It has been increasingly recognized that understanding the composition and function of the stratum corneum is essential for achieving safe and effective transdermal drug delivery. At the same time, intensive efforts have been made in order to select compounds capable of revers-ibly reducing the skin barrier resistance (5). Polar lipids such as CIS-unsaturated fatty acids have been shown to be effective enhancers for lipophilic or inter-mediate polarity drug molecules (6–8). Furthermore, they have been found less destructive to the skin than aggressive solvents such as dimethyl sulfoxide.

Nonionic surfactants are widely used in dermal formulations, primarily as stabilizers. Their effect on skin permeability has been determined for only a small number of drugs so far (9–14). The mode of action of nonionic surfactants as penetration enhancers is still unclear since, in most studies, no efforts have been made to distinguish between their direct effects on the skin barrier properties on the one hand and their effects on the thermodynamic activity of the penetrating species in the vehicle on the other. Lately, however, it has been demonstrated that both effects (termed "pull" and "push" effects, respectively) may operate jointly (15,16). First, it is quite likely that incorporating nonionic surfactants in topical preparations or transdermal patches will change the thermodynamic activity of the drug in the vehicle, and thereby lead to a positive or negative "push" effect. Second, some nonionic amphiphiles, especially those containing an oleyl chain, may conceivably penetrate into the highly ordered intercellular lipid structure of the stratum corneum and reduce its resistance by increasing lipid acyl chain mobility, for example (9,17), thus providing a "pull" effect.

In this study, the so-called stratum corneum silicone membrane sandwich model (18, 19) was used which permits the determination of "pull" effects of penetration enhancers (including water) on stratum corneum permeability, so that any push effects are excluded.

The potential skin irritancy of transdermal drug delivery systems or of their components is often a bottleneck in the development of these systems. Especially in the choice of penetration enhancers which is strongly limited by skin toxicity considerations. Primary irritancy often (but not always) arises from a direct interaction between the irritant and the viable skin cells. Special care must be taken with penetration enhancers, as they are usually applied under occlusive conditions at relatively high concentrations and may diffuse from the stratum corneum (their site of action) deeper down into the viable epidermis. The aim of the present work is to study the relationship between the molecular structures of various oleyl surfactants on the one hand and their skin irritancy and cell toxicity on the other.

II. MATERIALS AND METHODS

A. Materials

All reagents and chemicals were of the highest commercially obtainable purity. Oleyl surfactants containing ethylene oxide (EO) of various average chain lengths were obtained from ICI Chemicals (EO-2-oleyl ether, EO-10-oleyl ether), Servo b.v. (EO-5-oleyl ether, EO-5-oleyl ester) and Croda (EO-5-oleyl ether). Oleic acid was obtained from J. T. Baker (Holland). Oleyl alcohol from Fluka was distilled to obtain a purity of ~95%. The surfactants were used as a 0.14 M solution in propylene glycol from J. T. Baker, Holland. Nitroglycerin (1% ethanolic solution) was obtained from Merck. Polyethylene glycol 300 and 400 (EO-6 and EO-9, respectively) were obtained from Brocacef, Holland.

B. Skin Preparation

Full thickness human abdominal skin samples from cosmetic surgical corrections, was stored at 4°C (for a maximal period of 18 hours) before they were dermatomed (Padgett electro dermatome, model B) to obtain slices of about 120 μm thickness. The epidermal slices were then placed on a filter paper (stratum corneum side up), soaked in 0.2% solution of trypsine (Bovine pancreas type III, Sigma) in isotonic phosphate buffered saline (pH 7.4) and incubated for 24 hours, at 37°C. The stratum corneum was then carefully peeled off, rinsed with distilled water for several times and punched into 14 mm diameter disks. Each of the prepared stratum corneum samples was attached to a 18 mm diameter silicone membrane disk (Silastic™ 500-1, nonreinforced sheeting, 0.127 mm, Dow Corning, Michigan) using a thin layer of a silicon adhesive (Medical Adhesive X7-2920, Dow Corning). The samples were kept dry in a desiccator (for a maximal period of 3 months). Prior to any experiment, the stratum corneum was rehydrated for 48 hours in a constant humidity chamber at 95% Relative Humidity (over a saturated Na_2HPO_4 solution; the water weight fraction of the stratum corneum samples at equilibrium is 46 ± 2%). For the determination of the penetration enhancement effects, the rehydrated stratum corneum was pretreated with (i.e. submerged in) an 0.14 M surfactant solution in propylene glycol at 20°C, for 24 hours. After removing all residual material with a dry tissue, each skin sample was then covered with a second sticky silicone membrane and clamped between the donor and the acceptor chambers of a two chambered flow-through diffusion cell at 32°C. The diffusion area of the cells was 0.63 cm² and the volume of each chamber was 16 L. The donor phase, one liter of 0.05% nitroglycerin solution, was circulated through the donor chamber at a flow rate of 0.6 mL/min. The silicone membranes prevented excessive hydration of the stratum corneum and provided mechanical support: untreated stratum corneum took up only a limited amount of water throughout the diffusion experiments; the stratum corneum water content increased from 46 to 54% during 16 hours of diffusion (18). The acceptor perfusate (water) was pumped through the acceptor chamber at a flow rate of 5 mL/hr and collected periodically, by a fraction collector, at one hour intervals. Control experiments were carried out using the silicone double membrane only, without stratum corneum. For the determination of nitroglycerin in the acceptor perfusate, 50 L samples were injected directly into a reversed phase HPLC column (Chromspher C18 100 × 30 mm, chrompack) with a detector set at 201 nm. The mobile phase consisted of methanol/water (1:1 v/v) at a flow rate of 1.1 mL/min. Under these conditions, the retention time of nitroglycerin was 1.9 min.

C. Calculations

For multilaminar membranes under steady state conditions, the total resistance with respect to diffusable compounds equals the sum total of the resistances of separate laminae. Hence, the resistance (R) of the stratum corneum can be derived from the difference between the total diffusional resistance of the stratum corneum-silicone sandwich, R_t, and that of the double silicone membrane without the stratum corneum, R_m:

$$R_s = R_t - R_m \tag{1}$$

Since R is defined as the reciprocal P, the following equation also holds, permitting the calculation of the stratum corneum permeability, P_s:

$$P_s = (1/P_t - 1/P_m)^{-1} = (R_t - R_m)^{-1} \tag{2}$$

D. Cell Culture

SV-40 transformed keratinocytes (SVK_{14} cells) were cultured as described elsewhere (20,21). The culture medium was a mixture of Dulbecco's modification of Eagle's Essential Medium (DMEM) and Ham's F12 medium (3:1) supplemented with 5% fetal calf serum (FCS), 0.4 g/ml hydrocortisone, and 10^{-6} M isoproterenol.

E. Proliferation Inhibition Assay and Phase Contrast Microscopy

50,000 SVK_{14} cells were inoculated in a 6 well cluster (Costar) on day 0. On day 1, the medium was removed and the cells were refed with the culture medium to which increasing concentrations of the oleyl surfactants were added. On day 4, the cells were trypsinized and counted in a Rosenthal-Fuchs chamber. Each concentration was tested in duplicate. The number of cells with respect to the control (on a logarithmic scale) was plotted against the corresponding concentration of the enhancer in order to obtain a linear curve. The oleyl surfactant concentration at which the cell proliferation was inhibited to 50% of the untreated control (IC_{50}) was taken as a measure of cytotoxicity. Phase contrast micrographs of treated and untreated cultures were taken with an Olympus phase contrast microscope.

III. RESULTS AND DISCUSSION

A. Effects of Oleyl Surfactants on Stratum Corneum Permeability

Since the true effects of the penetration enhancers on the stratum corneum had to be determined while using the silicone membrane sandwich method, it was important that the penetration enhancer should not affect the permeability properties of the supporting silicone membranes. The data shown in Table 1 confirm that the effect of oleyl alcohol, which is one of the most effective penetration enhancers in this series, on the double silicone membrane is negligible.

In all cases, the flux of nitroglycerin across the stratum corneum-silicone membrane sandwich is lower than the flux across the silicone double membrane (empty sandwich) alone (Tables 1 and 2). It is clear that the rate-controlling barrier for the diffusion of nitroglycerin through the stratum corneum-silicone membrane sandwich is the stratum corneum itself.

Now consider the effects of the penetration enhancers as summarized in Table 2. Propylene glycol has only a small effect on the stratum corneum permeability:

Table 1 Enhancer Effect on Nitroglycerin Flux Through Double Silicone Membrane

Enhancer	Flux $(g/hr/cm^2)$	SEM	N^a	P $(cm/sec \times 10^6)$
Untreated	77.23	6.7	3	42.9
Oleyl alcohol, 0.14 M in propylene glycol	67.75	1.2	3	37.6

[a]Number of skin samples tested.

Table 2 Effects of Oleyl Surfactants on the Penetration of Nitroglycerin Through Human Stratum Corneum at 32°C

Enhancer[a]	Flux (g/hr/cm^2)	SD	N[b]	P_s[c] (cm/sec 10^{-6})	P_{sc} (cm/sec 10^{-6})	SD[d]	EF[e]
Untreated	6.9	0.6	3	3.83	4.2	0.4	
Propyleme glycol	8.3	1.0	3	4.6	5.1	0.7	1
EO-2-oleyl ether	14.1	2.6	3	7.83	9.6	2.1	1.9
EO-5-oleyl ether*	24.2	8.2	5	13.5	19.6	9.8	3.8
EO-10-oleyl ether	9.1	2.0	4	5.1	5.7	1.4	1.1
EO-5-oleyl ester	15.5	3.1	3	8.6	10.8	2.7	2.1
Oleic acid	33.3	4.5	3	18.5	32.5	8.6	6.4
Oleyl alcohol	24.4	5.2	3	13.6	19.8	6.3	3.9

[a]Pretreatments were performed with 0.14 M enhancer in propylene glycol for 24 hours.
[b]Number of stratum corneum samples tested.
[c]The permeability coefficient of the stratum corneum-silicone membrane sandwich for nitroglycerin.
[d]The stratum corneum permeability coefficient (calculated using Equation 2).
[e]The enhancement factor: (P_{sc} after surfactant treatment)/(P_{sc} propyplene glycol treated control).
*The surfactant was obtained from Servo bv. Similar results were found when Croda surfactant was used (21.9 ± 4.0 g/h/cm^2).

it causes a 1.2-fold increase. Therefore it can be considered as a suitable vehicle for the penetration enhancers.

The effects of the enhancers are expressed by the enhancement factor EF = (P_{sc} after surfactant treatment)/(P_{sc} propylene glycol treated control). For the EO-2$^-$, EO-5$^-$ and EO-10-oleyl ethers EF values of 1.9, 3.8, and 1,1 were obtained respectively. The enhancement effect of the EO-5-oleyl ester (EF = 2.1) is less than the effect of its ether analogue. Although the number of PEO-oleyl surfactants tested is too small to draw definite conclusions about the underlying mechanisms, the data suggest that under the conditions of this study, the enhancement effect by oxyethylene oleyl ethers maximizes at an optimal oxyethylene chain length or head group size between 2 and 10 oxyethylene units. If indeed one of the mechanisms by which oleyl surfactants enhance skin penetration is to increase degree of acyl chain disorder among the intercellular lamellar lipids (9, 17), then indeed an optimal headgroup size would be required to ensure (a) favorable partitioning of the surfactant into the intercellular lipid lamellae, and (b) sufficient perturbation of the local lipid arrangement.

Walters et al. (24) studied the effects of solutions of aqueous nonionic surfactants (0.1% w/v) of the PEO-alkyl ether type on the transport of methyl nicotinate across hairless mouse skin in vitro. They found an EF value for Brij96 of 1.8. In PEO-C_{16} ethers optimal penetration enhancement was observed at chain lengths between EO-6 and EO-14 (EF between 1.5–1.7) whereas the effect of EO-2 is very small (EF = 1.1).

There may be several reasons for the differences between the results obtained by Walters et al. and the results of the present study. In the first place, their experiments were conducted on hairless mouse skin that has permeability properties that differ from human skin and the physical structure of which deteriorates rapidly in these aqueous environments (25). Furthermore, Walters et al. observed that prolonged hydration already enhanced the stratum corneum permeability with respect to the very highly water soluble methyl nicotinate to such an extent (twofold) that after 24 hours no surfactant induced penetration enhancement effects were left. Hence relatively small effects of the surfactants may have been obscured by the large effects of the water on the skin.

Thirdly, an obvious reason for the differences might lie in differences in lipid composition between murin and human skin, as a result of which the partitioning and lipid structure perturbation by oleyl surfactants will depend differently on the headgroup properties.

In the present study both oleyl alcohol and oleic acid were found to be very effective penetration enhancers for the transdermal delivery of nitroglycerin: a 3.9- and 6.4-fold (Table 2) increase in penetration was observed, respectively, following the pretreatment of the stratum corneum with these compounds. The pretreatment with oleyl alcohol resulted in an increased steady state transdermal nitroglycerin flux (Fig. 1) while the pretreatment with oleic acid resulted in an even higher transdermal nitroglycerin flux over the first 10 hours, but after 10 hours the flux began to decline significantly. This might be explained by a gradual washout of oleic acid from the stratum corneum to the silicone membrane or the aqueous donor or acceptor phases. The water solubility of oleic acid is indeed higher than that of oleyl alcohol. Presumably, between 0 and 10 hours the enhancer concentration within the stratum corneum was still above a critical threshold.

B. Toxicity Screening

An important consideration in the testing and use of skin penetrant enhancers is to achieve a sensible balance between the desired effect (enhancement of drug flux) and any undesired side effects (skin irritation), the latter of which should be reduced as much as possible.

In order to provide for a well defined reproducible screening method, which permits the systematic investigation of the skin cell toxicity (a measure of primary

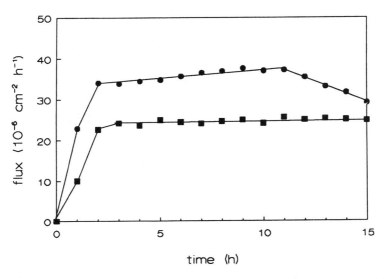

Figure 1 Typical graphs showing the flux of nitroglycerin from its 0.05% aqueous solution through human stratum corneum-silicone membrane sandwich following pretreatment with oleic acid (●) and oleyl alcohol (■).

skin irritancy) while avoiding the use of test animals, in vitro alternatives based on cultured human epidermal keratinocytes have been developed. In previous studies (22,23) three types of toxicity assay have been developed: (a) cell proliferation inhibition (fibroblasts and keratinocytes), (b) cell morphology changes, and (c) inhibition of fibroblast induced collagen contraction. The results of the three tests were found to be comparable and showed the same ranking order of cell toxicity for all the tested compounds: ethanol, propylene glycol, dimethylsulfoxide, dimethylformamide, polyoxyethylene-10-oleyl ether (in ranking order of cell toxicity) and N-alkyl-azacycloheptan-2-one derivatives. In this work toxicity screening was performed using a cell proliferation inhibition test on SV-40 transformed keratinocytes (SVK$_{14}$). Cell morphology was also studied using phase contrast microscopy. The results of the toxicity assays (Fig. 2) show increasing toxicity of the oleyl ethers with increasing ethylene oxide (EO) chain length. This effect might be attributed to increased damage to the exposed keratinocyte membranes. The IC$_{50}$ of the EO-5 and the EO-10 oleyl esters are equal and are an order of magnitude lower than those of their ether analogues. Since it is expected that the influence of the nature of the bond between the hydrophilic and hydrophobic moieties on the surface active properties will be relatively small, suggests that this 10 fold lower toxicity of the ester analogues

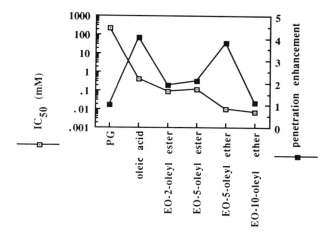

Figure 2 Skin cell toxicity and nitroglycerin skin penetration enhancement for oleyl-based surfactants.

may be the result of enzymatic hydrolysis of the ester bond. The breakdown of the surfactant leads to the formation of a polyoxyethylene fragment and oleic acid. Indeed, both oleic acid and polyethylene oxide are much less toxic than the corresponding surfactants (ester or ether), as shown in Figure 2. This phenomenon would make it possible to develop biodegradable skin penetration enhancers, that is, enhancers which remain largely intact and effective while in the stratum corneum, but would biodegrade as soon as they arrive in the more enzymatically active skin strata, such as the viable epidermis. The toxicity of the oleyl alcohol could not be determined due to its extremely low water solubility.

Figure 3 shows a correlation plot of the IC_{50} values versus enhancement factors for all the surfactants studied. In case of a perfect correlation between skin cell toxicity and drug flux enhancement, a hyperbola would be expected. This is clearly not the case, indicating that the two properties are not simply related to each other.

No changes in cell morphology could be observed at concentrations below the IC_{50}. However, a remarkable phenomenon was observed in the cell cultures containing oleic acid: as demonstrated in the phase contrast micrographs (Fig. 4), cells grown in a medium containing 2 mM oleic acid (Fig. 4b) contain lipid droplets (probably oleic acid) which accumulate on the cytosolic side of the nuclear envelope. The appearance of such lipid droplets may indicate that the cells deal with the excess amount of oleic acid "fed" to them, by storing it. No lipid droplets could be observed in control cultures (Fig. 4a).

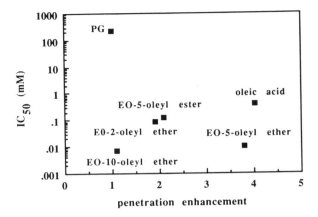

Figure 3 Non-correlation between penetration enhancement and skin cell toxicity.

IV. CONCLUSIONS

1. Oleic acid and oleyl alcohol are very effective penetration enhancers for the delivery of nitroglycerin through human stratum corneum.

2. It was shown that, compared with EO-10-oleyl ether, EO-2 and EO-5-oleyl ether solutions in propylene glycol significantly increase nitroglycerin transport through isolated human stratum corneum. In addition, EO-5-oleyl ether shows a greater enhancing effect than its ester analogues.

3. In the in vitro cell toxicity assay the EO-5- and EO-10 oleyl esters appear to be less toxic than their ether analogues, probably due to enzymatic degradation by the cultured skin cells. This observation immediately prompts the idea of developing biodegradable penetration enhancers.

4. The results of this study clearly show that highly effective penetration enhancers are not necessarily more toxic than less effective ones. In other words: there is no compelling reason for assuming a general correlation between enhancement properties on the one hand, and skin irritancy (primary cell toxicity) on the other.

ACKNOWLEDGMENTS

This work was partly supported by Squibb Derm, Biological Research Laboratory, Clwyd, United Kingdom.

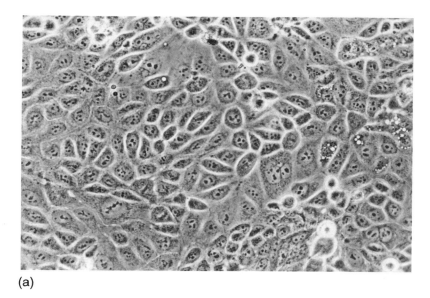

(a)

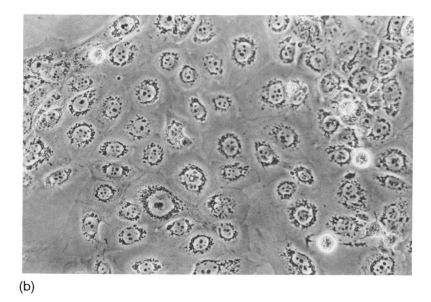

(b)

Figure 4   a) Control skin cell cultures and b) cultures grown in the presence of 2-mM oleic acid.

REFERENCES

1. Elias, P. M., Goerke, J., and Frind, D. S. Mammalian epidermis barrier layer lipids: composition and influence on structure. *J. Invest. Dermatol., 69*:535 (1977).
2. Wertz, P. W. and Dohning, D. T. Glycolipids in mammalians epidermis: structure and function in the water barrier. *Science, 217*:1262 (1982).
3. Ackermann, C., Flynn, G. L., and Smith, W. A. Ether-water partitioning and permeability through nude mouse skin in vitro. II. Hydrocortisone 21 n-alkyl ester, alkanols and hydrophilic compounds. *Int. J. Pharm., 36*:67 (1988).
4. Grubauer, G., Feingold, K. R., and Elias, P. M. Lipid content vs. lipid type as determinants of epidermal barrier function. *Skin Pharmacol., 1*:73 (1988).
5. Barry, B. W. Mode of action of penetration enhancers in human skin. *J. of Controlled Release, 6*:85 (1987).
6. Cooper, E. R. Increased skin permeability for lipophilic molecules. *J. Pharm. Sci., 73*:1153 (1984).
7. Hoelgaard, A., Moelgaard, B., and Baker, E. Vehicle effect on topical drug delivery. IV. Effect of n-methylpyrrolidone and polar lipids on percutaneous drug transport. *Int. J. Pharm. 43*:233 (1988).
8. Loftsson, T., Gildersleeve, N., and Bodor, N. The effect of vehicle additives on the transdermal delivery of nitroglycerin. *Pharm. Res., 4*:436 (1987).
9. Ashton, P., Hadgraft, J., and Walters, K. A. Effects of surfactants in percutaneous absorption. *Pharm. Acta Helv., 61*:228 (1986).
10. Walters, K. A., Walker, M., and Olejnik, O. Hydration and surfactant effects of methylnicotinate penetration through hairless mouse skin. *J. Pharm. Pharmacol., 37*:76 (1985).
11. Hwang, C. C. and Danti, A. G. Percutaneous absorption of flufenamic acid in rabbits: effect of dimethylsulfoxide and nonionic surface-active agents. *J. Pharm. Sci., 72*:857 (1983).
12. Ashton, P. and Hadgraft, J. Some effects of nonionic surfactants on topical availability. *J. Pharm. Pharmacol., 38*:70 (1986).
13. Hadgraft, J., Walters, K. A., and Wotton, P. K. Enhanced absorption through cadaver skin of sodium salicylate by long chain ethoxylated amines. *J. Pharm. Pharmacol., 38*:72 (1986).
14. Shen, W. W., Danti, A. G., and Bruscato, F. N. Effect of nonionic surfactants on percutaneous absorption of salicylic acid and sodium salicylate in the presence of dimethylsulfoxide. *J. Pharm. Sci., 65*:1780 (1976).
15. Kadir, R., Stempler, D., Liron, Z., and Cohen, S. The delivery of theophylline into excised human skin from alkanoic acids solution: a "push-pull" mechanism. *J. Pharm. Sci., 76*:774 (1987).
16. Kadir, R., Stempler, D., Liron, Z., and Cohen, S. Penetration of adeosine into excised human skin from binary vehicles: the enhancement factor. *J. Pharm. Sci., 77*:409 (1988).
17. Mak, V. H. W., Potts, R. O., and Guy, R. H. Oleic acid concentration and effect in human stratum corneum: non-invasive determination by attenuated total reflectance infrared spectroscopy in vivo. *J. Control Rel., 12*:67–75 (1990).

18. Tiemessen, H. L. G. M., Boddé, H. E., Mollee, H., and Junginger, H. E. A human stratum corneum-silicone membrane sandwich to simulate drug transport under occlusion. *Int. J. Pharm., 53*:119–127 (1989).

19. Tiemessen, H. L. G. M., Boddé, H. E., and Junginger, H. E. A silicone membrane sandwich method to measure drug transport through isolated human stratum corneum having a fixed water content. *Int. J. Pharm., 56*:87–94 (1989).

20. Taylor-Papadimitriou, J., Purkis, P., Lane, E. B., Mckay, I. A., and Chang, S. E. Effects of SV_{40}-transformation on the cytoskeleton and behavioural properties of human keratuinocytes, *Cell. Differ., 11*:169 (1982).

21. Ponec, M., Lavrijsen, S., Kempenaar, J., Havekes, L., and Boonstra, J. SV40-transformed (SVK_{14}) and normal keratinocytes: similarity in the expression of low-density protein, epidermal growth factor, glucocorticoid receptors, and the regulation of lipid metabolism, *J. Invest. Dermatol., 85*:476 (1985).

22. Ponec, M., Haverkort, M., Soei, Y. L., Kempenaar, J., and Boddé, H. E. Use of human keratinocyte and fibroblast cultures for toxicity studies of topically applied compounds. *J. Pharm. Sci., 79*:312–316 (1990).

23. Ponec, M., Haverkort, M., Soei, Y. L., Kempenaar, J., Brussee, H., and Boddé, H. E. Toxicity screening of N-Alkylazacycloheptan-2-one derivatives in cultured human skin cells: structure-toxicity relationships. *J. Pharm. Sci., 78*:738–741 (1989).

24. Walters, K. A., Walker, M., and Olejnik, O. Non-ionic surfactant effects on hairless mouse skin permeability characteristics. *J. Pharm. Pharmacol., 40*:525–529 (1988).

25. Van der Merwe, E. and Ackermann, C. Physical changes in hydrated skin. *Int. J. Cosmet. Sci., 9*:237–247 (1987).

10

Synergistic Effects in Percutaneous Enhancement

Birgitte Møllgaard

Pharmacia AS, Hillerød, Denmark*

I. INTRODUCTION

To use skin as an alternative route for drug administration, the drugs must be potent and have suitable physicochemical properties for efficient transdermal permeation to achieve therapeutic levels in the body. However, most drugs have suboptimal characteristics in this respect, and attempts to achieve full control of percutaneous absorption give rise to major problems, not only because of the relative impermeability of human skin, but also because of its considerably large biological variability.

One approach to render the skin more permeable is to administer a permeation enhancer along with the drug (for review, see 1–4). In the most simple form, the drug can be dissolved or dispersed in a solvent known to decrease the barrier function of the stratum corneum; for example dimethyl sulfoxide, ethanol, propylene glycol, and ethyl acetate, among others, have been used in this way. Another attempt is to use more lipophilic compounds, such as laurocapram (Azone) and derivatives thereof, long-chain alcohols, fatty acids and esters thereof, which probably penetrate the stratum corneum more slowly, but may have a more prolonged effect on the skin barrier resistance. However, it is most efficient to combine a simple solvent with a lipophilic component that by joint work delivers the drug at a requisite rate and degree into the skin.

A mixture of two or more solvents may affect the transport of a drug through the skin in different ways. Basically, the effects can be categorized as follows:

Current affiliation: Department of Pharmaceutical Development, H. Lundbeck A/S, Copenhagen-Valby, Denmark

(a) change in the thermodynamic activity (e.g., by increasing the degree of saturation in the vehicle and, hence, increasing the escaping tendency); (b) specific
interaction with the stratum corneum, either by increasing the drug solubility in
the stratum corneum (i.e., facilitate partitioning of drug from the vehicle into the
skin) or by altering the various pathways (i.e., the polar and nonpolar pathways) of
the stratum corneum.

It can be difficult to distinguish between the possible modes of action, and
several may be active at the same time. Different experimental setups have been
employed to identify the distinction between drug–vehicle interactions and
vehicle–skin interactions. These comprise (a) the use of saturated solutions of
drugs to maximize the thermodynamic activity, (b) the use of pretreatment of the
skin with the enhancer formulation before application of the drug, and (c) the use
of skin membranes derived from the stratum corneum. Examples of these methods
will be given in the following.

The purpose of this review is to excerpt from the literature examples in which
two or more permeation enhancers in mixture have been shown to act synergistically in percutaneous enhancement. A true synergistic effect is achieved when
the combination of penetration enhancer elicits a greater effect than the individual
components used alone. However, for practical reasons the definition is expanded
to comprise all examples for which two or more permeation enhancers in a
mixture have worked well together in increasing the transport of drugs into and
through the skin.

II. PENETRATION ENHANCERS NOT INCLUDED IN THIS CHAPTER

Several compounds will be discussed in detail in the individual chapters elsewhere
in this volume; therefore, they will not be commented on in the present chapter.
The compounds include: Azone and derivatives thereof, alkyl esters, surfactants,
terpenes, phospholipids, dimethyl sulfoxide and derivatives thereof.

III. PROPYLENE GLYCOL AS A VEHICLE

Propylene glycol (PG) is a commonly used solvent in topical formulations and an
efficacious cosolvent for other penetration enhancers (e.g., Azone, polar lipids,
and terpenes; 5–9). Thus, it is appropriate to sum up the current knowledge about
PG's mode of action in skin penetration enhancement.

Propylene glycol fulfills several requirements for an ideal penetration enhancer;
it is nonvolatile, has good solvent properties for many hydrophilic as well as
lipophilic drugs, and it has a transient enhancing effect on skin permeation under
suitable conditions. It has become an appropriate vehicle for a great variety of

drugs, for example, glucocorticoids (10), estradiol (11–15), metronidazole (5,14,15), and fluorouracil (12). The effect of PG as a penetration enhancer has been the subject of many discussions in the literature. It is well recognized that PG easily permeates both human skin (5,13,15) and rat skin (16). This observation led Kondo et al. to suggest that the enhancing effect of PG is caused by the constant change of the actual formulation, leading to a higher thermodynamic activity in the vehicle because of the disappearance of PG (16).

However, Barry et al. have shown that pretreatment of skin membranes with PG in vitro, 12 hr before application of a solvent-deposited dry drug film, increases the skin permeability of estradiol and fluorouracil, compared with the untreated skin. This must be the result of a direct effect of PG on the skin barrier function, probably owing to an increased drug solubility in the skin or an interaction with proteins of the stratum corneum, as verified by differential scanning calorimetry (DSC) (12,17). In another pretreatment study, PG did not increase the skin permeation, probably because of a prolonged time lag (i.e., 48 hr) between application of PG and the drug, estradiol (13).

Over the years, there has been some confusion about the effect of PG as a penetration enhancer. Thus, PG has alternately been called both an effective and an ineffective solvent used in the neat state. This discrepancy may be mainly due to differences in the research conditions. Consequently, in several instances, it has been observed that the effect of PG is most evident when the horny layer is not fully hydrated (i.e., under nonoccluded conditions; 10–12).

The effect of PG is highly influenced by other vehicle constituents. Therefore, addition of another glycol (e.g., glycerol) effectively reduced the effect of PG, whereas the permeation of estradiol was markedly enhanced by the addition of either hexadecanol or octadecanol (15). However, PG works very well with many components, and examples of these enhancer systems will be given in the following sections.

IV. FATTY ACIDS OR ALCOHOLS IN THE VEHICLE

Two-component systems, consisting of a hydrophilic solvent, such as propylene glycol, and a lipophilic molecule, such as fatty acids or alcohols, are very effective permeation enhancer systems for many drugs, including estradiol (12,18,22,28), progesterone (19), salicylic acid (6,20), acyclovir (7,21,22), narcotic analgesics (23), naloxone (24,25), hydrocortisone (19,22,26), 6-mercaptopurine (27), fluorouracil (12,18), triamcinolone acetonide (28), trifluorothymidine (22,28), nitroglycerin (22,29), retinoic acid (22), indomethacin (30,31), and metronidazole (8). Thus, these enhancer systems are well studied, and their ability to enhance permeation of both polar and nonpolar compounds is obvious.

However, the enhancing effect seems to be most pronounced for the more polar drugs. For example, addition of 2% oleic acid to propylene glycol had no effect on the permeability coefficient of estradiol, compared with propylene glycol in the neat state, whereas the same vehicle increased the permeability coefficient of acyclovir, a very polar compound, by a factor of about 140 (Table 1). On the other hand, by increasing the percentage of oleic acid in the vehicle by 10%, the permeability coefficient of 17β-estradiol was increased by a factor of 6 (22). Correspondingly, addition of either 5% oleic acid or 5% linoleic acid in propylene glycol had no effect on the permeation of another lipophilic compound (e.g., lidocaine; 21).

From the results in Table 1, it also appears that a choline ester (e.g., lauroyl-choline) acts synergistically with oleic acid. The effect of the ternary mixture of oleic acid, lauroylcholine, and propylene glycol on the permeation of both estradiol and acyclovir was much greater than the sum of the corresponding binary mixtures (e.g., oleic acid or lauroylcholine in propylene glycol; 22).

Metronidazole is a drug with intermediate polarity and, therefore, is susceptible to polar lipid–propylene glycol vehicles (8). Figure 1 illustrates the transport rate of metronidazole from vehicles containing an increasing percentage of polar lipids up to 10% in the PG vehicles. The results show that all of three polar lipids— linoleic acid, oleic acid, and oleyl alcohol—produce an enhanced drug permeation. [Direct comparisons are not possible because of varying permeation hours.] Addition of only a small amount of oleyl alcohol to the PG vehicle provides a rather large increase in the metronidazole transport. As the concentration of oleic acid or linoleic acid is increased, the drug transport is also increased, up to a point.

Table 1   Effect of Oleic Acid (OA) and Lauroylcholine Iodide (LCI) on the Permeability of 17β-Estradiol and Acyclovir Through Hairless Mouse Skin In Vitro From Saturated Solutions in Propylene Glycol (PG) Vehicles[a]

	17β-Estradiol		Acyclovir	
Vehicle	C_d[a] (mg/mL)	P/P_{PG}[b]	C_d (mg/mL)	P/P_{PG}[b]
PG	101	1.0	8.13	1.0
PG + 2% v/v OA	123	1.3	4.93	138.6
PG + 2% w/v LCI	95	6.9	5.29	ND[c]
PG + 2% v/v OA + 2% w/v LCI	128	14	5.08	404.5

[a]C_d is the solubility of drug in the vehicle at 35°C and P is the permeability coefficient.
[b]P_{PG} (17β-estradiol) = 4.91×10^{-6} cm/hr; P_{PG} (acyclovir) = 2.02×10^{-5} cm/hr.
[c]Not detectable.
Source: Ref. 22.

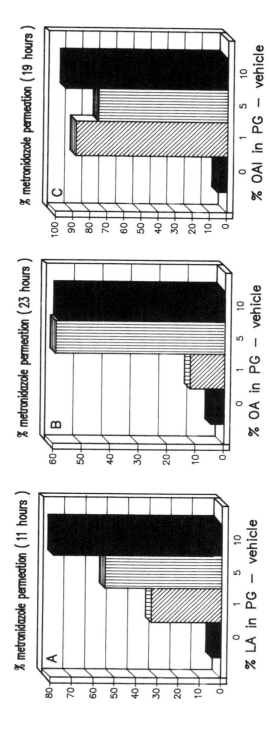

Figure 1 Effect of addition of polar lipids on the permeation of metronidazole in propylene glycol vehicle across human skin in vitro. LA, linoleic acid; OA, oleic acid; OAl, oleyl alcohol. (From Ref. 8)

233

For example, PG with 10% linoleic acid, gives a 30-fold increase in the transport rate (see Fig. 1).

Most of the studies on fatty acid penetration enhancers have focused on oleic acid, and to a lesser extent, linoleic acid. Both oleic acid and linoleic acid are unsaturated fatty acids with a *cis*-configuration. Accordingly, it has been proposed that the effects of these compounds are associated with the linked structure owing to the *cis* double bond (3,6,20). The enhancement effect of a series of octadecenoic acids was assessed by measuring the flux of salicylic acid through porcine stratum corneum. It was found that a greater flux is achieved with the *cis*- than with the corresponding *trans*-isomer, and that the enhancing effect increased with increasing distance of the *cis* double bond from the carboxylic group (20).

However, in a profound study on the structure–effect relation of fatty acid isomers, Aungst and coworkers found that the corresponding *trans*-isomers to oleic acid, elaidic acid, and to linoleic acid, linolelaidic acid, had substantially the same effect on the skin penetration of naloxone as the *cis*-isomers. Furthermore, they found that saturated acids, also, but to a much lesser extent, enhance the penetration rate, with an optimum at C_9–C_{12} chain length, for which the flux of naloxone was increased 20- to 40-fold. Branched saturated fatty acids were superior to unbranched compounds in only one case. Thus, isostearic acid (C_{18}), branched at a position distant from the carboxylic acid group, was significantly more effective in enhancing the naloxone flux than was the stearic acid. However, this was not true for the isostearic acid branched in a position proximal to the carboxylic acid group. This indicates the possibility that some branched fatty acid isomers may have an effect on skin permeation different from unbranched isomers, depending on the position or chain length of the branch (24,25).

Diols other than propylene glycol have been used in mixtures with oleic acid; for example, 1,2-butanediol and 1,2-hexanediol. But, although an effect of the mixed system on salicylic acid permeation compared with the solvent used alone was observed, the enhancing ability was much less than for propylene glycol as the base solvent (6). Correspondingly, oleic acid gave far less enhancement of the permeation of 17β-estradiol, triamcinolone acetonide, and trifluorothymidine, when propylene glycol was replaced by 2-ethyl-1,3-hexanediol (28).

It is now well accepted that the mechanism by which fatty acids in mixtures with, for example, propylene glycol increase the skin permeability involves an interaction with the intercellular lipids in the stratum corneum. Alteration of the lipid bilayers has been assessed using differential scanning calorimetry (DSC) and Fourier transformation infrared spectroscopy (FTIR) (3,17,20,32,33). These methods indicate that the enhancer system causes a disruption of the ordered lamellar structure of the biolayers in the stratum corneum, leading to an increased fluidization of the intercellular medium. It is likely that propylene glycol enhances the oleic acid penetration, and oleic acid promotes the propylene glycol permeation. This mutual effect could thus result in a more rapid diffusion of the drug molecules across the skin.

V. ESTERS OF FATTY ACIDS OR ALCOHOLS IN THE VEHICLE

Isopropyl myristate (IPM) is a commonly used oily liquid in topical preparations, and mixtures of IPM and PG have been effective vehicles for some drugs (e.g., nicorandil and nicardipine; 34,35).

In a comprehensive study on nicorandil permeation across hairless rat skin, Sato et al. (34) examined the effects of a series of binary mixtures of IPM and PG. Figure 2a shows the relationship between the IPM content and the pseudo–steady state flux. The flux was markedly increased by addition of 1% IPM, compared with that of the neat PG vehicle, and was kept approximately constant up to 50% IPM. However, to maximize thermodynamic activity, the drug was applied in saturated solutions. The solubility of nicorandil varied with the IPM content and, to compensate for this, the permeability coefficient can be estimated (i.e., the flux divided by the drug solubility in the vehicle). Figure 2b shows the approximate relation between the IPM content and the permeability coefficient of nicorandil. The results clearly demonstrate the paradox of using either flux or the permeability coefficient to evaluate the vehicle effect. Thus, from the permeability coefficient relationship, 10% IPM–PG seems to be equivalent to neat IPM. However, from the flux relationship, it is obvious that the 10% IPM–PG delivers 20–30 times more nicorandil through the skin per hour than neat IPM. The difference between the 10% IPM–PG vehicle and the neat PG vehicle, as seen with full-thickness skin, vanished when the skin was deprived of the stratum corneum by stripping. Therefore, it was suggested that IPM had a direct effect on the stratum corneum. The influence of different isopropyl esters, with varying chain length (C_3, C_5, C_7, C_{13}, and C_{15}) on nicorandil permeation was also investigated in mixtures with PG. Isopropyl myristate showed an intermediate effect, whereas isopropyl butyrate and isopropyl hexanoate were twice as effective.

In another study with adenosine, IPM in mixtures with propionic acid was used as a vehicle. The permeability coefficient of adenosine was increased with increasing content of IPM. Thus, the permeability coefficient of adenosine was increased fivefold by addition of 25% IPM, compared with neat propionic acid (36).

Several homologues of midrange n-alkyl fatty acid esters in a mixture with alcohol have been evaluated as potential enhancers of skin permeability. In the series, ranging from C_6 through C_{12}, optimal enhancement of minoxidil transport across hamster skin occurred with the methyl nonanoate (C_9) and methyl caprate (C_{10}). Thus methyl caprate produced a sevenfold increase in the amount of minoxidil absorbed, compared with neat alcohol as a vehicle, and the methyl

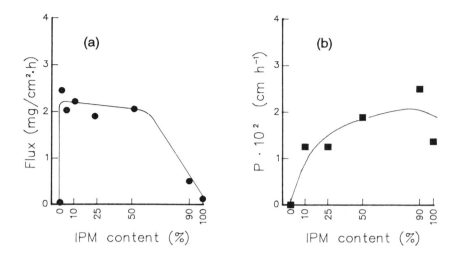

Figure 2 Effect of isopropyl myristate content in isopropyl myristate–propylene glycol vehicles on the permeation rate of nicorandil (a) and permeability coefficient of nicorandil (b) in hairless rat skin. (Data from Ref. 34)

esters were more effective than the corresponding ethyl and propyl esters (37). Besides minoxidil, methyl caprate enhanced the skin permeability of $1\alpha,25$-dihydrooxycholecalciferol, erythromycin, hydrocortisone, triamcinolone acetonide, and testosterone. At a fixed concentration of 10% in alcohol, methyl caprate produced a 7-, 21-, 8-, 5-, and 13-fold increase, respectively, in skin penetration of the drug through hamster ear skin (37).

To elucidate the enhancing effects of fatty alcohol–lactic acid esters, cetyl lactate was selected as a candidate to increase the percutaneous absorption of indomethacin through rat skin in vivo. Addition of 3% cetyl lactate to propylene glycol greatly increased the bioavailability of indomethacin by a factor of 170. It was suggested that cetyl lactate had a direct effect on the barrier function of the stratum corneum, as the PG vehicle without cetyl lactate and the PG vehicle with cetyl lactate yielded the same percutaneous absorption of indomethacin through skin from which the stratum corneum had been stripped (38).

VI. PYRROLIDONES AND UREAS IN THE VEHICLE

Many compounds identified as components of the natural moisturizing factor of stratum corneum have been evaluated as potential penetration enhancers. Most promising results have been obtained by using naturally occurring fatty acids or analogues thereof, as previously mentioned, but also pyrrolidones and urea have been investigated to some extent. The most widely studied derivatives of the naturally occurring pyrrolidone carboxylic acid are 2-pyrrolidone and N-methyl-pyrrolidone (NMP), which have been effective in enhancing the permeation of, among others, hydrocortisone; a polar model compound, mannitol (19); and indomethacin (39).

The effect of including 5% NMP in a hydrophilic vehicle, propylene glycol, and a lipophilic vehicle, isopropyl myristate, on metronidazole permeation has been investigated using full-thickness human skin in vitro. It appeared that the delivery of metronidazole was not unaffected by including NMP in propylene glycol, whereas NMP alone and in a mixture with isopropyl myristate promoted the drug permeation three- to fourfold, compared with neat propylene glycol. The marked difference in drug permeation from vehicles based on propylene glycol and isopropyl myristate cannot be due to differences in the thermodynamic activity in the vehicles, as the drug solubility in the vehicles is almost similar (Table 2). The permeation of metronidazole is linearly correlated with the permeation of the enhancer itself, NMP; therefore, it is assumed that the degree of NMP permeation plays a predominant role in drug transport through the skin (Fig. 3; 8).

The skin permeability of very large molecules, such as insulin, is extremely low, but improved permeation by means of penetration enhancer systems has been reported (40,41). Thus, in vitro transdermal absorption of insulin was improved when NMP was incorporated in aqueous PG through pig skin and rat skin vehicles. The maximum penetration efficacy depended on optimal concentrations of both NMP and propylene glycol. N-Methylpyrrolidone showed maximum efficacy at a concentration of about 10%, and the optimum concentration of PG was 40%. The use of the vehicle alone or of the penetration enhancer without the vehicle resulted in very low efficiency, whereas the combination of the vehicle and the penetration enhancer resulted in a pronounced effect (40,41).

Table 2 Comparison of 23 hr Permeation of Metronidazole From Various Vehicles Across Human Skin In Vitro

Vehicle	Enhancement ratio	Solubility of metronidazole $(mg \cdot g^{-1})$
A (PG)	1.0	18
B (NMP)	2.7	187
C (NMP/PG)	0.95	22
D (NMP/IPM)	3.8	25

Source: Ref. 8

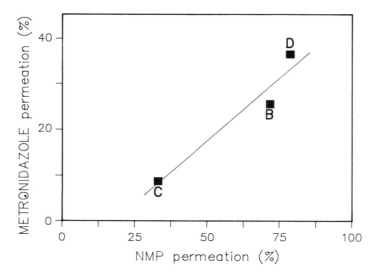

Figure 3 Comparison of a 23 hr permeation across human skin in vitro of metronidazole and *N*-methylpyrrolidone in percentage of amount applied from various vehicles. B, neat *N*-methylpyrrolidone vehicle; C, *N*-methylpyrrolidone–propylene glycol vehicle; D, *N*-methylpyrrolidone–isopropyl myristate vehicle. (Data from Ref. 8)

    Well-known penetration enhancers, such as Azone and decylmethyl sulfoxide, contain a medium-length hydrocarbon chain of C_{12} and C_{10}, respectively. Therefore, with the purpose of simulating their effect on the skin permeability, urea derivatives containing one or two similar alkyl groups, 1-dodecylurea and 1,3-didodecylurea, together with a derivative with two aryl groups, 1,3-diphenylurea, were synthesized (42). In Figure 4 the activity of the urea analogues is clearly demonstrated in terms of the enhancement ratios; that is, the ratio between the permeability coefficient of fluorouracil before and after application of the penetration enhancer system. The vehicles alone (i.e., liquid paraffin, dimethylisosorbide, and propylene glycol) and urea saturated in the vehicles produce no significant increase in the permeability coefficient of fluorouracil. Also no significant difference exists in the penetration activities of the three urea analogues in a given vehicle. However, the choice of a cosolvent for the urea analogues clearly affects the efficacy. In particular, when applied as a saturated solution in propylene glycol, the enhancement ratios of the urea derivatives are significantly greater than when applied saturated in dimethylisosorbide or liquid paraffin (42).

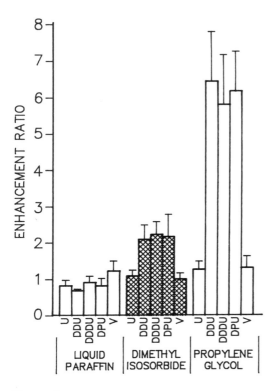

Figure 4 The mean enhancement ratios of urea and the analogues from the three vehicles on fluorouracil permeation across human epidermal membranes. U, urea; DDU, 1-dodecylurea; DDDU, 1,3-didodecylurea; DPU, 1,3-diphenylurea; V, vehicle alone. (From Ref. 42)

VII. CONCLUSION

Many compounds act as penetration enhancers because of their ability to pass into the skin and, in so doing, reversibly decrease its resistance to drug passage. The range of enhancers discovered so far indicates that many commonplace substances in the pharmaceutical or cosmetic industries might be effective. Propylene glycol, a solvent widely used in topical formulations, is highly effective as a cosolvent for many potent penetration enhancers. However, propylene glycol is not generally applicable as a cosolvent. For example, N-methylpyrrolidone is active only in very high concentrations in propylene glycol, whereas lower concentrations are needed in isopropyl myristate. The use of penetration enhancers in high concentrations will increase the risk of dermal toxicity.

In the past, the risks of irritative or contact allergic effects of penetration enhancers have received only little attention, and it has been more or less implied that local toxicological effects are inseparably linked to the effect as a penetration enhancer. However, in a structure–effect study of fatty acid isomers in propylene glycol vehicles, no distinct correlation between the naloxone skin penetration enhancement and the irritation potential of the vehicles was found. The importance of this is that some penetration enhancers can increase the skin permeability, but not at the expense of causing irritation (25).

Another area that is receiving growing attention is the possible biotransformation of drugs and other compounds during their passage through the skin. Current knowledge about the metabolizing capacity of skin has been exploited to increase the bioavailability of drugs by designing prodrugs that, after diffusion into and through the skin, undergo enzymatic reconversion into the parent active drug molecules. Another approach to increase the bioavailability of drugs that are subject to degradation in the skin would be to administer a compound along with the drug that inhibits the enzyme activity. The possible interaction between the penetration enhancers and the enzyme systems of skin await future investigation.

REFERENCES

1. Woodford, R. and Barry, B. W. Penetration enhancers and the percutaneous absorption of drugs: An update. *J. Toxicol. Cutan. Ocular Toxicol.* 5:167–177 (1986).
2. Cooper, E. R. and Berner, B. Penetration enhancer. In *Transdermal Delivery of Drugs, Vol. 2*. Kydonieuss, A. F. and Berner, B. (eds.). CRC Press, Boca Raton, p. 57 (1987).
3. Barry, B. W. Action of skin penetration enhancers—the lipid protein partitioning theory. *Int. J. Cosmet. Sci.* 10:281–293 (1988).
4. Walters, K. A. Penetration enhancers and their use in transdermal therapeutic systems. In *Transdermal Drug Delivery*. Hadgraft, J. and Guy, R. H. (eds.). Marcel Dekker, New York, p. 197 (1989).
5. Wotton, P. K., Møllgaard, B., Hadgraft, J., and Hoelgaard, A. Vehicle effect on topical drug delivery. III. Effect of Azone on the cutaneous permeation of metronidazole and propylene glycol. *Int. J. Pharm.* 24:19–26 (1985).
6. Cooper, E. R. Increased skin permeability for lipophilic molecules. *J. Pharm. Sci.* 73:1153–1156 (1984).
7. Cooper, E. R., Merritt, E. W., and Smith, R. L. Effect of fatty acids and alcohols on the penetration of acyclovir across human skin in vitro. *J. Pharm. Sci.* 74:688–689 (1985).
8. Hoelgaard, A., Møllgaard, B., and Baker, E. Vehicle effect on topical drug delivery. IV. Effect of N-methylpyrrolidone and polar lipids on percutaneous drug transport. *Int. J. Pharm.* 43:233–240 (1988).
9. Barry, B. W. and Williams, A. C. Human skin penetration enhancement: The synergy of propylene glycol with terpenes. *Proc. Int. Symp. Controlled Release Bioactive Mater.* 16:33–34 (1989).

10. Bennett, S. L., Barry, B. W., and Woodford, R. Optimization of bioavailability of topical steroids: Non-occluded penetration enhancers under thermodynamic control. *J. Pharm. Pharmacol.* 37:298–304 (1985).

11. Møllgaard, B. and Hoelgaard, A. Permeation of estradiol through the skin—effect of vehicles. *Int. J. Pharm.* 15:185–197 (1983).

12. Goodman, M. and Barry, B. W. Lipid–protein-partitioning (LPP) theory of skin enhancer activity: Finite dose technique. *Int. J. Pharm.* 57:29–40 (1989).

13. Møllgaard, B. and Hoelgaard, A. Enhancement of cutaneous estradiol permeation by propylene glycol and dimethyl sulfoxide. *Arch. Pharm. Chem. Sci. Ed.* 12:71–78 (1985).

14. Møllgaard, B. and Hoelgaard, A. Vehicle effect on topical drug delivery. I. Influence of glycols and drug concentration on skin transport. *Acta Pharm. Suec.* 20:433–442 (1983).

15. Møllgaard, B. and Hoelgaard, A. Vehicle effect on topical drug delivery. II. Concurrent skin transport of drugs and vehicle components. *Acta. Pharm. Suec.* 20:443–450 (1983).

16. Kondo, S., Yamanaka, C., and Sugimoto, I. Enhancement of transdermal delivery by superfluous thermodynamic potential. III. Percutaneous absorption of nifedipine in rats. *J. Pharmacobiodyn.* 10:743–749 (1987).

17. Goodman, M. and Barry, B. W. Action of penetration enhancers on human stratum corneum as assessed by differential scanning calorimetry. In *Percutaneous Absorption Mechanisms—Methodology, Drug Delivery*, 2nd ed. Bronaugh, R. L. and Maibach, H. I. (eds.). Marcel Dekker, New York, pp. 567–593 (1989).

18. Goodman, M. and Barry, B. W. Action of penetration enhancers on human skin as assessed by the permeation of model drugs 5-fluorouracil and estradiol. I. Infinite dose technique. *J. Invest. Dermatol.* 91:323–327 (1988).

19. Barry, B. W. and Bennett, S. L. Effect of penetration enhancers on the permeation of mannitol, hydrocortisone and progesterone through human skin. *J. Pharm. Pharmacol.* 39:535–546 (1986).

20. Golden, G. M., McKie, J. E., and Potts, R. O. Role of stratum corneum lipid fluidity in transdermal drug flux. *J. Pharm. Sci.* 76:25–28 (1987).

21. Møllgaard, B., Hoelgaard, A., and Baker, E. Vehicle effect on topical drug delivery—effects of N-methylpyrrolidone, polar lipids and Azone on percutaneous drug transport. *Proc. Int. Symp. Controlled Release Bioactive Mater.* 15:209–210 (1988).

22. Loftsson, T., Somogyi, G., and Bodor, N. Effect of choline esters and oleic acid on the penetration of acyclovir, estradiol, hydrocortisone, nitroglycerin, retinoic acid and trifluorothymidine across hairless mouse skin in vitro. *Acta Pharm. Nord.* 1:279–286 (1989).

23. Mahjour, M., Mauser, B. E., and Fawzi, M. B. Skin permeation enhancement effects of linoleic acid and Azone on narcotic analgesics. *Int. J. Pharm.* 56:1–11 (1989).

24. Aungst, B. J., Rogers, N. J., and Shefter, E. Enhancement of naloxone penetration through human skin in vitro using fatty acids, fatty alcohols, surfactants, sulfoxides and amides. *Int. J. Pharm.* 33:225–234 (1986).

25. Aungst, B. J. Structure–effect studies of fatty acid isomers as skin penetration enhancers and skin irritants. *Pharm. Res.* 6:244–247 (1989).

26. Mirejovsky, D. and Takruri, H. Dermal penetration enhancement profile of hexa-methylenelauramide and its homologues: In vitro versus in vivo behavior of enhancers in the penetration of hydrocortisone. *J. Pharm. Sci.* 75:1089–1093 (1986).
27. Waranis, R. P., Siver, K. G., and Sloan, K. The solubility parameter of vehicles as a predictor of relative vehicle effects on the diffusion of 6-mercaptopurine. *Int. J. Pharm.* 36:211–222 (1987).
28. Loftsson, T., Gildersleeve, N., Soliman, R., and Bodor, N. Effect of oleic acid on diffusion of drugs through hairless mouse skin. *Acta Pharm. Nord.* 1:17–22 (1989).
29. Loftsson, T., Gildersleeve, N., and Bodor, N. The effect of vehicle additives on the transdermal delivery of nitroglycerin. *Pharm. Res.* 4:436–437 (1987).
30. Kaiho, F., Nomura, M., Makabe, E., and Kato, Y. *Chem. Pharm. Bull.* 35:2928–2934 (1987).
31. Chien, Y. W., Xu, H., and Huang, Y. Transdermal controlled administration of indo-methacin: Enhancement of skin permeability. *Pharm. Res.* 5:103–106 (1988).
32. Golden, G. M., Guzek, D. B., Harris, R. R., McKie, J. E., and Potts, R. O. Lipid thermotropic transitions in human stratum corneum. *J. Invest. Dermatol.* 86:255–259 (1986).
33. Barry, B. W. Mode of action of penetration enhancers in human skin. *J. Controlled Release* 6:85–97 (1987).
34. Sato, K., Sugibayashi, K., and Morimoto, Y. Effect and mode of action of aliphatic esters on the in vitro skin permeation of nicorandil. *Int. J. Pharm.* 43:31–40 (1988).
35. Seki, T., Sugibayashi, K., Juni, K., and Morimoto, Y. Percutaneous absorption enhancer applied to membrane permeation-controlled transdermal delivery of nicardipine hydro-chloride. *Drug Design Deliv.* 4:69–75 (1989).
36. Kadir, R., Stempler, D., Liron, Z., and Cohen, S. Penetration of adenosine into excised human skin from binary vehicles: The enhancement factor. *J. Pharm. Sci.* 77:409–413 (1988).
37. Chukwumerije, O., Nash, R. A., Matias, J. R., and Orentreich, N. Studies on the efficacy of methyl esters of *n*-alkyl fatty acids as penetration enhancers. *J. Invest. Dermatol.* 93:349–352 (1989).
38. Kaiho, F., Koike, R., Nomura, H., Hara, H., Maruoka, K., Mohi, M., and Kato, Y. Enhancing effect of cetyl lactate on the percutaneous absorption of indomethacin in rats. *Chem. Pharm. Bull.* 37:1114–1116 (1989).
39. Sugibayashi, K., Nemoto, M., and Morimoto, Y. Effect of several penetration enhancers on the percutaneous absorption of indomethacin in hairless rats. *Chem. Pharm. Bull.* 36:1519–1528 (1988).
40. Priborsky, J., Takayama, K., Nagai, T., Waitzová, D., and Elis, J. Combination effect of penetration enhancers and propylene glycol on in vitro transdermal absorption of insulin. *Drug Design Deliv.* 2:91–97 (1987).
41. Priborsky, J., Takayama, K., Nagai, T., Waitzová, D., Elis, J., Makino, Y., and Suzuki, Y. Comparison of penetration-enhancing ability of laurocapram, *N*-methyl-2-pyrrolidone and dodecyl-L-pyroglutamate. *Pharm. Weekbl. Sci. Ed.* 10:189–192 (1988).
42. Williams, A. C. and Barry, B. W. Urea analogues in propylene glycol as penetration enhancers in human skin. *Int. J. Pharm.* 36:43–50 (1989).

11

Supersaturated Solutions as Topical Drug Delivery Systems

Adrian F. Davis

SmithKline Beecham Consumer Brands, Weybridge, Surrey, United Kingdom

Jonathan Hadgraft

The Welsh School of Pharmacy, University of Wales, Cardiff, Wales

I. INTRODUCTION

This chapter describes the background to, and the use of, supersaturated solutions in topical drug delivery. First it is necessary to discuss why these systems have potential to improve topical drug delivery.

The effect of formulation, or vehicle, on drug bioavailability is much greater in topical drug delivery than in any other route of administration. The vehicle interacts with the drug and the skin to influence both rate and extent of absorption. With the exception of a few small volatile materials, topical drug delivery is slow owing to the relatively low permeability of the stratum corneum, the rate-limiting outer layer of the skin. Thus, in one aspect, supersaturated solutions, with their ability to increase percutaneous absorption beyond the limiting value of saturated solutions, have the potential to improve percutaneous absorption and clinical performance.

The combination of vehicle effects on both the drug and the skin and the intrinsic differences in skin permeability, both between subjects and between different body sites on a single subject, results not only in low, but variable, topical drug bioavailability being the standard for many current formulations. Studies on topical bioavailability in humans show approximately 40-fold differences from vehicle effects (1) and several hundredfold differences from variability in skin permeability within and between subjects (2). Despite clear acknowledgment of this variation in the development of transdermal devices with the incorporation of rate-controlling membranes, variable absorption remains, in general, the current standard for both local and regional topical delivery. Thus, in a further aspect, supersaturated solutions in combination with carefully selected low-concentrations, have the potential to provide efficacy, but with improved control of percutaneous absorption.

Clearly, any topical delivery system with the potential to enhance and control topical drug delivery is of interest. This chapter reviews the potential of vehicles using supersaturated solutions in topical drug delivery.

II. DRUG–VEHICLE INTERACTIONS IN TOPICAL DRUG DELIVERY

A. Theoretical Model of Higuchi

Figure 1 after Higuchi (3), shows a simple model relevant to percutaneous absorption when the rate-controlling barrier is in the outer layer of the skin and the vehicle does not interact with the skin. Under these conditions F, flux per unit area, is given by

$$F = \frac{D}{L} \times C_{\text{skin}} \qquad [1]$$

where C_{skin} is the concentration of the solute within the outer layer of the stratum corneum and D and L are the diffusion coefficient of the solute in, and the effective thickness of, the stratum corneum barrier, respectively.

Equation 1 assumes absolute sink conditions into the lower layers of the skin. Furthermore,

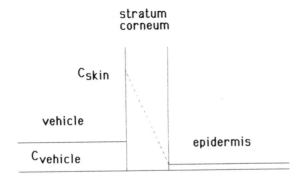

Figure 1 Schematic representation of the "Higuchi" model of percutaneous penetration.

$$C_{skin} = C_{vehicle} \times P_c \qquad [2]$$

where $C_{vehicle}$ is the concentration of solute in the vehicle and P_c is the partition coefficient of the solute between the vehicle and the stratum corneum. C_{skin} is the driving force for the diffusional process of percutaneous absorption.

Equation 2 is of fundamental importance in topical vehicle design, as it predicts that flux will be dependent on both concentration of solute in the vehicle and equally the physicochemical properties of the vehicle as these influence partitioning into the skin.

Topical vehicle design, in the past, has suffered from an overemphasis of the importance of concentration at the expense of vehicle optimization. As a result, many current formulations are poorly bioavailable; that is, they contain concentrations that are high compared with the fractional amount absorbed.

Under stable, equilibrium conditions, flux will be at a maximum when the outer layer of the skin is saturated and, by definition, this will occur when the vehicle is also saturated with solute. From Eq. 2, it is apparent that there is an inverse relation between the saturated solubility of the solute in the vehicle and the partition coefficient between that vehicle and the skin, such that for all saturated systems, their product is a constant, the saturated solubility of the solute in the stratum corneum (4).

$$C_{vehicle\,(saturated)} \times P_c = constant \qquad [3]$$

Equations 2 and 3 are the basis for the statement commonly found in the literature that all saturated vehicles of the same permeant will give the same flux, independently of concentration, provided that vehicle components do not alter the barrier function of the skin and that significant depletion of the permeant from the vehicle does not occur.

Equation 1 may be rewritten (3):

$$F = \frac{a \times D}{L\gamma} \qquad [4]$$

where a is the thermodynamic activity of the solute in the vehicle and γ is its activity coefficient in the membrane.

As all saturated solutions of the same solute, by definition, have the same chemical potential—that of the solid state—Eq. 4 also predicts they will give rise to the same flux. However, Eq. 4 also predicts the potential of supersaturated states to increase membrane flux beyond that from saturated systems.

B. Optimization Using Saturated Vehicles

From Eq. 2, both the concentration of drug in the vehicle and the partition coefficient of the drug between the vehicle and the membrane are important in optimization of membrane flux. At equilibrium, these parameters are optimized

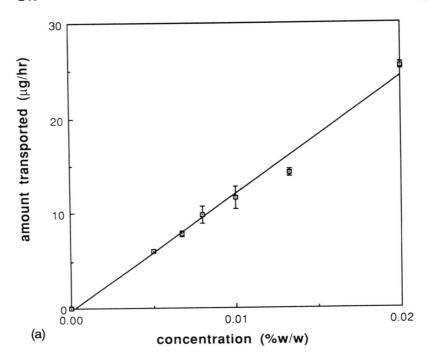

(a)

Figure 2 (a) Transport of hydrocortisone acetate from 0.005% to 0.02% w/w in a single vehicle: mean, $n = 3 \pm$ standard error. (b) Transport of 0.02% w/w hydrocortisone acetate from different propylene glycol–water vehicles: mean, $n = 3 \pm$ standard error. (c) Transport of hydrocortisone acetate from 0.005% to 0.08% w/w saturated vehicles: mean, $n = 3 \pm$ standard error. (From Ref. 5)

with the use of vehicles in which the drug is saturated. Figure 2 shows the in vitro flux of hydrocortisone acetate across a model polydimethylsiloxane membrane (5). Figure 2a shows the linear relation between flux and concentration for a fixed vehicle, thus, a constant partition coefficient. Figure 2b shows the corresponding linear relation between flux and partition coefficient for a fixed concentration. Figure 2c shows that membrane flux is the same for all saturated solutions, independent of concentration.

In a series of now classic publications on fluocinolone acetonide and its acetate ester, Syntex researchers showed that in vitro release, using a simple membrane–receptor phase (6) and human skin (7) and in vivo vasoconstrictor response (7) were dependent on both drug concentration and vehicle composition, and that flux was at a maximum from saturated systems.

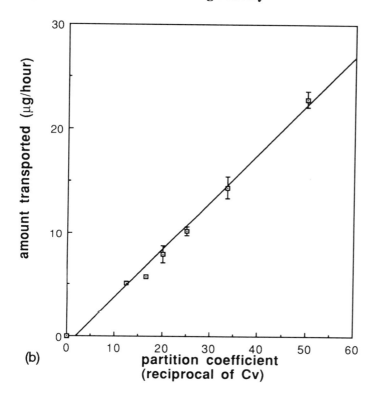

(b)

Since this early work many publications, using in vitro–release (8–12), in vivo human pharmacodynamics (1,11–14) and clinical study (15), have confirmed these findings.

Thus, and despite the complexity of human skin and the known interactions between topical vehicles and the skin membrane, drug–vehicle interactions are important in topical drug delivery, and achievement of saturation is of prime importance in vehicle design. Given the importance of drug–vehicle interactions and the potential of nonequilibrium high thermodynamic states to increase flux, these supersaturated states are reviewed in the next section.

III. SUPERSATURATION

A. Physicochemistry of Supersaturated Solutions

James (16) defines a *solution* as a molecular dispersion of a solute in a solvent. Under equilibrium conditions, a solution is capable of a continuous variation in

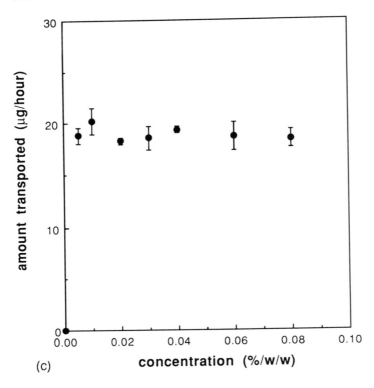

(c)

Figure 2 (Continued)

composition within limits. At the lower limit, the solution is represented by the pure solvent and, at equilibrium, the upper limit occurs when the solvent is incapable of dissolving any more solute and a second phase of undissolved solute is present. A solution in equilibrium with undissolved solute is known as a *saturated solution*. In saturated solutions, the thermodynamic activity of the solute is equal to that of the pure solute.

If the pure solute is a solid under the conditions of interest, this may be present in more than one crystalline form or polymorph. These polymorphs will have different melting points and enthalpies of fusion, which will contribute to different saturated solubilities of the polymorphic forms. Thus, one form may give rise to solutions that are deemed supersaturated relative to other forms. Normally, "supersaturated" solutions formed from higher-energy polymorphs will undergo phase changes to produce the solid lower-energy polymorph in equilibrium with its saturated solution. Amorphous solids without any regular crystalline structure will give rise to the highest levels of solubility, which may be considered super-saturated relative to all solid crystalline forms.

In the same way that polymorphic or amorphous solids can be used to generate solutions that are supersaturated relative to the equilibrium suspension state, supersaturated states may also be generated using the dependence of solubility on temperature, pH, and solvent composition, and utilizing changes in these. These are discussed in more detail in Section IV.

In terms of topical drug delivery and Eq. 2, supersaturated systems may be considered to be solutions in which the concentration in solution is high, compared with the value predicted from the stable equilibrium partition coefficient of the system or vice versa. Either way, the product of these terms exceeds the normal value, the outer layer of the skin is supersaturated, and the driving force for percutaneous absorption is increased.

B. Crystal Growth and Effects of Additives

A solution that contains concentrations of solute in excess of the saturated solubility of a lower-energy solid state will undergo a phase change to form a suspension of the lower-energy solid in equilibrium with its saturated solution. This process is known as recrystallization.

Excess solute in solution (i.e., supersaturation) will not, in itself, cause crystallization to occur. Crystallization in addition to supersaturation requires formation of nuclei of critical size and then crystal growth around the nuclei. Those who have used crystallization (e.g., in purification) will know of the importance of nucleation, in that solutions that have remained "stable" will suddenly recrystallize within seconds. The formation of a critical nucleus occurs by a process of random collision, the critical size depending upon the degree of supersaturation, among other factors.

Several theories exist to explain the process of crystal growth, and the mechanism is not fully understood and is likely to differ between systems. In diffusion theory, diffusion across a stagnant layer is proposed to be rate-controlling and, thus, crystal growth is seen as a reverse dissolution process. Bulk diffusion may be an important factor in control of crystallization in viscous systems. Miyazaki et al. (17) have proposed that the ability of sodium carboxymethylcellulose to inhibit the polymorphic transition of chlor-tetracycline may be due to an increase in viscosity. However, effects on microviscosity, rather than effects on macroviscosity as brought about by water-swellable polymers, are likely to be more important in inhibition of crystal growth.

The surface adsorption–diffusion theory, as developed by Frank (18), is most widely recognized and explains the remarkable effect of additives on inhibition of

Davis and Hadgraft

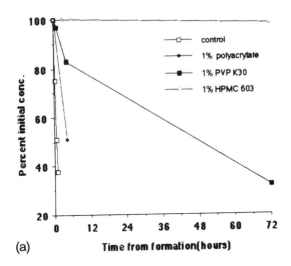

(a)

Figure 3 (a) Effect of polymer additives on concentration of hydrocortisone acetate in solution over time from 0.02% w/w eightfold supersaturated solutions of hydrocortisone acetate formed at $t = 0$. (b) Transport across polydimethylsiloxane membrane from supersaturated solutions measured over 60 min. (1) Transport 1 hr after formation of supersaturation; (2) transport 72 hr after formation of supersaturation. Note that relative transport at both 1 and 72 hr from the control and solutions with polymer additive is comparable with concentration in solution at these times in (a). (Adapted from Ref. 44)

crystal growth. A molecule landing on the flat surface of a crystal has only a single binding surface and, thus, dissolution may occur. For the molecule to be incorporated into the crystal surface, diffusion across the surface to a step or kink site is needed where binding occurs at multiple surfaces. Additives, especially polymers, that inhibit crystal growth are believed to do so by binding to, and thereby blocking, step and kink growth sites or by binding to the crystal surface to inhibit surface diffusion to growth sites (19).

Figure 3 shows the effects of polymer additives on the rate of crystal growth from highly supersaturated solutions of hydrocortisone acetate. Figure 3a shows hydrocortisone acetate concentrations in solution and Figure 3b release rates across a polydimethylsiloxane membrane with time. Similar results from the two analyses confirm that the polymers are not simply acting as solvents, but are stabilizing the supersaturated solutions. All of the polymers studied showed marked effects on crystal growth, with the 1% hydroxypropylmethylcellulose systems showing complete inhibition of crystal growth over 3 days, compared

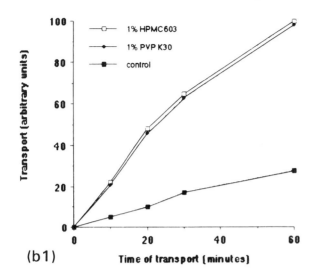

(b1)

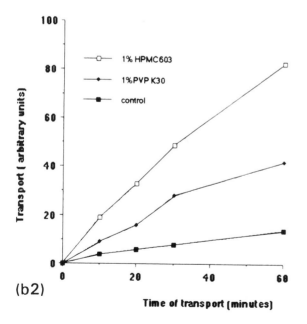

(b2)

with a 30 min half-life in the untreated system. More recent studies with this system show that crystal growth is not measurable after 1 month.

The ability of polymer additives to stabilize supersaturated solutions over useful periods is the key to the practical use of supersaturation in topical drug delivery. Examples of this will be apparent in the review of the literature on supersaturation in topical drug delivery.

In addition to polymer additives, compounds that are similar to the crystal molecule have been used to inhibit crystal growth by incorporation into and partial blocking—poisoning—of step and kink sites (20).

IV. USE OF SUPERSATURATION IN TOPICAL DRUG DELIVERY

A. Use of Changes in Vehicle Composition

Coldman et al. (21) were the first authors to demonstrate that volatile solvent systems could be used to generate supersaturated states and lead to increase in percutaneous flux. With an in vitro human skin model, they studied the penetration of fluocinolone acetonide and its acetate ester from solution vehicles containing the volatile solvent isopropanol combined with the less volatile solvent propylene glycol or nonvolatile isopropyl myristate. Relatively poor penetration was observed under conditions of occlusion, whereas under open conditions loss of the volatile components led to supersaturation and up to tenfold increase in flux. As the percentage volatile solvent was increased, the degree of supersaturation and flux also increased, up to the point at which precipitation of the steroid occurred. At this point, a rapid decrease in flux was seen. These early results clearly demonstrate the potential of supersaturation to increase membrane flux and also the critical requirement for physical stabilization of the supersaturated state.

Since this early work, others have confirmed these findings. Theeuwes (22) produced supersaturated solutions of hydrocortisone alcohol by evaporation of acetone from acetone–water solutions and studied their transport in vitro across an ethylene–vinyl acetate copolymer membrane. Fluxes were increased from the supersaturated solutions directly proportional to the degree of saturation. Seeding of the supersaturated solutions caused precipitation and a decrease in flux to the normal saturated solution value. Tanaka et al. (23) showed that evaporation of ethanol from an ethanol–propylene glycol–water gel resulted in supersaturation of hydrocortisone butyrate propionate and a corresponding increase in in vitro flux across a polydimethylsiloxane membrane. An interesting feature of this work is the demonstration that loss of water competes with the effect of loss of ethanol and reduces the degree of supersaturation. This is predicted from the relative solubilities of hydrocortisone butyrate propionate in ethanol, propylene glycol, and water and is a further demonstration that increase in flux is due to increase in degree of saturation and not solely to increase in concentration.

Recently, Chiang et al. (24), using an in vitro human skin model, have shown that loss of ethanol from ethanol–propylene glycol–water solutions leads to supersaturation of minoxidil and subsequent increase in percutaneous flux. As found by Coldman (22), these authors also reported that increase in supersaturation results in increased flux until crystallization occurs, at which point there is a corresponding marked decrease in flux.

Kondo et al., as others (25–27), have been impressed with the remarkable ability of solid solutions of solutes in polymer dispersions not only to generate but, especially, to maintain supersaturated solutions by virtue of inhibition of nucleation and crystal growth and have applied these findings to topical drug delivery design. In a series of papers, Kondo et al. (28–30) used a range of methodologies, from an in vitro synthetic membrane model through to in vivo animal studies, to demonstrate the potential for use of volatile solvent systems to enhance topical drug delivery. Kondo (28) studied the transport of saturated and supersaturated solutions of nifedipine across an ethylene–vinyl acetate membrane in vitro. Despite a 10,000-fold difference in nifedipine concentration in solution, the flux from saturated suspension systems was approximately constant. In vitro, supersaturated solutions formed by evaporation of acetone resulted in increased flux, and maximum flux was obtained when the supersaturated states were stabilized with various polymers. Kondo et al. (29) used solutions of ethanol and diethyl sebacate as volatile and nonvolatile solvents to study in vitro flux across synthetic membrane and rat skin and in vivo absorption in the rat from supersaturated solutions of nifedipine. By optimization of the ethanol/diethyl sebacate ratio, to achieve maximum increase in thermodynamic activity, in vitro flux through the synthetic membrane or through rat skin was increased by up to fourfold. In vivo, as measured by area under the plasma level/time curve, topical bioavailability was also increased by up to fourfold from the supersaturated solution. Finally, Kondo et al. (30) used binary and ternary solutions of acetone, propylene glycol, and isopropyl myristate to form supersaturated solutions of nifedipine, stabilized with polymers, to evaluate their percutaneous absorption in rats. Figure 4, shows the ability of supersaturated solutions stabilized with polymer additives to increase markedly the topical bioavailability of nifedipine. Throughout their studies, Kondo et al. demonstrated, by pretreating skin with volatile solvent, by use occluded conditions, and by removal of solvent before application, that increase in penetration was due to increase in thermodynamic activity, rather than to the effects of the volatile solvents on the skin barrier function.

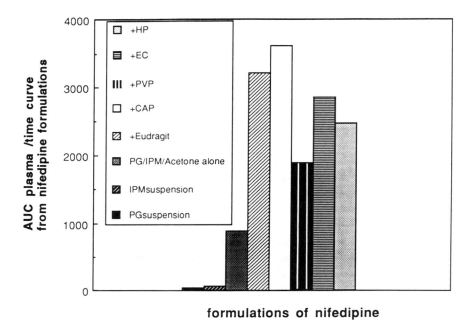

Figure 4 Percutaneous absorption of nifedipine from saturated suspensions and supersaturated solutions applied to rat skin in vivo. Effects of polymers on absorption of nifedipine from PG/PM/acetone supersaturated solution. (Data adapted from Ref. 30)

Other changes to vehicle composition may also result in generation of supersaturated states and increase in membrane flux. Thus, Kondo et al. (31) have suggested that the enhancing effect of N,N-diethyl-m-toluamide on nifedipine percutaneous absorption are caused by the formation of supersaturated solutions of nifedipine owing to loss of this solvent from the vehicle into the skin, rather than to direct effects on the skin barrier. Thus, absorption of solvents may lead to supersaturation of solute in the residual phase. Coldman et al. (32) have proposed that, under certain circumstances, the penetration enhancer effect of dimethyl sulfoxide (DMSO) may, in part, be due to uptake of water from the skin, reducing the solubility of solutes in the resultant vehicle phase, such that large increases in thermodynamic activity occur.

The use of microemulsion systems to generate supersaturated states for use in transdermal delivery has recently been reviewed by Muller (33). Change in composition of the microemulsion owing to uptake of water from the skin or loss of volatile components is used to increase the thermodynamic activity of penetrants. Water uptake into subsaturated microemulsions of β-blockers increases their thermodynamic activity and onset and peak response in an in vivo pharmacodynamic model (34). The inclusion of relatively high levels of surfactants may also contribute, owing to effects on the barrier function, to increase in percutaneous absorption seen with microemulsion systems.

It is likely that change in vehicle composition, to increase thermodynamic activity of the solute in the residual vehicle, occurs in many marketed formulations and is necessary for adequate, although generally low, percutaneous absorption and efficacy.

B. Use of Amorphous States

Solid solutions or molecular dispersion systems were first produced by Chiou and Riegelman in an attempt to increase the dissolution rate of poorly water-soluble drugs (35). Depending on the conditions of the dissolution system used, dissolution of solid dispersions will often result in generation of supersaturated states (25–27). As often, these supersaturated states will be maintained for a considerable period by the antinucleant and anticrystal growth effects of the polymeric dispersed phase, it is not surprising that such systems have been investigated for their ability to increase percutaneous absorption. Similarly, amorphous states prepared by grinding with carrier or by deposition on carrier have also been studied.

Morita and Horita (36) prepared amorphous hydrocortisone acetate by grinding with crystalline cellulose or by forming dispersions by coprecipitation from ethanol with polyvinylpyrrolidone. In vitro dissolution studies showed formation of supersaturation from the coprecipitate, and in vivo vasoconstrictor studies in volunteers demonstrated a general trend for increase in blanching with increase in amorphous nature of hydrocortisone acetate from both ground mixture and the coprecipitate. The authors conclude that chemical activity and biological activity are correlated.

Szeman et al. (37) prepared a ground mixture of tolnaftate with β-cyclodextrin polymer and showed this to be more amorphous than the original crystalline material, by differential scanning calorimetry. Although not commented on by the authors, this material showed typical supersaturation behavior on dissolution. In a percutaneous absorption study in mice, the ground mixture gave rise to a two- to threefold increase in skin and blood levels over either tolnaftate alone or tolnaftate in simple mixture with β-cyclodextrin polymer.

Norman (38) prepared coprecipitates of hydrocortisone with polyvinylpyrolidone (1:10). Supersaturated solutions, up to 12 times the degree of saturation prepared by dissolution of the coprecipitate in water, showed increase in flux across a cellulose membrane, proportional to the degree of saturation compared with a saturated control.

Campigli et al. (39) formed dispersions of indomethacin on fumed silicon dioxide by a fusion process to form high-thermodynamic activity states and increase percutaneous absorption. Amorphous material and alpha and gamma polymorphs were suspended in polydimethylsiloxane oil, and in vitro transport was compared across polydimethylsiloxane and human epidermal membrane. Transport was up to 100% greater from the amorphous state than from the crystalline forms. Although this increase is not large, experimental conditions, especially the physical stability of the supersaturated states in the polydimethylsiloxane oil, are likely to have been important.

The requirement to increase flux in transdermal drug delivery has led to much recent interest in the use of supersaturated states generated within polymer systems. Dittgen and Bombor (40) describe the use of polymer films in which supersaturated drug solutions are stabilized. Films containing isosorbide dinitrate or nitroglycerin are produced by dissolving the drug and mixing this with a suitable polymer in dispersion (e.g., Eudragits) and then drying to form a film. Modest degrees of saturation, up to approximately two times are formed, but are claimed to be stable on long-term storage. Similar systems have been described in a series of patents assigned to Sekisui Chemicals (41). For example, patent J6 3093-715-A describes the formation of supersaturated films of isosorbide dinitrate by mixing the drug with an ethyl acetate solution of 2-ethylhexyl acrylate–vinylpyrrolidone copolymer and drying. Supersaturated states at more than 1.5 times saturated solubility are produced that are claimed to be physically stable over long-term storage. In patent J6 3307-819-A similar systems are claimed in which the drug is contained within the polymer at more than twice the saturated solubility. Here, higher degrees of supersaturation lead to crystallization after manufacture, and the plaster is heated just before use to dissolve the drug. On cooling, high degrees of supersaturation are formed that are stable over the required period. These plasters give rise to higher plasma levels than can be achieved from saturated suspensions of the drug in an otherwise similar form.

Recently, Merkle (42) has reported on studies to minimize drug–carrier interactions within transdermal devices. Minimizing interaction (i.e., increasing the thermodynamic activity of the drug in the carrier) leads to increase in drug release. Merkle proposes the use of highly supersaturated drug preparations, with thermodynamic activity far beyond that of the crystalline form, as alternative strategy to the use of penetration enhancers in transdermal delivery.

Finally, in this section, Japanese patent J6 3297-320-A assigned to Nitto Electric (43) describes the use of a composite plaster in which a water-free drug–polymer dispersion phase is separated from a water gel by a water-impermeable membrane. In use, the membrane is removed and the two phases are brought into contact. This ingenious device uses dissolution of a drug–polymer dispersion system in water to generate a supersaturated state. Figure 5 shows that plasma levels of indomethacin are approximately four times greater following topical application to humans of the supersaturated plaster than from a proprietary gel formulation.

The review of this section serves to highlight the role of polymers in stabilizing supersaturated states and the natural synergy of polymeric devices, especially transdermal devices, with supersaturated states.

C. Use of Mixed Cosolvent Systems

The use of mixed cosolvent systems to generate supersaturated states for use as topical drug delivery systems has been of special interest to the authors (5,44).

Figure 6 shows the process schematically. Depending on the relative polarities of the solute and the components of the cosolvent system, saturated solubility

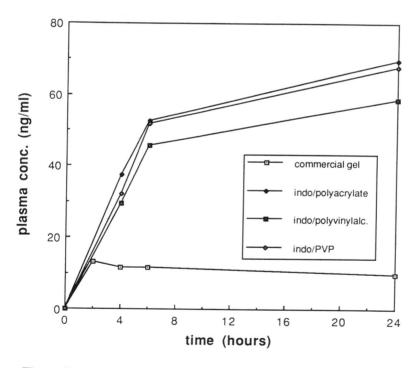

Figure 5 Plasma levels of indomethacin following application of a saturated commercial gel and three experimental supersaturated gels to human back skin. (Data adapted from Ref. 43)

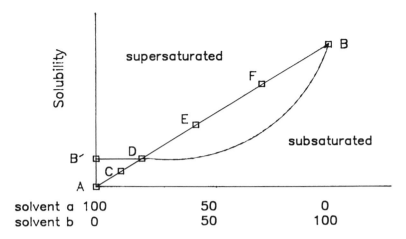

Figure 6 Saturated solubility of a solute in a binary cosolvent system. Effects of mixing: B'B is the saturated solubility curve of solute in binary cosolvent system ab. System B (saturated solute in solvent b) is mixed with system A (no solute in solvent a) to produce subsaturated, saturated, or supersaturated solutions exemplified by C, D, and E, F, respectively.

plots will often show an exponential increase with solvent composition as shown in Curve B'B of Figure 6. A basic property of these systems is that, by mixing suitable solute–cosolvent systems, subsaturated, saturated, or supersaturated solutions can be formed. Figure 6 shows that mixing system A (no solute in 100% solvent a) with system B (saturated solute in solvent b) will result in systems C (subsaturated), D (saturated), and E and F (both supersaturated), depending on the ratio of A to B used. In practice, systems A and B may themselves be mixed cosolvents, and system B need not necessarily be saturated with solute.

Figure 7 shows an example using hydrocortisone acetate in a simple water–propylene glycol cosolvent system (5). (Table 1 gives the composition of solutions A–G.) The donor solution, equivalent to system B in Figure 6, was 0.08% w/w of hydrocortisone acetate in 88% propylene glycol–12% water. System A was 100% water containing 0.5% hydroxypropylmethylcellulose, to inhibit crystal growth, and was mixed with system B in the ratios shown in Table 1 to produce supersaturated systems C–G. The curve A–H in Figure 7 is the degree of supersaturation and is given by the value on the line AB divided by the value on B'B at various cosolvent compositions.

Figure 8a shows the in vitro transport of hydrocortisone acetate from the donor solution B and supersaturated solutions C–G across a polydimethylsiloxane membrane, plotted against concentration and Figure 8b plotted against degree of

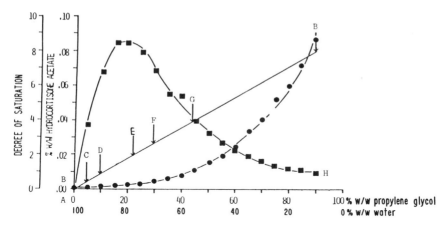

Figure 7 Generation of supersaturated solutions (line AB) of hydrocortisone acetate by mixing cosolvent systems A and B (see Table 1). Curve AH is the degree of supersaturation of the solutions. (Adapted from Ref. 44)

Table 1 Composition of Solutions Used in Mixed Cosolvent Systems[a]

| | Parts of each solution mixed | | | |
| | System B | System A | | |
Solution	Hydrocortisone acetate 0.08% w/w in 90:10 propylene glycol/water	Water plus antinucleant	Resultant concentration (% w/w)	Resultant degree of saturation (saturated = 1)
B	1	0	0.080	0.9
G	1	1	0.040	4.0
F	1	2	0.027	6.8
E	1	3	0.020	8.0
D	1	7	0.010	7.0
C	1	15	0.005	4.0

[a]See Figures 8 and 9.

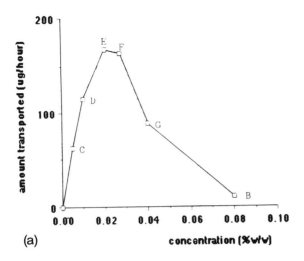

(a)

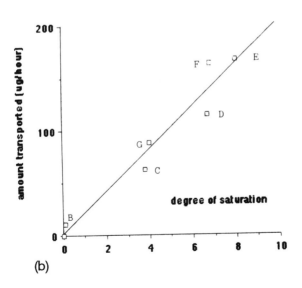

(b)

Figure 8   In vitro transport across a polydimethylsiloxane membrane: (a) as a function of concentration; (b) as a function of degree of saturation (see Table 1). (Adapted from Ref. 5)

saturation. Transport is correlated with the degree of saturation, but not with the concentration, and a plateau of transport is seen with the ratio of B/A of 1:3, which forms a 0.02% w/w hydrocortisone acetate eightfold the degree of saturation system.

Figure 9 shows in vitro transport of hydrocortisone acetate from 0.02% w/w solutions of from one (saturated) to eight times saturated formed by mixing appropriate cosolvent systems. Transport is clearly linearly related to the degree of saturation.

The overemphasis of concentration in topical vehicle design has been mentioned earlier, as has the fact that many current topical formulations are poorly bioavailable; that is, they contain high concentrations of active agent compared with the fractional amount absorbed. The topical bioavailability of hydrocortisone acetate in humans is between 1 and 2% of the dose applied (45,46) which referred to a standard concentration of 1%, equates to 0.02% w/w. Figure 10 shows the

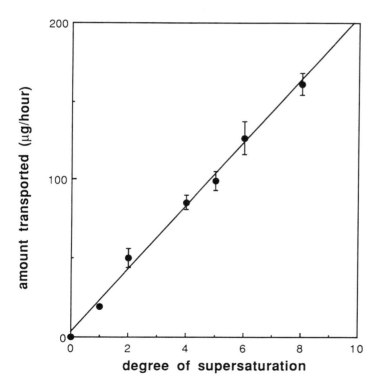

Figure 9 In vitro transport across a polydimethylsiloxane membrane from 0.02% w/w solutions of hydrocortisone acetate from one to eight times saturated.

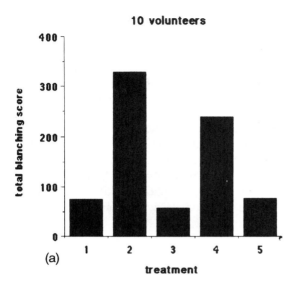

(a)

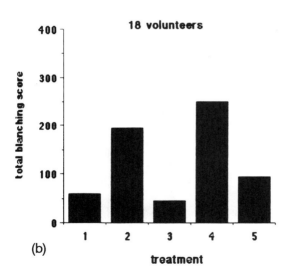

(b)

Figure 10 Bioequivalence of 0.02% w/w supersaturated hydrocortisone acetate (HA) with conventional 1% w/w HA cream. Studies (a) and (b) vasoconstrictor, blanching, in volunteers; studies (c) and (d) surfactant-induced erythema in volunteers. Treatments: 1, untreated; 2, 0.02% w/w supersaturated HA in gel; 3, gel base; 4, 1% w/w HA in cream; 5, cream base; 6, 0.02% w/w saturated HA in gel. (Adapted from Ref. 47.)

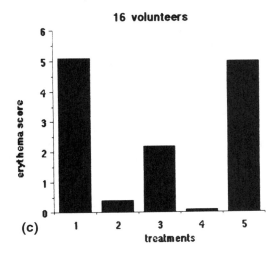

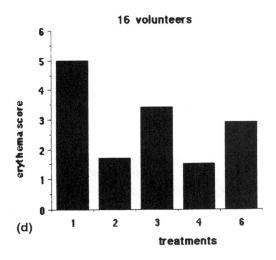

results of studies in volunteers undertaken to establish the bioequivalence of 0.02% w/w eightfold supersaturated solutions of hydrocortisone acetate in gel form with standard hydrocortisone acetate cream, 1% w/w (47). The results of both vasoconstrictor and surfactant-induced dermatitis studies clearly show bioequivalence of the formulations, with statistically significant difference between them and the control formulas. The main benefit in use of low-concentration, supersaturated topical formulations is in transferring control of percutaneous absorption from the skin to the vehicle. For example, the potential for overdosing and local and systemic adverse effects that occurs when high-concentration formulations are applied to permeable skin sites is abolished by use of carefully designed low- concentration, supersaturated systems.

Mixed cosolvents may be used to generate supersaturated solutions within ointment and cream vehicles, without the use of high levels of volatile components that may have drying and irritant effects on the skin. However these systems require specialized packaging that will deliver the two phases separately for mixing in situ on the skin.

V. SUMMARY

The theoretical basis for the use of supersaturation in topical drug delivery was first established by Higuchi, and since then, many studies reviewed here, have shown the benefits in transport across model membranes and human skin, both in vitro and in vivo, and in human pharmacology studies.

It is likely that many marketed formulations inadvertently take advantage of supersaturation. In alcoholic lotions and gels, the effects are predictable, but for more complex systems in which, for example, loss of solvents into the skin or uptake of water from the skin, lead to increase thermodynamic activity in the residual vehicle, effects may not have been anticipated.

Topical drug delivery has to face the formidable barrier properties of the skin, and any strategy to enhance delivery—flux—is of interest.

Supersaturation appears to offer an advantage over traditional "enhancers" in that the enhancement is specific to the compound of interest, there is no breakdown of barrier function, and absorption of other compounds (e.g., excipients) is not enhanced.

The use of antinucleant and anticrystal growth agents is the key to the practical use of supersaturation in topical drug delivery. Progress on use of transdermal drug delivery remains relatively slow owing to the problems of low flux with many compounds of potential interest. Use of supersaturation to drive flux from polymeric systems seems a natural synergy and one that is actively being investigated.

Pioneers in transdermal delivery quickly addressed the problem of wide differences in permeability of the skin, both between and within subjects, by the introduction of rate-controlling membranes. Strangely, variability has not been seen as an important issue in intradermal (i.e., topical or regional) delivery. Variability is worse when "infinite" doses of drug are used as with many current formulations. Here, the diffusion coefficient of the skin is the major factor controlling the actual dose of drug absorbed. The relevant pharmacokinetics have not been reviewed here, but it is our opinion that supersaturation in combination with low, yet rationally derived, concentrations will lead to significant improvement in control of percutaneous absorption and set new standards for future topical products.

REFERENCES

1. Lippold, B. C. and Schneemann, H. The influence of vehicles on the local bioavailability of betamethasone-17-benzoate from solution- and suspension-type ointments. *Int. J. Pharm.* 22:31–43 (1984).
2. Feldman, R. J. and Maibach, H. I. Regional variation in percutaneous penetration of ^{14}C cortisol in man. *J. Invest. Dermatol.* 48:181–183 (1967).
3. Higuchi, T. Physical chemical analysis of percutaneous absorption process from creams and ointments. *J. Soc. Cosmet. Chem.* 11:85–97 (1960).
4. Poulsen, B. J. Diffusion of drugs from topical vehicles: An analysis of vehicle effects. *Adv. Biol. Skin* 12:495–509 (1972).
5. Davis, A. F. and Hadgraft, J. Effect of supersaturation on membrane transport: 1. Hydrocortisone acetate. *Int. J. Pharm.* 76:1–8 (1991).
6. Poulsen, B. J., Young, E., Coquilla, V., and Katz, M. Effect of topical vehicle composition on the in vitro release of fluocinolone acetonide and its acetate ester. *J. Pharm. Sci.* 57:928–993 (1968).
7. Ostrenga, J., Steinmetz, C., and Poulsen, B. J. Significance of vehicle composition 1: Relationship between topical vehicle composition, skin penetrability, and clinical efficacy. *J. Pharm. Sci.* 60:1175–1179 (1971).
8. Flynn, G. L. and Smith, R. W. Membrane diffusion III: Influence of solvent composition and permeant solubility on membrane transport. *J. Pharm. Sci.* 61:61–66 (1972).
9. Turakka, L. and Ala-Fossi, N. Influence of propylene glycol on the release of hydrocortisone and its acetate ester from carbopol hydrogels. *Acta Pharm. Fenn.* 96:15–21 (1987).
10. Dugard, P. H. and Scott, R. C. A method of predicting percutaneous absorption rates from vehicle to vehicle: An experimental assessment. *Int. J. Pharm.* 28:219–227 (1986).
11. Moes-Henschel, V. and Jaminet, F. Percutaneous absorption of corticosteroids from formulations of equal thermodynamic activity. *J. Pharm. Belg.* 31:367–375 (1976).
12. Moes-Henschel, V. and Jaminet, F. Influence of the vehicle composition on the release and percutaneous penetration of corticosteroids. *J. Pharm. Belg.* 30:390–404 (1975).
13. Hadgraft, J., Hadgraft, J. W., and Sarkany, I. The effect of thermodynamic activity on the percutaneous absorption of methyl nicotinate from water glycerol mixtures. *J. Pharm. Pharmacol.* 25(suppl.):122–123P (1973).
14. Woodford, R. and Barry, B. W. Optimization of bioavailability of topical steroids: Thermodynamic control. *J. Invest. Dermatol.* 79:388–391 (1982).
15. Malzfeldt, E., Lehmann, P., Goetz, G., and Lippold, B. C. Influence of drug solubility in the vehicle on clinical efficacy of ointments. *Arch. Dermatol. Res.* 281:193–197 (1989).

16. James, K. C. *Solubility and Related Properties*, Vol. 28. Drugs and the Pharmaceutical Sciences. Marcel Dekker, New York (1986).
17. Miyazaki, S., Nakano, M., and Arita, T. Effects of additives on the polymorphic transformation of chlortetracycline hydrochloride crystals. *Chem. Pharm. Bull.* 24: 2094–2101 (1976).
18. Frank, F. C. The influence of dislocations on crystal growth. *Discuss. Faraday Soc.* 5:48–54 (1949).
19. Holder, G. A. and Thorne, J. Inhibition of crystallisation by polymers. *Polymer Preprints Am. Chem. Soc. Div. Poly. Chem.* 20:766–769 (1979).
20. Carless, J. E., Moustafa, M. A., and Rapson, H. D. C. Effect of crystal form, cortisol alcohol and agitation on crystal growth of cortisone acetate in aqueous suspension. *J. Pharm. Pharmacol.* 20:639–642 (1968).
21. Coldman, M. F., Poulson, B. J., and Higuchi, T. Enhancement of percutaneous absorption by use of volatile:nonvolatile systems as vehicles. *J. Pharm. Sci.* 58:1098–1102 (1969).
22. Theeuwes, F., Gale, R. M., and Baker, R. W. Transference: A comprehensive parameter governing permeation of solutes through membranes. *J. Membr. Sci.* 1:3–16 (1976).
23. Tanaka, S., Takanashima, Y., Murayama, H., and Tsuchiya, S. Studies on drug release from ointments: V. Release of hydrocortisone butyrate propionate from topical dosage forms to silicone rubber. *Int. J. Pharm.* 27:29–38 (1985).
24. Chiang, C.-M., Flynn, G. L., Weiner, N. D., and Szpunar, G. J. Bioavailability assessment of topical delivery systems: Effect of vehicle evaporation upon in-vitro delivery of minoxidil from solution formulations. *Int. J. Pharm.* 55:229–232 (1989).
25. Kala, H., Traue, J., Moldenhauer, H., and Zessin, G. Production and characterisation of spray-dried microcapsules. *Pharmazie.* 36:106–111 (1981).
26. Hasegawa, A., Nakagawa, H., and Sugimoto, I. Application of solid dispersions of nifedipine with enteric coating agents to prepare a sustained-release dosage form. *Chem. Pharm. Bull.* 33:1615–1619 (1985).
27. Hasegawa, A., Kawamura, R., Nakagawa, H., and Sugimoto, I. Physical properties of solid dispersions of poorly-water soluble drugs with enteric coating agents. *Chem. Pharm. Bull.* 33:3429–3435 (1985).
28. Kondo, S. and Sugimoto, I. Enhancement of transdermal delivery by superfluous thermodynamic potential. 1. Thermodynamic analysis of nifedipine transport across the lipoidal barrier. *J. Pharmacobiodyn.* 10:587–594 (1987).
29. Kondo, S., Yamasaki-Konishi, H., and Sugimoto, I. Enhancement of transdermal delivery by superfluous thermodynamic potential. 11. In-vitro–in-vivo correlation of percutaneous nifedipine transport. *J. Pharmacobiodyn.* 10:662–668 (1987).
30. Kondo, S., Yamanaka, C., and Sugimoto, I. Enhancement of transdermal delivery by superfluous thermodynamic potential. III. Percutaneous absorption of nifedipine in rats. *J. Pharmacobiodyn.* 10:743–749 (1987).
31. Kondo, S., Mizuno, T., and Sugimoto, I. Effects of penetration enhancers on percutaneous absorption of nifedipine. Comparison between *DEET and Azone. J. Pharmacobiodyn.* 11:88–94 (1988).
32. Coldman, M. F., Kalinovsky, T., and Poulsen, B. J. The in-vitro penetration of fluocinolone through human skin from different volumes of DMSO. *Br. J. Dermatol.* 85:457–460 (1971).

33. Muller, B. W. Supersaturated systems in transdermal delivery. *Second Int. Symp. Dermal and Transdermal Delivery New Insights and Perspectives.* APV Symposium Nov. 11–13 (1991).

34. Kemken, J., Zeigler, A., and Muller, B. W. Investigation into the pharmacodynamic effects of dermally administered microemulsions containing β-blockers. *J. Pharm. Pharmacol. 43*:679–684 (1991).

35. Chio, W. L. and Riegelman, S. Pharmaceutical applications of solid dispersion systems. *J. Pharm. Sci. 60*:1281–1302 (1971).

36. Morita, M. and Horita, S. Effect of crystallinity on the percutaneous absorption of corticosteroid. II. Chemical activity and biological activity. *Chem. Pharm. Bull. 33*:2091–2097 (1985).

37. Szeman, J., Ueda, H., Szejtli, J., Fenyvesi, E., Watanabe, Y., Machida, Y., and Nagai, T. Enhanced percutaneous absorption of homogenised tolnaftate/β-cyclodextrin polymer ground mixture. *Drug Design Deliv. 1*:325–332 (1987).

38. Norman, F. H. In *Design of Biopharmaceutical Properties Through Prodrugs and Analogs.* Roche, E. B. (ed.). Apha Series, pp. 198 (1977).

39. Campigli, V., Di Colo, G., Nannipieri, E., and Serafini, M. F. Silicon dioxide as support for amorphous and metastable crystalline forms of indomethacin. Correlation between drug thermodynamic activity and percutaneous absorption. *Il Pharmaco 43*:57–70 (1987).

40. Dittgen, M. and Bombor, R. Process for the production of a pharmaceutical preparation. German patent DD 217 989 A1.

41. Sekisui Chemical Industries KK. Patent J6 3093-714-A: Dermal absorption plaster— has adhesive layer containing super-saturated medicine on a previously heated plaster impervious to the medicine. J6 3093-715-A: Dermal absorption plaster—comprising adhesive layer containing solid medicine on substrate surface which is impervious to the medicine. (See also J6 3307-818-A; J6 3307-819-A).

42. Merkle, H. P. Transdermal delivery systems. *Methods Find. Exp. Clin. Pharmacol. 11*:135–153 (1989).

43. Nitto Electric Industry Ind. KK. Patent J6 3297-320-A: Composite plaster sheet—comprising water-impermeable sheet layer containing water-soluble pharmaceutical active ingredient and aqueous gel layer of e.g., polyacrylic acid.

44. Davis, A. F. US patent 4,940,701. Topical drug release system.

45. Feldmann, R. J. and Maibach, H. I. Percutaneous penetration of steroids in man. *J. Invest. Dermatol. 52*:89–94 (1969).

46. Feldmann, R. J. and Maibach, H. I. Percutaneous penetration of hydrocortisone with urea. *Arch. Dermatol. 109*:58–59 (1974).

47. Marks, R., Dykes, P. J., Gordon, J., Hanlan, G., and Davis, A. F. *Percutaneous penetration from a low dose supersaturated hydrocortisone acetate formulation.* British Society of Investigative Dermatology Annual Meeting. Sheffield, September 1992.

12

Infrared Spectroscopy of Stratum Corneum Lipids

In Vitro Results and Their Relevance to Permeability

Russell O. Potts

Cygnus Therapeutic Systems, Redwood City, California

Michael L. Francoeur

Pharmetrix, Inc., Menlo Park, California

I. INTRODUCTION

The technique of infrared (IR) spectroscopy, and most notably Fourier transform (FTIR) spectroscopy, has been used extensively to study the phase behavior of lipid membranes. The reader is referred to the review of Casal and Mantsch (1) for a comprehensive survey of the use of FTIR spectroscopy to evaluate phospholipid membranes.

The lipids of the stratum corneum (SC) also can be studied by FTIR techniques. Unlike other membrane systems in which samples are suspended in water, however, SC samples are evaluated as intact sheets. In these studies, the intense IR absorption associated with water does not compromise the spectra of SC, even for highly hydrated samples. A sheet of SC is obtained by trypsin digestion (2) and treated under the desired experimental conditions before sealing between two windows, made of IR transparent material such as ZnS. The sandwiched sample is then mounted in a temperature-controlled heating–cooling mantle in the IR spectrometer. The signal from a thermocouple in direct contact with the sample serves as feedback to a personal computer that is programmed to regulate the rate and extent of temperature change. This computer also communicates with the FTIR instrument workstation to automatically coordinate temperature changes and spectral data acquisition. Because of the thin (10 to 20 μm) cross section of the SC, a significant amount of IR radiation passes through the sample, while some of the IR energy is absorbed, causing various molecular vibrations. Analysis of the absorbed radiation over the IR energy range provides spectra with characteristic peaks associated with specific vibrational modes.

A typical FTIR spectrum of porcine SC is shown in Figure 1. This spectrum looks like other hydrated biological samples with separate peaks from lipids, proteins, and water. Of particular interest for the study of lipid biophysics are the peaks caused by C-H stretching vibrations. These absorbances occur near 2920 and 2850 cm^{-1} for the asymmetric and symmetric C-H vibrations, respectively. Upon heating the SC, both C-H stretching peaks broaden and shift to higher wavenumbers. A plot of the shift in C-H symmetric stretching frequency ($v_s(CH)_2$) over a continuous range of temperature is shown in Figure 2. These results show that there is a modest increase in $v_s(CH)_2$ from about 30° to 60°C and from about 80°C to the highest temperatures measured. In contrast, there is an abrupt increase in $v_s(CH)_2$ from about 60° to 80°C. Similar sigmoidal curves of $v_s(CH)_2$ versus temperature have been obtained for a variety of phospholipid systems and reflect lipid phase transition(s). For example, data obtained for dipalmitoyl phosphotidylcholine (DPPC) exhibited a similar, although even more abrupt increase in $v_s(CH)_2$ at 41°C, corresponding to a gel-to-liquid crystal transition (1). Note that

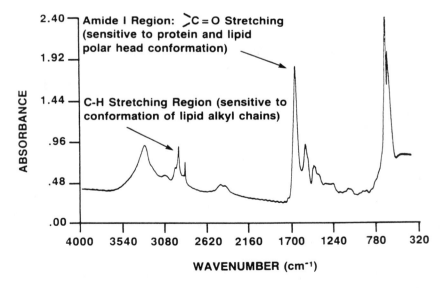

Figure 1   The infrared (IR) spectrum of porcine SC.

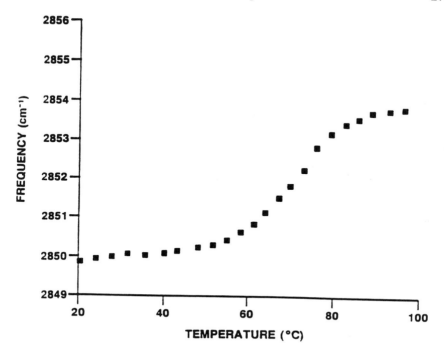

Figure 2   The change in the C-H symmetric stretching frequency $[\nu_s(CH_2)]$ as a function of temperature for porcine SC.

for a highly homogeneous sample, such as pure DPPC, the transition occurs over a narrow temperature range. In contrast, the data of Figure 2 show that the transition in SC is broad, primarily owing to the heterogeneous nature of the constituent lipids.

The assignment of the C-H stretching peaks to SC lipids is further corroborated by results from differential scanning calorimetry (DSC) experiments. The IR and DSC thermal profiles for porcine SC are shown in Figures 3a and 3b, respectively. The DSC results show that the intact SC has two thermal transitions with midpoints (T_m) near 60° and 70°C. However, upon reheat only a single endotherm at about 60°C is observed, with an enthalpy that is equal to the sum of the two original transitions. The IR data for an identical sample (see Fig. 3a) show that the initial heat results in a transition that spans the range seen for the two lipid transitions in DSC. In addition, the IR results show an inflection near 70°C, suggestive of two transitions in the range of 50°–80°C. After reheat, the transitions seen with both the IR and DSC techniques occur over a narrower range, with

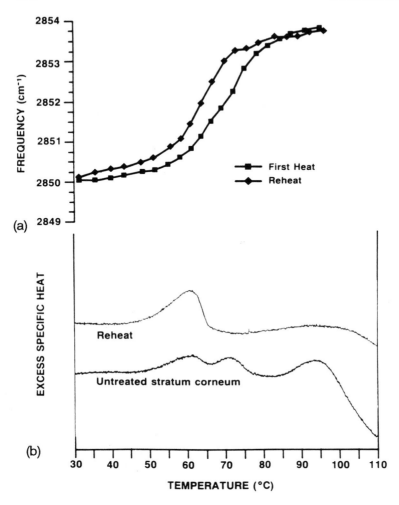

Figure 3 (a) The change in the C-H symmetric stretching frequency $[\nu_s(CH_2)]$ as a function of temperature for porcine SC. (b) The DSC thermal profile for identically treated porcine SC.

a lower T_m. The correlation between the IR and DSC data (see Figs. 3a and 3b) at temperatures below about 80°C is quite good, and the DSC data appear to be a first derivative of the IR results.

Additional evidence for the assignment of the C-H stretching peaks comes from the results of lipid-extraction experiments. Removal of extracellular SC lipids by chloroform–methanol extraction leads to a dramatic decrease in intensity (>95%) for the C-H stretching peaks (2). Furthermore, as shown by a comparison of the data in Figures 3 and 4, the lipids extracted from the SC show a temperature-dependence similar to the intact sample. The data obtained for extracted lipids (see Figs. 4a and 4b) again show a parallel between DSC and IR data. Taken together, these results indicate that both techniques are sensitive to the lipid transitions that occur in the extracellular lipids of the SC.

The molecular basis for the shift in the C-H stretching frequency is well described (1). A qualitative explanation of the effect is offered here. In particular, the shift to higher frequency (or wave number) results when methylene groups along the alkyl chain adopt an increased number of gauche (nonlinear) con-formers. In the minimum free-energy state, lipid alkyl chains conform to an all-*trans*-configuration. As shown in Figure 5, when adjacent carbons adopt such a configuration, every fourth methylene group along the chain is *trans* across the intervening carbon–carbon bond. Consequently, the C-H bonds experience mini-mal steric hindrance from neighboring groups. As the temperature is increased, gauche conformers begin to occur where the first and fourth methylene along the chain are no longer maximally separated. As a consequence, C-H stretching is sterically hindered and, thus, more energy is required to stretch this bond, making the vibration occur at higher frequency.

The magnitude of the shift in $v_s(CH)_2$ is directly related to the ratio of the number of gauche to *trans* conformers (a process called *rotamer disordering*) (1). Thus, the frequency shift provides a measure of the lipid alkyl chain conforma-tional disorder, in general, and the number of gauche conformers, in particular. The remarkable similarity between IR data shown here for SC lipids and those of other biomembranes suggests that, even though the lipids of the SC are composi-tionally different from other biomembranes, they all contain long alkyl chains that undergo rotamer disordering upon heating. Clearly, the precise temperature and width of the transition depends critically upon the particular lipid; however, the underlying biophysics remains the same.

II. STRATUM CORNEUM PERMEABILITY

A. The Effect of Temperature and Permeant Size

In several lipid membrane systems, permeability and biophysical properties are correlated (3). These results show, for example, that the permeability of small nonelectrolytes and ions increases as lipids with short or unsaturated alkyl chains are incorporated into the membranes, or as the temperature is increased (4,5). Results obtained from temperature-dependent changes in water vapor perme-ability suggest that a similar correlation exists for porcine SC (6,7). Water vapor

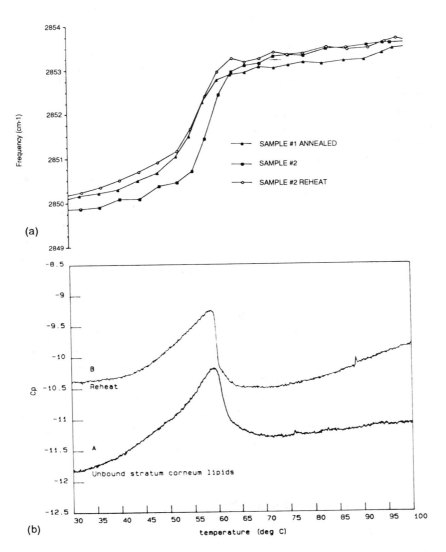

Figure 4 (a) The change in the C-H symmetric stretching frequency $[\nu_s(CH_2)]$ as a function of temperature for lipids extracted from porcine SC. (b) The DSC thermal profile for identically treated lipids extracted from porcine SC.

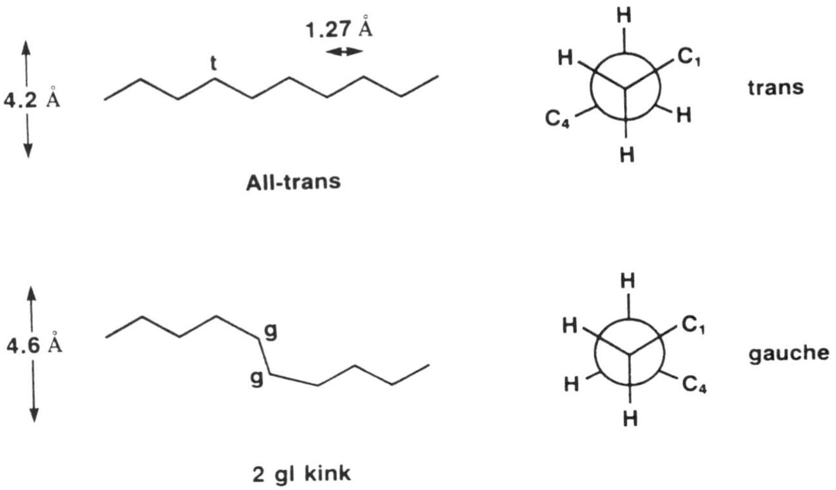

Figure 5 A schematic representation of *trans*- and gauche-conformers in an alkyl chain.

permeability was measured for two important reasons. First, although unstirred layer effects can be appreciable in liquid-phase diffusion experiments, they are negligible in vapor studies. Thus, temperature-dependent changes in permeability are not due to changes in unstirred layer effects. Second, vapor experiments were performed using saturated aqueous salt solutions in the donor and receptor compartments to maintain constant thermodynamic activity of water. In these experiments, NaCl was used to provide a constant 75% relative humidity (RH), which was unchanged from 10° to 90°C. Changes in permeability, therefore, cannot be attributed to changes in the thermodynamic activity of water.

The permeability coefficient (P) and $v_s(CH)_2$ values for porcine SC samples, measured at 10°C intervals from 20° to 90°C, are plotted in Figure 6. A linear regression analysis of these data shows a high correlation ($r>0.999$) between P and $v_s(CH)_2$ over a broad range for both variables. These results strongly suggest a functional relation between water permeability and the IR spectral shift. Although it is possible that this correlation reflects a fortuitous relation between two activated processes, this seems unlikely, since the data show that P and $v_s(CH)_2$ are correlated at all temperatures measured, including those above and below the SC lipid-phase transition. This requires that both processes share a common T_m and display a similar temperature dependence on either side of the transition temperature, an unlikely chance event.

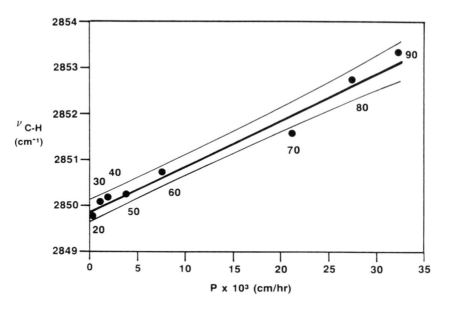

Figure 6 The water permeability coefficient (P) of SC vs $v_s(CH_2)$ for samples heated from 22° to 90°C. The 95% confidence interval obtained from that analysis is also shown. No experimental point differs significantly ($p>0.95$; t-test) from the predicted value.

The shift in $v_s(CH)_2$ results from an increased number of gauche conformers in the lipid alkyl chain. Thus, the results shown in Figure 6 imply that water permeability through SC and the number of gauche conformers in the SC lipids are functionally related. This conclusion is consistent with two related mechanisms that were postulated for the permeation of water through biological membranes, involving the formation of free-volume defects. Lieb and Stein proposed that permeant molecules were transported by randomly "jumping" from donor to acceptor "holes" within the membrane (8). Alternatively, Traüble proposed that water permeation through lipid bilayers involves the propagation of water-carrying "kinks" along the alkyl chain (9). Furthermore, he postulated that the kinks occurred owing to the random (e.g., thermal) formation of gauche conformers in an otherwise primarily *trans* lipid alkyl chain. The data presented in Figure 6 suggest that water permeation through the SC is highly correlated with the number of gauche conformers (as measured by $v_s(CH)_2$). Although not distinguishing between the water jump or kink propagation hypotheses, these results, nevertheless, provide strong evidence that water permeation through a lipid membrane is dependent on the formation of gauche conformer, free-volume holes.

A schematic representation of these free-volume holes can be seen in Figure 5. Upon the formation of a gauche-*trans*-gauche (g-t-g') kink along the alkyl chain, the lateral spacing between the hydrocarbon chains increases by about 10% relative to the all-*trans*-configuration. As a consequence, free-volume holes of about 50 Å^3 are created, especially in the region immediately adjacent to the g-t-g' linkage (10). [Note that the volume of a water molecule is less than 20 Å^3.] As described in the foregoing, this leads to increased membrane permeability. In addition, the average chain length and, hence, membrane thickness decreases as g-t-g' conformers are formed. Once again, membrane permeability should increase, since permeability and membrane thickness are inversely related. Results obtained with DPPC membranes, for example, suggest that, in the gel-to-liquid crystal transition, the bilayer thickness decreased by about 10%, whereas the free volume increased by about 2% (10). Changes in free volume and thickness also occur at other temperatures, albeit with a lower temperature-dependence. Thus, the occurrence of gauche conformers can directly increase the membrane permeability by the formation of transient holes or reduction in the membrane thickness. It is important to realize that gauche conformers fluctuate rapidly. When integrated over time, however, a finite average number of gauche conformers exist. That time-average is what is measured by the FTIR results presented here.

The correlation of water transport through the SC with free-volume effects suggests that the size of the permeant may be an important parameter in skin permeability. For passive transport through the SC (or any lipid membrane), the *permeability coefficient* (P) is defined in Eq. 1 as the product of the diffusion coefficient (D) and the partition coefficient (K), divided by the diffusion path length (δ).

$$P = \frac{DK}{\delta}$$

[1]

Rearranging Eq. 1,

$$\frac{P}{K} = \frac{D}{\delta}$$

[2]

shows that the ratio of P divided by K is proportional to the diffusion coefficient, assuming that δ is constant. Many investigators have plotted log P vs log K for a series of structurally related permeants and found a straight line with an intercept proportional to log D/δ.

Although K reflects the partitioning of permeant between an applied aqueous phase and the transport domain within the SC, this is experimentally difficult to measure. Thus, many researchers use octanol/water partition coefficients (K_{oct}) as an estimate of K (11). Several investigators have measured P through SC for a series of n-alkanols and water (12,13). The data for human tissue are shown in Table 1, along with values for K_{oct}. Also shown in the last column of Table 1 are the molecular volumes of each compound, as determined by the method described by Bondi (14). Figure 7 shows a plot of log (P/K_{oct}) vs molecular volume for these permeants. These data show a remarkable inverse correlation, suggesting that log D and the molecular volume of the permeant are functionally related. These results also demonstrate the strong dependence of diffusion on the molecular volume of the permeant (D decreases as an **exponential** function of increasing molecular volume). Kasting et al. showed a similar correlation for a broad range of compounds, with relative molecular masses (M_r) from 100 to over 400 dal (15).

A similar inverse correlation between log(P/K_{oct}) (or log D) and molecular volume was demonstrated for other lipid systems and reflects the strong volume dependence of transport through these membranes (3). Furthermore, the functional relation between log D and molecular volume can be derived from a statistical mechanical description of diffusion by a free-volume mechanism (16). The results presented here show that transport through the skin is dependent on the molecular volume of the permeant. When taken together with the strong correlation between P and an IR measure of increased free-volume within the lipid hydrocarbon chains, these combined results suggest that transport through the SC is a lipid-mediated, free-volume effect.

Interestingly, the slope of log(P/K_{oct}) vs molecular volume obtained here for SC is similar to other lipid membranes (3), suggesting that volume-dependent diffusion is rather similar in these apparently disparate systems. Although the

Table 1 The Permeability Coefficient (P) of Water and n-Alkanols Through Human Epidermis, Along With Values for the Octanol/Water Partition Coefficient (K_{oct}) and Molecular Volume (MV)

Permeant	Log P (cm/sec)	Log K_{oct}	MV (Å^3/molecule)
Water	−6.9	−1.4	12.7
Methanol	−6.9	−0.73	36.2
Ethanol	−6.7	−0.32	55.6
Propanol	−6.4	0.34	76.4
Butanol	−6.2	0.88	87.3
Pentanol	−5.8	1.4	104.3
Hexanol	−5.4	2.0	121.3
Heptanol	−5.1	2.5	138.4
Octanol	−4.9	3.1	156.4

Source: Permeability data from Ref. 13; molecular volumes calculated according to Ref. 14.

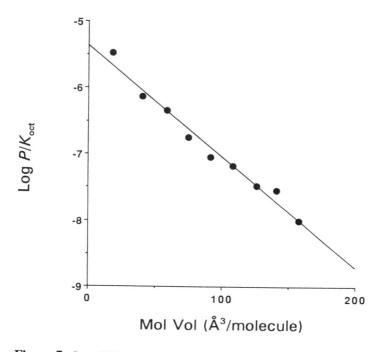

Figure 7 Log (P/K_{oct}) vs molecular volume of a series of alkanols and water. The data were obtained from transport through human SC. (Data from Ref. 13)

slopes are similar among these membranes, the log (P/K_{oct}) data for the SC are uniformly displaced by about −4. In other words, these results show that, although P/K_{oct} has a similar molecular volume-dependence in a number of lipid membranes, P/K_{oct} is about 10,000-fold less for transport through the SC. Equation 2 suggests that the lower value of P/K_{oct} for the SC must reflect either a smaller intrinsic diffusion coefficient or a greater diffusion path length when compared with other lipid membranes. Since volume-dependent changes in the diffusion are quite similar among these membranes and SC, it seems reasonable that the diffusion coefficient (D) is also similar. Thus, these results suggest that the diffusion path length is much greater in the SC. A similar conclusion was obtained by Hadgraft and Ridout, who compared transport through model lipids and human SC (17). Independent experimental results obtained by Potts and Francoeur (18) likewise suggest that only the diffusion path length differs significantly between the SC and other lipid membranes.

The free-volume hypothesis also explains the anomalously high permeability of water, methanol, and other small, polar permeants. For example, the log P vs log K_{oct} data from Table 1, plotted in Figure 8, show that ethanol, methanol, and water, all have greater permeabilities than predicted by an extrapolation of data from the higher molecular mass homologues, using Eq. 1. This extrapolation suggests that for the more polar molecules, permeation is independent of partitioning, consistent with transport through an aqueous pore (12). Predictions based on Eq. 1, however, assume that D is constant, regardless of the permeant. In contrast, the dependence of log D on molecular volume shows that small permeants are transported more rapidly than large molecules. Thus, the apparently anomalous permeabilities of small (and polar) molecules may simply reflect a strong volume-dependence of diffusion in a lipid milieu, rather than the existence of a continuous aqueous pore. Interestingly, the molecular volume of all three permeants is less than 50 Å^3, the calculated volume created by a g-t-g' link (10).

In summary, the results of FTIR experiments show that the extracellular lipids of porcine SC undergo phase transitions between about 60° and 80°C.

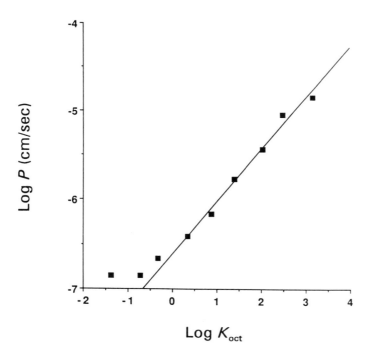

Figure 8   Log P vs log K_{oct} for the results presented in Figure 7.

Furthermore, temperature-dependent increases in water vapor permeability and the C-H stretching frequency are highly correlated. The spectral shift is due to increased gauche conformers in the lipid alkyl chain. Thus, these findings argue that water permeability through the SC is dependent on conformational changes in the lipid alkyl chain. These results also suggest that water transport through the SC depends on free-volume fluctuations in the lipid alkyl chains. Finally, permeability data obtained for a number of compounds demonstrate that transport through the SC decreases exponentially with the increasing molecular volume of the permeant. These combined results suggest that permeant size is a strong determinant of SC transport.

B. The Use of Deuterated Lipids to Study Penetration Enhancers

The mechanism(s) of penetration enhancement were also studied using FTIR techniques. One of the principal advantages of this approach is the ability to separately monitor endogenous lipids and enhancers using deuterated compounds. Fully or partially deuterated lipids have been employed, in conjunction with IR or Raman spectroscopy, to probe the biophysical properties of a variety of phospholipid-based membranes (19–22). These systems ranged from simple phospholipid vesicles, to phospholipid–protein complexes, to intact viable cells. The advantage of using deuterated lipids is predicated on the fact that the isotopic substitution of deuterium for hydrogen shifts the C-H stretching bands into the spectral region, which is essentially free from other protein or lipid absorbances. As with the C-H signal, the C-D symmetric stretching frequency ($v_s(CD_2)$) is sensitive to the conformational order of the lipid hydrocarbon chains (23,24). A frequency value of approximately 2090 cm^{-1} is indicative of lipid chains that are highly ordered with a low population of gauche conformers. As described earlier, a shift to higher frequencies is associated with increased conformational freedom and flexibility of the hydrocarbon chain, leading to a reduction in lamellar thickness and segmental order, with a value near 2098 cm^{-1} being the upper limit for $v_s(CD_2)$.

Recently, Ongpipattanakul et al. (25) used perdeuterated oleic acid (^{2}H-OA) to investigate the molecular nature of this penetration enhancer's interaction with the constituents of the SC. As shown in Figure 9, the absorption bands from the ^{2}H-OA are distinct from the C-H stretching signal of endogenous SC lipids. This particular spectrum is obtained from porcine SC treated with ^{2}H-OA at a final oleic acid concentration of 60 μg/mg SC. If treated and normal SC are hydrated to a constant weight at 75% RH, and then scanned by the FTIR spectrometer as a function of temperature, the $v_s(CH_2)$ profile shown in Figure 10 is obtained. The untreated SC yields a typical sigmoid-shaped curve indicative of gel-to-liquid crystal phase transition with an apparent T_m (inflection point) at approximately

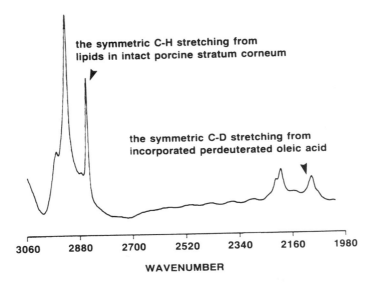

the symmetric C-H stretching from
lipids in intact porcine stratum corneum

the symmetric C-D stretching from
incorporated perdeuterated oleic acid

| 3060 | 2880 | 2700 | 2520 | 2340 | 2160 | 1980 |

WAVENUMBER

Figure 9 The infrared spectrum of porcine SC treated with perdeuterated oleic acid.

70°C (see also Fig. 2). The addition of oleic acid to the SC does not appreciably change the shape of the frequency–temperature profile, but does lower the inflection point by about 8°C. Furthermore, above the T_m, frequency values for the oleic acid-treated SC are higher, indicating a greater degree of disorder for those SC lipids.

This decrease in T_m for the SC lipids after treatment with oleic acid can be partly explained by thermodynamic principles. The transition temperature is a function of the relative enthalpy (ΔH) and entropy (ΔS) contributions from the respective gel and liquid crystalline phases. At equilibrium ($\Delta G=0$), T_m will be equal to $\Delta H/\Delta S$, where $\Delta S = S_{final} - S_{initial}$. Since previous calorimetric results (26) showed that there is little change in ΔH following treatment with oleic acid, the decrease in T_m may be partially attributed to an increase in ΔS. This inference is supported by the observation that $\nu_s(CH_2)$ is the same for both treated and normal SC below the T_m, yet significantly higher for the oleic acid-treated sample above the T_m. In other words, there is no change in the conformational order along the SC lipid alkyl chain in the presence of oleic acid until all the chains are melted. Although the conformational order, as indicated by $\nu_s(CH_2)$ does not define the total entropy of the SC lipids, it is certainly a contributing factor to S_{final}.

The increase in SC lipid conformational order (or entropy) above the phase-transition temperature can be a direct consequence of at least two different

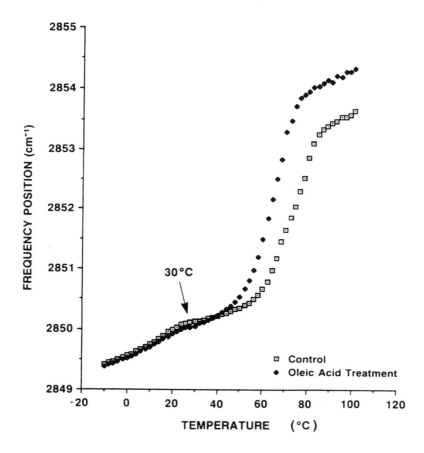

Figure 10 The symmetric CH_2 stretching vibration frequency $[\nu_s(CH_2)]$ vs temperature for control and ^2H-oleic acid-treated porcine SC.

phenomena. The methylene groups nearest the polar interface of phospholipid bilayers are known to be significantly more ordered than the rest of the alkyl chain, even in the liquid crystalline state (27,28). If a similar situation exists for the SC lipids, it can be postulated that oleic acid must exert its disordering effect primarily on the methylene groups most proximal to the polar headgroup. The second possibility is that oleic acid may increase the total fraction of SC lipids that have undergone a gel-to-fluid phase transition. In either event, S_{final} will be increased. Inspection of the methyl stretching region of the IR spectrum provides additional insight into these two possible mechanisms. As shown in Figure 11, the

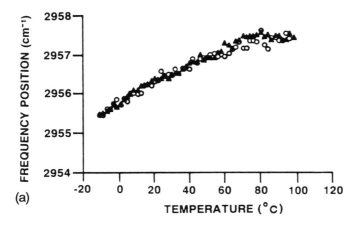

(a)

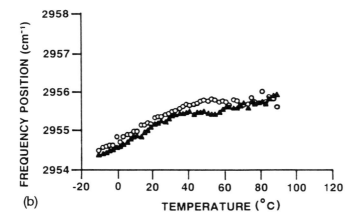

(b)

Figure 11 The temperature dependence of (a) the asymmetric methyl stretching frequency for intact SC and (b) extracted lipids. Control and ^{2}H-oleic acid-treated samples are represented by open and closed symbols, respectively.

asymmetric methyl stretching frequency exhibits no phase transition behavior for either intact SC or extracted lipids. Similar results were obtained for other lipid systems (29). Furthermore, oleic acid treatment has no effect on the thermal behavior of either intact SC or extracted lipids. These results are in marked contrast with those obtained for methylene groups (see Fig. 10), suggesting that

intensities range between 0 and 3.0 W/cm^2, the intensity used being influenced by the therapeutic indications.

C. Pulsed or Continuous Mode

Therapeutic ultrasound equipment can generate both continuous and pulsed ultrasound energy. In pulsed mode the frequency of the ultrasound waves remains unaltered, but the transducer output is interrupted; therefore, the total output in unit time is reduced. Pulsed ultrasound allows high intensities to be used without increasing skin temperature. Pulse mode duty cycles of 1:1, 1:4, and 1:8 are commonly available.

D. Time of Exposure

The total time of exposure to ultrasound is commonly 5–10 min. It varies according to the functional abnormality of the condition being treated and the area of the treatment site.

E. Coupling Agent

Ultrasound energy is almost 100% reflected at both the transducer–air interface and air–tissue interface and is rapidly attenuated in air; therefore, in ultrasound therapy, a coupling medium is used to exclude air from the region between the transducer and the treatment site. Ideally, a coupling medium should have an absorption coefficient similar to that of water. A good-coupling medium should retain a gel consistency at body temperature to maintain contact between the ultrasound source and the skin. The efficiencies of a range of available ultrasound couplants have been tested (3–6). Warren et al. (6) reported that "no practical difference exists in the transmissitivites of the common coupling agents."

Unlike ultrasound-coupling media formulated specifically for that purpose, topical pharmaceutical products are not formulated in a way such that their efficiency as ultrasound couplants is optimized. The findings of a recent investigation indicate that there is great variation in the coupling efficiency of topical preparations (7). Preparations containing large amounts of solid material, such as creams and ointments, do not permit the transmission of ultrasound, whereas formulations containing little or no undissolved material (such as gels and some creams) are more efficient coupling agents. The number of suitable medicinal products available for use with ultrasound, therefore, is greatly limited. The present data (7) indicate that gel formulations provide the most suitable ultrasound-coupling media (Table 1). Therefore, if ultrasound is to be used with topical pharmaceuticals, or transdermal systems, there is a need for the formulation of appropriate active ingredients in gel forms.

Table 1 Transmission of Ultrasound Energy Through Topical Pharmaceutical Products

Class	Product	Active ingredients	% Transmission relative to water (±SE)		
			0.75 MHz	1.5 MHz (1.5 W total output)	3.0 MHz
1. Ultrasound coupling agents	Aquasonic 100		89.2 ± 0.43	88.6 ± 0.51	98.14 ± 0.32
	Duffield US. Coupling cream		7.07 ± 0.61	18.40 ± 1.14	63.60 ± 2.33
	Movelat gel		91.20 ± 0.38	82.93 ± 0.54	103.87 ± 0.49
2. Preparations for relief of soft-tissue inflammation	Algesal cream	Diethylamine salicylate	0.00 ± 0.00	0.00 ± 0.00	0.00 ± 0.00
	Aroldene cream	Diethylamine salicylate, capsicum, menthol, rectified camphor oil	35.74 ± 0.49	36.80 ± 0.93	41.60 ± 0.25
	Balmosa cream	Camphor, capsicum, menthol, methyl salicylate	0.00 ± 0.00	9.88 ± 1.04	51.87 ± 0.74
	Bayolin cream	Benzyl nicotinate, glycol salicylate, heparinoid	12.93 ± 0.16	59.47 ± 0.32	91.33 ± 0.72
	Benques Balsam	Menthol, methyl salicylate	0.00 ± 0.00	6.13 ± 0.25	2.67 ± 0.55
	Cremalgin Balm	Capsicum, glycol salicylate, methyl nicotinate	0.00 ± 0.00	0.00 ± 0.00	0.00 ± 0.00
	Difflam cream	Benzydamine hydrochloride	0.53 ± 0.13	14.27 ± 0.72	32.50 ± 0.81
	Intralgin gel	Benzocaine, sailcylamide	87.33 ± 0.29	11.40 ± 0.54	120.27 ± 0.50
	Movelat cream	Corticosteroids, heparinoid, salicylic acid	32.97 ± 1.75	48.13 ± 2.31	68.53 ± 0.57
	Transvasin cream	Benzocaine, ethyl and hexyl nicotinate, tetrahydrofurfuryl salicylate	2.00 ± 0.00	30.67 ± 0.99	78.53 ± 1.03
3. Topical cortico-steroids	Adcortyl cream	Triamcinolone acetonide	0.00 ± 0.00	3.18 ± 0.13	22.84 ± 1.12
	Betnovate cream	Betamethasone valerate	0.00 ± 0.00	5.07 ± 0.16	41.07 ± 0.16
	Cobadex cream	Hydrocortisone, dimethicone	54.67 ± 0.78	66.67 ± 0.00	75.33 ± 0.29
	Dermovate cream	Clobetasol propionate	0.00 ± 0.00	0.00 ± 0.00	0.00 ± 0.00
	Dioderm cream	Hydrocortisone	7.47 ± 0.57	31.07 ± 0.95	43.47 ± 0.67
	Diprosone cream	Betamethasone dipropionate	1.47 ± 0.44	11.07 ± 0.95	14.67 ± 0.59

Source: Ref. 7.

F. Contact Time

It has been reported (8,9) that a contact time of 5–6 min may be required for efficient phonophoresis. This allows sufficient drug to penetrate the superficial layers of the skin before ultrasound application. However, Hadgraft et al. (10) have shown phonophoretically enhanced nicotinate penetration in which the drug was applied as a finite dose to a delineated skin site that had been previously treated with continuous-output ultrasound (3 MHz; 1 W/cm^2) for 5 min, indicating that a presoak period may not be required for all drug species.

IV. BIOPHYSICAL EFFECTS OF ULTRASOUND

Attenuation of the ultrasound beam by living tissues may produce structural and functional changes by way of mechanical mechanisms and thermal effects.

A. Mechanical Effects

Microstreaming is the term used for the circulation of fluid induced by radiation forces. Microstreaming may produce high viscous stresses that can change cell membrane structure and function, either reversibly or irreversibly, depending on their magnitude (11). Provided damage to the cell membrane does not occur, microstreaming could be of therapeutic value by facilitating the movement of calcium and other ions and metabolites across the cell membrane. Beneficial responses to changes in intracellular calcium ions, including synthesis (e.g., of collagen), secretion (e.g., of chemotactic agents and wound factors), motility changes (e.g., of pericytes, fibroblasts, and endothelial cells, all of which could accelerate repair processes), may result (12). Changes in membrane permeability to sodium ions could be involved in the altered electrical activity that ultrasound can induce in nerves, a possible mechanism involved in the relief of pain associated with ultrasound therapy (13).

Another mechanical effect of ultrasound that has been reported is micromassage. Essentially, this involves the mechanical distortion of tissues at the cellular level as a result of the positive and negative pressure changes in the ultrasound beam. Several biological effects are reported to result from the micromassage. These include alterations in cell membrane structure and in membrane proteins.

B. Thermal Effects

Absorption of ultrasound energy causes a rise in temperature in the tissue. The rise in temperature is proportional to the absorption coefficient (i.e., the extent to which a tissue will absorb energy from the beam). The absorption coefficient varies from tissue to tissue and with the frequency of the incident ultrasound beam. Dunn et al. (14) reported that the absorption coefficient of bone is ten times greater than muscle, which in turn absorbs 2.5 times more than fat (measured at 1.0 MHz). Over the frequency range of therapeutic ultrasound, this variation is approximately linear (i.e., the absorption coefficient at 3.0 MHz is three times that at 1.0 MHz).

V.   REPORTED STUDIES OF PHONOPHORESIS

Phonophoresis was first reported nearly 40 years ago, and since then several clinical reports have been published concerning a wide range of drugs. As a result, phonophoresis has become an accepted therapeutic treatment (15). However, it was not until recently that researchers have begun to examine the evidence available to quantify the efficacy of phonophoresis.

A.   In Vitro Investigations

Several in vitro investigations have been reported that have used both synthetic membranes and tissue samples.

Julian and Zentner (16) investigated the influence of ultrasound on the permeation of hydrocortisone through cellulose and of benzoic acid through polydimethyl siloxane (Silastic) membranes. Ultrasound produced a 23% increase in the permeability coefficient of benzoic acid through Silastic membrane. They showed that by stirring the aqueous diffusion layers, membrane–solution interfacial temperature, membrane integrity, and diffusant stability were not responsible for the observed increases in permeability.

Other workers have demonstrated phonophoretically enhanced diffusion of sodium and potassium chloride through cellophane membranes (17). These workers suggested that the effect was mainly due to acoustically induced microcurrents within the diffusing solution, decreasing the thickness of the diffusion layer and, thereby, increasing the diffusion process. However, creating similar currents in the solution by means of mechanical stirring, resulted in a smaller increase in diffusion. Therefore, either ultrasound provided more effective stirring or other factors were important.

Gatev (18) studied the passage of hydrocortisone through isolated frog skin. Higher concentrations of hydrocortisone migrated under the influence of ultrasound than with controls. However, this effect was noted only at high ultrasound intensities and when high concentrations of drug were employed. Under these conditions, the effect was proportional to the exposure time and the intensities used.

Safiulina and Proskurova (19) have also demonstrated phonophoretically enhanced diffusion of hydrocortisone. By doubling the ultrasonic exposure time, the diffusion of hydrocortisone through frog skin and cellophane membranes was increased by 5–10%.

It has recently been reported that ultrasound can increase the penetration of ibuprofen through human skin in vitro (20).

However, all the in vitro studies of phonophoresis reported involve the use of glass diffusion cells, which limits their ability to reproduce in vivo conditions. In vivo, ultrasound energy applied to the skin surface is gradually attenuated (converted into heat) as it passes through the soft tissues. At the soft tissue–bone interface the ultrasound wave is reflected and may interact with the incident wave, which may cause standing waves. In a standing wave, regions of high and low intensity are fixed in space relative to the interface, with high-intensity points separated by half a wavelength. In clinical practice, the formation of standing waves within the tissues is minimized by constantly moving the transducer during treatment. The in vitro diffusion cells now used in studies possess glass bases; therefore, ultrasound waves are reflected from the glass surface at the base of the cell, producing standing waves within the cell, especially since the aqueous fluids, unlike normal tissue, will not attenuate the ultrasonic energy. A novel diffusion cell suitable for investigation of the influence of ultrasound on percutaneous absorption has recently been described (Fig. 1; 21). The cell has been used to show increased penetration of methyl and ethyl nicotinates through excised animal skin under the influence of ultrasound. The use of this apparatus should provide a method for further in vitro research into phonophoresis.

B. In Vivo Investigations

Phonophoresis was first reported in 1954, by Fellinger and Schmid (22), who successfully administered ultrasound in conjunction with hydrocortisone ointment in the treatment of polyarthritis of the digital joints of the hand. Griffin and Touchstone (23–26) have investigated phonophoresis using swine tissue. Ultrasound-driven cortisol was recovered from skeletal muscle and nerve tissue. Reported data showed that swine muscle and nerve tissue exposed to low-intensity, long-duration phonophoretically applied hydrocortisone (10.1 W/cm^2 for 51 min; 1.0 MHz) exhibited much higher cortisol levels than did similar tissue exposed to high-intensity, short-duration phonophoresis (0.3 W/cm^2 for 17 min; 1.0 MHz) (25).

Kosin (27) treated rats with dermatitis using a steroid ointment, with and without ultrasound (0.2 W/cm^2), and showed enhanced antiproliferative effects of the drug with ultrasound.

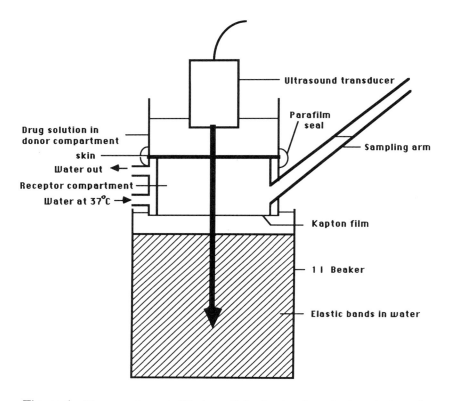

Figure 1 Diagram of novel diffusion cell for in vitro investigation of phonophoresis (21). The receptor compartment base is composed of Kapton film, which allows ultrasound to be transmitted into water contained in a 1 L beaker. Elastic bands in this beaker dissipate the ultrasonic energy, so avoiding back-reflection into the diffusion cell. Drug can be placed in the donor compartment either in solution form (as shown) or as a formulated ointment, cream, or gel. Percutaneous absorption across the skin barrier can be monitored by removing aqueous buffer samples through the sampling arm of the thermostated receptor compartment. Mixing of receptor compartment contents can also be carried out through the sampling arm.

Hydrocortisone has been the most widely studied drug in the ultrasonic–phonophoretic field. Hydrocortisone phonophoresis has been used to successfully treat many skin conditions [e.g., chronic psoriasis (28), kraurous vulvae, and pruritus vulvae essentiallis (29,30)] as well as several clinical conditions, including facial nerve neuritis (31,32), vasomotor rhinitis (33), allergic rhinitis (34), and rheumatoid arthritis (35).

Enhanced local anesthetic activity has been reported following treatment with phonophoretically administered local anesthetic drugs. Novak (36) showed that the concentration of lidocaine in rabbit muscle tissue was much higher when the tissues had been subjected to ultrasound during application of lidocaine (for example, 180% increase in drug concentration in tissue excised 30 min after treatment). Cameroy (37) reported that carbocaine anesthesia "is vastly enhanced in both rapidity and effectiveness" when the drug is applied with ultrasound (1.0 W/cm^2 for 30 sec). In a clinical trial involving healthy volunteers, McElnay and coworkers (8) indicated that there was slightly faster onset time for local anesthesia when ultrasound was administered in conjunction with a lidocaine cream, compared with control values (no ultrasound), although the differences were not statistically significant. The influence of ultrasound on the percutaneous absorption of lidocaine and prilocaine from Emla cream has been investigated in healthy volunteers (38). The effect of both 1:1 pulsed-output ultrasound (1.5 MHz and 3.0 MHz at intensity 1.0 W/cm^2 for 5 min) and continuous-output ultrasound at a range of frequencies (0.75, 1.5, and 3.0 MHz, each at intensity 1.5 W/cm^2 for 5 min) were compared with a placebo control (massage without ultrasound for 5 min). Loss of sensation caused by lidocaine and prilocaine was used to monitor the percutaneous absorption of the drugs. Ultrasound led to an increased rate of drug absorption, as determined by onset of anesthesia; however, this increase was not statistically significant (Fig. 2a). The extent of drug absorption, as determined by duration of anesthesia, was increased by a statistically significant degree (see Fig. 2b). The 1.5 MHz (1:1 pulsed-output) and 3.0 MHz (continuous-output) ultrasound were the most effective frequencies in improving the rate of percutaneous absorption, whereas the 1.5 and 3.0 MHz (1:1 pulsed-output) ultrasound treatments were the most effective frequencies in improving the extent of drug absorption. These results suggest that pulsed-output ultrasound may provide the most effective conditions in the technique of phonophoresis with that topical formulation.

In a clinical study involving 50 patients with soft-tissue injuries treated with 3% w/w benzydamine hydrochloride cream, it was noted that incidental use of ultrasound therapy together with the drug caused more "rapid and dramatic improvement" of symptoms (39). More recently, Haig (40) heralded ultrasound therapy with benzydamine cream as a new form of treatment for soft-tissue injuries. This was based on the clinical assessments of 119 patients with soft-tissue injuries. The extent to which mobility, pain, swelling, and tenderness were relieved was recorded following treatment with a combination of benzydamine cream or placebo cream and ultrasound (1 or 3 MHz at 0.5 W/cm^2 for 5 min). No measurement was made to determine whether ultrasound actually enhanced the absorption of the drug. A further investigation by independent researchers of the influence of ultrasound on the percutaneous absorption of

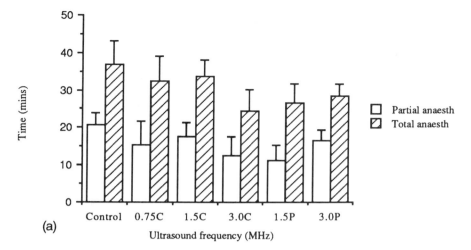

(a)

Figure 2 (a) Time to onset of anesthesia ±SE and (b) duration of anesthesia ±SE following application of Emla cream (lidocaine/prilocaine) with a range of ultrasound parameters (0 MHz, control; 0.75 MHz, 1.5 MHz, 3.0 MHz at 1.5 W/cm², continuous-output; 1.5 MHz, 3.0 MHz at 1.0 W/cm², 1:1 pulsed-output). (Data from Ref. 38)

benzydamine showed no significant enhancement of drug penetration over a range of ultrasound frequencies (41). However, benzydamine was applied to the skin in an alcohol gel base in this latter study. The alcohol itself may have enhanced drug penetration, thereby masking any enhancement effect provided by the ultrasound treatment.

Although many of the studies of phonophoresis have involved anesthetic and anti-inflammatory agents, a range of miscellaneous drugs have also been examined. Phonophoretic administration of phenylbutazone, α-chymotrypsin, and other nonsteroidal anti-inflammatory drugs was reported to be successful in the treatment of musculoskeletal disorders (42–44). Phonophoresis using a number of drugs has been successful in the treatment of chronic tonsillitis (45), chronic pharyngitis (46), and vocal cord nodes and polyps (47). Ultrasonic treatment with a lotion containing urea, tannic acid, zinc oxide, and menthol has been proposed in the treatment of oral and genital herpes simplex virus type 2 (48,49). Phonophoresis of antibiotics, including tetracycline (50) and biomycin (51), has been reported for the therapy of several skin conditions. A summary of the reported in vivo percutaneous phonophoresis studies is given in Table 2.

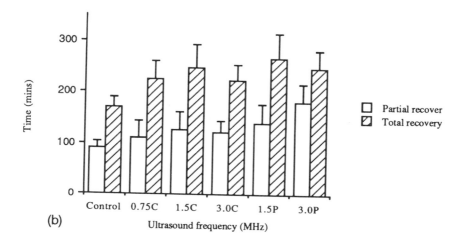

(b)

VI. MECHANISM OF ACTION OF PHONOPHORESIS

The mechanism by which ultrasound enhances the percutaneous absorption of compounds, has not yet been defined. Summer and Patrick (52) proposed that ultrasound moves a particle in an oscillatory motion about a rest position, but this phenomenon, in itself, does not explain the transport of drugs through tissue. Ultrasound may produce structural and functional changes in biological tissue by way of mechanical mechanisms and thermal perturbation effects not yet understood.

No correlation has been found between a given ultrasound dose to the skin and changes in skin temperature or blood flow (53). Therefore, any beneficial effects of ultrasound cannot be attributed to increased blood flow in cutaneous, subcutaneous, and muscle tissue.

Mechanical stress may result from *cavitation* in biological systems. This is the formation of small gaseous inclusions that expand and collapse with ultrasound. Cavitation may play a role in increased cell permeation, causing rapidly reversible cell damage (54). Although this may be important for enhanced drug transport into cell suspensions (55), no cavitation has been reported in tissues exposed to therapeutic levels of ultrasound (intensities <3 W/cm^2) (56).

A recent theory suggests that ultrasound affects the permeability of stratum corneum lipid structures to mediate phonophoretic drug delivery.

Table 2 Reported Studies of Therapeutic Ultrasound Combined With Drug Application to the Skin

Drug	Application	Ref.	Type of study	Frequency (MHz)	Intensity (W/cm^2)	Mode	Regimen	Outcome
Corticosteroids Hydrocortisone	Temporomandibular joint dysfunction	63	C	*	1.0–1.5	CW	8 min	Improvement
	Polyarthritis—digital joints	22	C	*	2.0–4.0 W (total output)	*	5–15 min	Improvement
	Bursitis and posttraumatic	64	B	0.8–1.0	0.4–1.5	*	5–10 min	Successful
	lesions of muskuloskeletal	65	C	1.0	1.0–2.0		5–6 min	Successful
	system	66	C	0.87	0.5–0.8		5 min	Successful
		67	B	*	0.8–3.0		5–10 min	Successful
	Epicondylitis/bursitis	68	B	1.0	2.0	*	6 min	Improvement
	Chronic arthritis	69	A	1.0	1.5	*	5 min/25 in.^{2} of skin	Successful
	Rheumatoid arthritis	40	C	3.0–5.0	0.1–0.2	*	*	Improvement
	Chronic psoriasis	28	C	3.0–12.0	0.2–0.8	*	*	Improvement
	Kraurosis vulvae lichen, Sclerotrophicus/pruritus vulvae essentiallis	29, 30	C	5.0–10.0	0.5–1.2	*	*	Improvement
	Facial nerve neuritis	31	C	3.0–5.0	0.2–0.4	*	10–15 min	Improvement
		32	B	3.0–5.0	0.2–0.4	*	*	Improvement
	Vasomotor rhinitis	33	C	5.0	0.15–0.4	*	*	Improvement
	Allergic rhinitis	34	C	5.0	0.2–0.4	*	5 min intransal	Improvement
	Rheumatoid arthritis	70	D	*	0.8	*	*	Inhibition
	Vocal cords nodes and polyps	47	C	5.0	0.2–0.4	*	*	Improvement
Hydrocortisone and cuprenil	Schleroderma	71	C	10.0	0.4–0.6	*	*	Improvement

Drug	Subjects/condition	Ref.	Study type			Mode	Duration	Effect
Fluocinolone acetonide	Healthy volunteers	9	A	0.87	2.0	CW	5 min	Significant increase in percutaneous absorption
	Dermatitis	72	D	*	*	*	*	Morphological changes in skin
	Dermatitis	73	D	5.0	0.2	*	*	Aided normalization of biochemical and structural processes of skin
Local anaesthetics								
Carbocaine	Bone fractures	37	C	*	1.0	*	30 sec	Enhanced local anesthesia
Lidocaine	Healthy volunteers	8	A	0.87	2.0	CW	5 min	Slight enhancement of local anesthesia (not significant)
Lidocaine	Rabbit	36	D	*	2.0	*	5 min	Increased drug penetration
Lidocaine/prilocaine	Healthy volunteers	38	A	0.75–3.0	1.0–1.5	CW/P	5 min	Enhanced local anesthesia
Analgesic/anti-inflammatory								
Benzydamine hydrochloride	Soft-tissue injuries	39	A	*	*	*	*	More rapid effect
	Soft-tissue injuries	40	B	1.0–3.0	0.5	*	5 min	Significant improvement of symptoms
Phenylbutazone	Healthy volunteers	41	A	1.0–3.0	0.2–2.0	CW	5 min	No significant effect
	Arthrosynovitis	42	A	*	*	*	*	Improvement
Antibiotics								
Tetracycline	Cow udders	50	D	10.0	1.0–2.0	*	*	Enhanced drug penetration
Biomycin	Hidradenitis	51	C	5.0–15.0	0.8–1.0	*	*	Improvement
Others								
Nicotinate esters	Healthy volunteers	57	A	3.0	1.0	CW	5 min	Enhanced drug penetration
Interferon	Chronic pharyngitis	46	B	2.064	0.2–0.4	*	5 min × 8–10 sessions	Improvement
Zinc, urea, and tannic acid	Oral and genital herpes	48, 49	A	1.1	1.0	*	60 sec	Improvement

Key: A, controlled study; B, comparative study; C, descriptive report; D, experimental study; *, not specified; CW, continuous output.

In a recent study, nicotinate esters were used to provide some insight into the possible mechanism of action of phonophoresis (57). The influence of ultrasound (3.0 MHz at 1.0 W/cm^2 for 5 min) on the percutaneous absorption of methyl, ethyl, and hexyl nicotinates was compared with placebo controls (massage with each of the gels without ultrasound for 5 min). Laser Doppler velocimetry was used to monitor the vasodilation caused by the nicotinates, which provided a measure of the percutaneous absorption of the drugs. It was also established that massage with ultrasound alone did not influence blood flow within the experimental protocol. Ultrasound led to significant enhancement of the percutaneous absorption of methyl and ethyl nicotinates (increase compared with control data was about 59 and 79%, respectively). In some cases, no response was noted in the absence of ultrasound, whereas a marked vasodilative response was seen when ultrasound was used. Percutaneous absorption of hexyl nicotinate was also enhanced, although to a smaller degree (21%). Ultrasound-mediated enhancement of percutaneous absorption was greater for the more aqueous-soluble methyl and ethyl nicotinates than for the more lipid-soluble hexyl nicotinate. The authors proposed that, although further work is required to substantiate the hypotheses, the data obtained in this investigation suggest that ultrasound may interact with the structured lipids located in the intercellular channels of the stratum corneum. In the same way that some penetration enhancers act by fluidizing the lipids (58–61), the ultrasound energy may act to facilitate diffusion through the lipid domains. If this is true, it would be expected that the more polar the molecule, the greater the degree of enhancement. It can be proposed that the absorption of methyl and ethyl nicotinates was enhanced because diffusion through the intercellular lipid channels is the rate-limiting process. For hexyl nicotinate, the rate-limiting step is partitioning from the lipid-rich stratum corneum environment. This appeared to be relatively unaffected by ultrasound.

Variability between subjects exists in the effect of ultrasound on the percutaneous absorption of the drugs, and this was certainly shown to be true with nicotinates in the foregoing study. A possible explanation for this may be that there are variations in the integrity of the stratum corneum lipid structure among subjects. The stratum corneum lipids of some individuals may possess a natural fluidity and, therefore, are less influenced by ultrasound energy, whereas those of others may be more rigid in structure and, therefore, are subject to fluidization by ultrasound energy. If this is indeed true, variations in the natural fluidity of stratum corneum lipids would have important implications for the variation in percutaneous absorption of drugs and the influence of some penetration enhancers (that act by fluidizing stratum corneum lipids).

Further experiments are currently being undertaken to verify the ultrasound-mediated stratum corneum lipid fluidization hypothesis. Preliminary investigations involving ultrasound treatment administered before methyl nicotinate application have shown an enhancement of percutaneous absorption of the drug (10). This suggests that ultrasound energy affects the structure of the skin and, therefore, supports the proposed hypothesis.

VII. FUTURE DEVELOPMENTS

From the published work to date, it appears that phonophoresis may be used to enhance both localized and systemic drug delivery. Variables affecting drug delivery by this technique include length of treatment, output frequency, power level, and pulse duration. An understanding of these variables is important for the optimization of phonophoretic drug delivery.

Use of both pulsed and continuous-wave ultrasound has been reported in the literature. Continuous-output ultrasound provides a combined mechanical and thermal effect. The pulsed mode provides an equivalent mechanical effect. Benson et al. (21) indicated that pulsed-output ultrasound provided the most effective conditions for maximum increase in rate and extent of drug absorption.

The pulse mode, typically 2–3 msec on and 10–20 msec off, allows higher intensities to be used. Moreover studies investigating the optimum pulse duration for phonophoresis are needed.

It has been reported that depth of penetration is inversely proportional to the frequency of ultrasound used. High frequencies are needed to focus ultrasound in the upper layers of the skin. It has been suggested that a frequency of 16 MHz, 0.2 W/cm^2 would be better localized in the stratum corneum, leading to better perturbation (62).

Increasing the duration of treatment would also produce a greater effect. The optimum tolerated duration and frequency of ultrasound need to be further investigated.

REFERENCES

1. ter Harr, G. *Physiotherapy 73*:110–113 (1987).
2. ter Harr, G. *Physiotherapy 64*:100–103 (1978).
3. Bantjes, A. and Klomp, R. *Physiother. Sport 3*:9–13 (1979).
4. Docker, M. F., Foulkes, D. J., and Patric, M. K. *Physiotherapy 68*:124–125 (1982).
5. Reid, D. C. and Cummints, G. E. *Physiother. Can. 25*:5–9 (1973).
6. Warren, C. G., Koblanski, J. N., and Sigelmann, R. A. *Arch. Phys. Med. Rehabil.* 57:218-222 (1976).
7. Benson, H. A. E. and McElnay, J. C. *Physiotherapy 74*:587–588 (1988).
8. McElnay, J. C., Matthews, M. P., Harland, R., and McCafferty, D. F. *Br. J. Clin. Pharmacol. 20*:421–424 (1985).
9. McElnay, J. C., Kennedy, T. A., and Harland, R. *Int. J. Pharm. 40*:105–110 (1987).

10. Hadgraft, J., McElnay, J. C., and Murphy, T. M. Proceedings of the International Conference on Prediction of Percutaneous Penetration. Manchester, England (1989).
11. Lehmann, J. F. and Guy, A. W. In *Interaction of Ultrasound and Biological Tissues*. Reid, J. M. and Sikov, M. R. (eds.). DHEW Publication (FDA), pp. 141–152 (1972).
12. Dyson, M. *Physiotherapy 73*:116–120 (1987).
13. Madsen, P. W. and Gersten, J. W. *Arch. Phys. Med. Rehab. 42*:645–649 (1961).
14. Dunn, F., Edmonds, P. B., and Fry, W. J. In *Biological Engineering*. Schwan, H. P. (ed.). McGraw-Hill, New York, pp. 205–336 (1969).
15. Wassworth, H. and Chanmugam, A. P. P. In *Electrophysical Agents in Physiotherapy*. Science Press, New South Wales (1983).
16. Julian, T. N. and Zentner, G. M. *J. Pharm. Pharmacol. 38*:871–877 (1986).
17. Lenart, I. and Auslander, D. *Ultrasonics 18*:216–218 (1980).
18. Gatev, S. *Eksp. Med. Morfol. 11*:231–236 (1972).
19. Safiulina, S. N. and Proskurova, G. I. *Vopr. Kurortol. Fizioter. Lech. Fiz. Kult. 35*:293–295 (1970).
20. Brucks, R., Nanavaty, M., and Jung, D. *Pharm. Res. 6*:697–701 (1989).
21. Benson, H. A. E. PhD Thesis, The Queen's University of Belfast, United Kingdom (1988).
22. Fellinger, K. and Schmid, J. In *Klinik und Therapie des Chronischen Gelenkhuematismus*. Maudrich, Vienna, pp. 549–552 (1954).
23. Griffin, J. E. and Touchstone, J. C. *Am. J. Phys. Med. 42*:77–85 (1963).
24. Griffin, J. E., Touchstone, J. C., and Liu, A. C.-Y. *Am. J. Phys. Med. 44*:20–25 (1965).
25. Griffin, J. E. and Touchstone, J. C. *Phys. Ther. 48*:1336–1344 (1968).
26. Griffin, J. E. and Touchstone, J. C. *Am. J. Phys. Med. 51*:62–78 (1972).
27. Kosin, W. M. *Zdrevookhr. Beloruss. 4*:81–82 (1976).
28. Belts, E. A. and Bondarenko, M. M. *Vestn. Dermatol. Venerol. 45*:70–72 (1971).
29. Burgudjeva, T. *Akush. Ginekol. 10*:287–291 (1971).
30. Burgudjeva, T. *Akush. Ginekol. 10*:477–482 (1971).
31. Gristitein, A. B., Tolmacheva, A. N., and Kriptulov, V. V. *Vopr. Kurortol. Fizioter. Lech. Fiz. Kult. 36*:528–530 (1971).
32. Antropova, M. I. *Zh. Nevropatol. Psikhiatr. 74*:506–511 (1974).
33. Nikolaevskaia, V. P. *Nov. Med. Priborostr. 3*:32–35 (1969).
34. Kornienko, A. M. *Vestn. Otorinolaringol. 1*:55–57 (1974).
35. Artemonova, V. A. and Nikitina, T. P. *Vopr. Kurortol. Fizioter. Lech. Fiz. Kult. 42*:29–33 (1977).
36. Novak, E. J. *Arch. Phys. Med. Rehabil. 45*:231–232 (1964).
37. Cameroy, B. M. *Am. J. Orthop. 8*:47 (1966).
38. Benson, H. A. E., McElnay, J. C., and Harland, R. *Int. J. Pharm. 44*:65–69 (1988).
39. Chatterjee, D. S. *J. Int. Med. Res. 5*:450–458 (1977).
40. Haig, G. *Res. Clin. Forums 10*:49–55 (1988).
41. Benson, H. A. E., McElnay, J. C., and Harland, R. *Phys. Ther. 69*:113–118 (1989).
42. Brondol, W. *Arch. Orthop. 73*:532–540 (1960).
43. Famaey, J. P. *J. Belg. Rheumatol. Med. Phys. 30*:129–141 (1975).
44. Wanet, G. and Dehon, N. *J. Belg. Rheumatol. Med. Phys. 31*:49–58 (1976).
45. Babich, V. S. *Voenn Med. Zh. 12*:40–43 (1974).

46. Tsyganov, A. I., Feigin, N. P., Povolotsky, Y. L., Gumenyuk, P. V., and Tarasyuk, M. V. *Vestn. Otorinolaringol.* 7:32–34 (1979).
47. Vasilenko, Y. S. and Nikolaevskaya, V. P. *Vestn. Otorinolaringol.* 3:59–62 (1975).
48. Fahim, M., Brawner, T. A., Millikan, L., Nickell, M., and Hall, D. G. *J. Med.* 9:245–264 (1978).
49. Fahim, M., Brawner, T. A., and Hall, D. G. *J. Med.* 11:143–167 (1980).
50. Parikov, V. A. *Veterinariia* 43:88–91 (1966).
51. Indkevich, P. A. *Vestn. Dermatol. Venerol.* 44:75–77 (1971).
52. Summer, W. and Patrick, M. K. *Ultrasonic Therapy.* Elsevier, New York (1964).
53. Paaske, W. P., Hovind, H., and Sejrsen, P. *Scand. J. Clin. Lab. Invest.* 31:389–394 (1973).
54. Fischer, E., White, E. A., Hendricks, S. L., Chevalier, B. A., and Chevalier, R. B. *Am. J. Phys. Med.* 33:184–297 (1954).
55. Kremkau, F. W. *Br. J. Cancer* 45(Suppl.):226–232 (1982).
56. Griffin, J. E. *J. Am. Phys. Ther. Assoc.* 46:18–26 (1966).
57. Benson, H. A. E., McElnay, J. C., Harland, R., and Hadgraft, J. *Pharm. Res.* 8:204–209 (1991).
58. Beastall, J. C., Hadgraft, J., Palin, K. J., and Washington, C. *J. Pharm. Pharmacol.* 39(Suppl.):23P (1987).
59. Beastall, J. C., Hadgraft, J., and Washington, C. *Int. J. Pharm.* 43:207–213 (1988).
60. Goodman, M. and Barry, B. W. *J. Pharm. Pharmacol.* 37(Suppl.):80P (1985).
61. Goodman, M. and Barry, B. W. *J. Pharm. Pharmacol.* 38(Suppl.):71P (1986).
62. Bommanan, D., Okuyama, H., Stauffer, P., and Guy, R. *Proc. Int. Symp. Controlled Release Bioactive Mater.* 17:31–32 (1990).
63. Wing, M. *Phys. Ther.* 62:32–33 (1982).
64. Aldes, J. H., Jadeson, W. J., and Grabinski, S. *Amer. J. Phys. Med.* 33:79–83 (1954).
65. Coodley, E. L. *Am. Pract.* 2:181–187 (1960).
66. Mane, O. and Thorseth, K. *Acta Orthop. Scand.* 33:347–349 (1963).
67. Newman, M. K., Kill, M., and Frampton, G. *Am. J. Phys. Med.* 37:206–209 (1958).
68. Kleinkort, J. A. and Wood, F. *Phys. Ther.* 55:1320–1324 (1975).
69. Griffin, J. E., Echternach, J. L., Price, R. E., and Touchstone, J. C. *Phys. Ther.* 47:594–601 (1967).
70. Tsitlanadaze, V. G. *Soobshch. Akad. Nauk. Ciruz. SSR.* 63:237–240 (1971).
71. Dovzhanskaya, V. S. *Vestnik. Dermatol. Venerol.* 10:50–51 (1980).
72. Kosin, W. M. *Zdrevookhr. Beloruss.* 4:81–82 (1976).
73. Chirkin, A. A. and Kosin, W. M. *Voprosy. Med. Khim.* 22:448–459 (1976).

14

Iontophoretic Drug Delivery

Philip G. Green

Zyma SA, Nyon, Switzerland

Michael Flanagan and Braham Shroot

CIRD Galderma, Valbonne, France

Richard H. Guy

University of California–San Francisco, San Francisco, California

I. INTRODUCTION

The controlled delivery of drugs by the transdermal route is increasingly considered as a means of achieving therapeutic systemic blood levels. However, this mode of administration is presently applicable for only few drugs of appropriately balanced lipophilicity (1). Such molecules are typically small, relatively lipophilic, but with a certain degree of water solubility. For charged, polar molecules, administration by the cutaneous route is particularly difficult owing to the intrinsic lipophilicity of the outermost layer of the skin, the stratum corneum. Several methods have been employed to facilitate the permeation of such molecules, including selective penetration enhancers (2,3) and ion pairing (4–8). However, both methods have been useful for only a few molecules. Iontophoresis is another technique that has been used to enhance the delivery of charged and neutral polar molecules through the skin. This method employs an electrical potential gradient, as a driving force, to increase the cutaneous transport of molecules. The use of iontophoresis is particularly appealing, since it offers the possibility of systemic delivery in a controlled fashion and is potentially effective for any charged molecule.

The technique was in use during the 19th century, and was extensively investigated (9). Recently, the technique has undergone a renaissance of interest as the potential of transdermal drug delivery has been recognized. This is demonstrated by the increase in iontophoretic publications and patents in the scientific literature

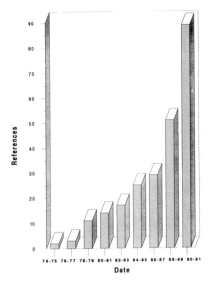

Figure 1 Iontophoresis references found in Derwent world patent file between 1974 and 1991.

(Fig. 1). Currently, however, iontophoresis is approved by the US Food and Drug Administration (FDA) only as a diagnostic test for cystic fibrosis (10) and for the treatment of hyperhydrosis (11,12).

The recent interest in iontophoresis is, in part, linked to the increased production of therapeutically active peptide drugs from the expanding biotechnology industry. Such drugs are typically charged and, therefore, are candidates for delivery by iontophoresis. In this chapter, we will briefly outline some basic principles and current research. In addition, we will draw on our own, and others', research findings to identify several factors that determine the efficiency and limitations of drug delivery by this technique.

II. BASIC PRINCIPLES

A. The Iontophoretic Device

An iontophoretic device basically consists of a power supply connected to an anode and a cathode. Simplistically speaking, when a charged drug is dissolved in the electrolyte surrounding the electrode of similar polarity and an electromotive force is applied, the molecules are repelled into the subjacent tissue (Fig. 2). For

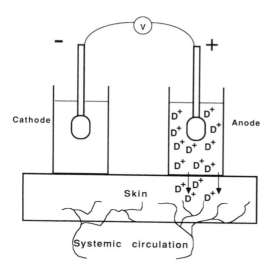

Figure 2 Schematic diagram of the iontophoretic process showing electrorepulsion of drug cation, D^+, from the anode compartment into the skin.

neutral molecules, the mechanism of iontophoretic delivery is intrinsically linked with electroosmotic water flux (see Sect. II.D).

B. Porous Pathways

The major contribution to the impedance of the skin appears to reside in the stratum corneum. This conclusion is supported by the negligible resistance to ion flow that is presented by skin stripped of its stratum corneum (13). When a potential gradient is established across intact skin, ions will flow through routes of lowest impedance. These routes have been identified with various porous pathways (14–18) (e.g., sweat glands, sebaceous glands, hair follicles, and so-called skin imperfections). Burnette and Ongpipattanakul (18) elegantly demonstrated that the iontophoretically driven movement of a negatively charged, fluorescent, dye (fluorescein) occurred through skin "pores." In these experiments, a solution of fluorescein was placed in the receptor chamber (dermal side) of a skin diffusion cell; the anode was placed in the donor compartment, the cathode in the receptor. Current was applied, and the dye moved through the skin from the dermal to the epidermal side. The pathways of dye transport were located at discrete sites (pores) on the skin surface using a microscope with a fluorescent attachment. Microelectrodes were then scanned across the skin surface to record the potential difference as a function of position: the potential difference was significantly elevated at positions directly above the pore centers.

C. Skin Permselectivity

The skin is believed to be negatively charged at pH values above 4 (19) owing to the presence of a preponderance of carboxylic acid functionalities in the barrier layer (20). Consequently, the skin is expected to behave as a permselective membrane, favoring cation transport, but hindering the movement of anions. Since the major route for drug flux under iontophoresis appears to occur through pores, it is the charge associated with these pathways that is important. It follows that the configuration of the charged groups will determine the relative polarity of each pore (21). Pikal has suggested that hairless mouse skin contains three types of pores (22), negative, positive, and neutral, and that the negative subset is preponderant. Subsequently, it was demonstrated, both theoretically (23) and experimentally (24), that the iontophoretic enhancement of molecules of various size and charge could be described adequately with a model based on a heterogeneous array of pores.

A very clear demonstration of the permselectivity of the skin to cation transport comes from experiments (25) showing that the transport number (the proportion of total current carried by a particular ion) of Na^+ across excised human skin, at pH 7.4, is about double that of Cl^-.

D. Electroosmosis

The application of iontophoresis also enhances the transport of neutral molecules across the skin (17,25–29). Gangarosa et al. employed cathodal and anodal iontophoresis to facilitate the in vivo penetration of several uncharged molecules into the skin (26) and demonstrated that penetration was greater from the anode than from the cathode. Neutral molecules move, under the influence of a potential gradient, by convective flow, which is the result of electroosmotic and osmotic forces (20). Both forces arise because of the permselectivity of the skin. The electroosmotic term derives from the fact that, under an applied current, the skin favors the transport of Na^+ over Cl^- (the transport number of Na^+ through excised cadaver skin at pH 7.4 has been determined to be > 0.5; 25,30). As a result, there is a net movement of water from anode to cathode, and this momentum is transferred to the neutral drug molecules.

The osmotic flow contribution is established as follows: Consider an excised skin membrane separating anode and cathode compartments, which both contain saline solutions at identical concentrations. Application of current induces Na^+ to move from anode to cathode, Cl⁻ to move in the opposite direction. Because t_{Na^+} > t_{Cl^-}, and electroneutrality must be maintained, there is a net increase in [NaCl] in the cathodal compartment, and a net decrease in the anodal chamber. Accordingly, this disparity causes an osmotic flow of water from anode to cathode. The importance of the osmotic flux term has not been examined in detail. However, Pikal has stated recently that its contribution to the total volume flow is rather insignificant (22).

Pikal and Shah measured bulk water flow across hairless mouse skin under iontophoretic conditions (pH 8.3, 35°C, 1.0 mA/cm²) and found that it flowed, from anode to cathode, at a rate in the order of microliters per hour per square centimeter (23). From this data one would expect that cathodal iontophoresis would retard the passage of a neutral molecule. However, Gangarosa et al. have shown that is possible to facilitate the penetration of the neutral molecules water, thymidine, and 9-β-D-arabinofuranosyladenine across excised skin using cathodal iontophoresis (26). In addition, we have also demonstrated the effectiveness of cathodal iontophoresis in facilitating the permeation of tritiated water (Fig. 3) and alanine (Fig. 4) across hairless mouse skin. These observations may be due to electrically induced skin changes and a resulting decrease in barrier function. An alternative hypothesis invokes a mechanism by which neutral molecules are "cotransported," along with Cl⁻, within closely bound hydration sheaths.

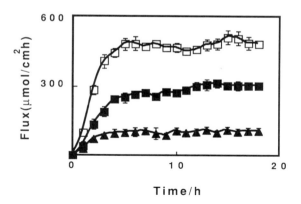

Figure 3 Iontophoretic flux of water across hairless mouse skin in vitro. (a) Passively (closed triangles), (b) from the cathode (closed squares), and (c) from the anode (open squares). Each data point represents the mean (±SD) of four determinations. Electrode chamber contained 1 μCi/mL tritiated water in pH 7.4 HEPES-buffered saline. Iontophoresis was performed at 0.36 mA/cm².

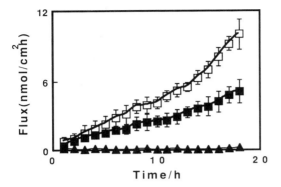

Figure 4 Iontophoretic flux of alanine across hairless mouse skin in vitro. (a) Passively (closed triangles), (b) from the cathode (closed squares), and (c) from the anode (open squares). Each data point represents the mean (±SD) of four determinations. Electrode chamber contained 10 mM alanine in pH 7.4 HEPES-buffered saline. Iontophoresis was performed at 0.36 mA/cm². (From Ref. 68)

III. EXPERIMENTAL DESIGN

A. Diffusion Cells

Several in vitro diffusion cells have been employed in iontophoretic studies (31–34). Typically, such cells consist of anode and cathode compartments separated by excised skin in a vertical configuration. The drug solution is placed in the "driving" electrode compartment in contact with the stratum corneum side of the skin (donor chamber); the electrode of opposite polarity is immersed in electrolyte on the dermal side (receptor chamber). The design can be simply modified to allow quantification of volume flows during iontophoresis (23,24). Such systems, though, are not wholly representative of the in vivo situation, since they involve placement of an electrode effectively "under" the skin. A different type of cell, which more faithfully reflects in vivo experiments, has been developed by Glikfeld et al. (34). In this design, the electrodes are placed on the same side of the skin (Fig. 5). The two electrode compartments are separated electrically and physically by a glass wall. Consequently, the path of current flow is from the driving electrode compartment across the skin into the receiver chamber, and then from this chamber and back *out* across the skin again to the electrode of opposite polarity. Communication between electrodes along the surface of the skin has been shown to be negligible (34). A similar design was also proposed by Bellantone et al. (32). In their cell, the skin membrane was large

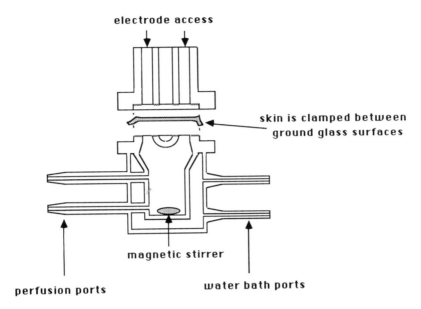

electrode access

skin is clamped between
ground glass surfaces

magnetic stirrer

perfusion ports

water bath ports

Figure 5 In vitro iontophoretic diffusion cell.

enough to overlap the edges of the diffusion cell. One electrode was placed in the donor compartment, the other was attached to the stratum corneum side of the skin that protruded from the rim of the diffusion cell. The effect of different cell configurations on the iontophoretic delivery of benzoate was examined, and the results implied that the overall delivery was independent of cell design. Therefore, it now appears that reliable data can be acquired from both of the major types of cell design. The advantages of the cell with electrodes on the same (surface) side of a single piece of skin are (a) the significance of lateral transport can be assessed, and (b) the usefulness of iontophoresis for subcutaneous, noninvasive sampling can be examined (see Sect. V.B).

B. Electrodes

When a potential difference is applied across the skin, ions move between the electrodes. The permselectivity of the skin leads to the preferential transport of cations and a charge imbalance in the electrolyte surrounding each electrode. To maintain electroneutrality, reactions at the electrodes must create or remove the necessary ions. With inert electrodes, such as nickel, stainless steel, or platinum, the anode fulfills its responsibility by producing hydronium ions from the oxidation of water; the cathode, on the other hand, produces hydroxide by reduction of water. Electrolysis of water in iontophoretic systems is undesirable, since it creates highly mobile current-carrying species (i.e., H^+ and OH^-). Such ions can compete with similarly charged drug ions and, thereby, reduce the transport number of that drug. In addition, the accompanying (and potentially large) pH fluctuations can damage the skin (and cause, for example, irritation) and degrade the drug. Reversible electrodes such as silver/silver chloride, are considered more desirable for iontophoresis experiments (25,35,36). The Ag/AgCl electrodes do not electrolyze water because the electrode potential necessary is higher than that for the electrode reactions of silver and silver chloride. The sequence of electrical events that occur within an iontophoretic system consisting of Ag/AgCl anode and cathode in solutions of NaCl electrolyte is outlined in Figure 6. The Na^+ ion is repelled from the anode compartment and enters the skin, leaving a charge imbalance in the solution surrounding the positive electrode. This is resolved by Cl^-, which is attracted to the anode, combining with Ag^0 to form solid AgCl, and releasing an electron to the electrical circuit:

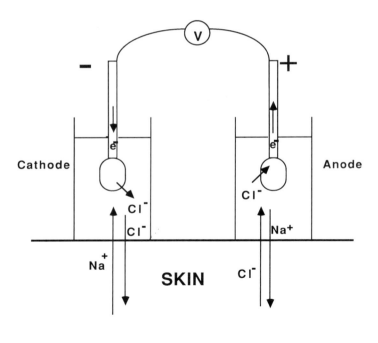

Figure 6   Schematic diagram of iontophoretic system showing electrode reaction.

$$Ag^0(s) + Cl^-(aq) \rightarrow AgCl(s) + e^-$$

In the cathodal compartment, the negative electrode attracts Na^+ through the skin into the receptor phase. Again, a charge imbalance is created, which is then resolved by dissociation of AgCl(s) from the electrode using an electron from the circuit:

$$AgCl(s) + e^- \rightarrow Ag^0(s) + Cl^-(aq)$$

Thus, the net transfer of one $Na^+(aq)$ and one $Cl^-(aq)$ from anode chamber to cathode chamber is effected. Although the reverse movement of Cl^- balances, to a certain extent, the foregoing process, the permselectivity of the skin to Na^+ (by a factor of about 2:1) dictates the *net* flow of ions as stated (and the net osmotic flow of solvent in the same direction).

An alternative method to minimize pH variations within iontophoretic systems has been devised by Sanderson et al. (37,38). In this approach, the anode, for example, is surrounded by an anion-exchange material so that the generated cations, such as H^+, are unable to reach the drug solution and inhibit the transport efficiency of the drug.

A novel electrode system to delivery molecules iontophoretically in vivo has been devised by Schaefer et al. (39). This device consists of two electrode pads, one of which contains the drug, the other contains only the electrolyte. Dissimilar metals are made to contact the surface of the pads and are connected to one another by conducting wire. The electromotive force that is then generated between the electrodes, provides the driving force for the iontophoresis.

C. Skin

Many different animal models have been used in vitro for iontophoretic drug delivery studies, including hairless mouse (23,25,28,31,32,34), hairless guinea pig (40), hairless rat (29,41), and fuzzy rat (27). In vivo experiments have been performed in the pig (36,42), monkey (43), dog (38), and rabbit (44,45). Human skin has been used both in vitro (18,36) and in vivo (46,47). Kasting and Bowman (30) observed that excised human skin has a lower electrical resistance than the tissue in vivo, but that Na^+ permeability in vitro was similar to that in vivo (48). In the same report, it was also shown that human skin could be stored frozen, for up to 2 months, without significantly affecting Na^+ permeability. The iontophoretic flux of simple ionic species has been reported to be independent of the type of skin used (36); furthermore, there are several studies in which in vivo and in vitro results compare well (30,36,48). However, it has been noted that the iontophoretically induced volume flow through hairless mouse skin is significantly less than that through human skin under identical experimental conditions. This may be due to the lower net negative charge supported by the animal skin (23). The transport path length across the skin, which is a key determinant of the passive steady state flux (49), should be less important in iontophoresis, since it is the current level that dictates the flux of ions. However, the thicker the skin section, the larger its electrical resistance is likely to be and, under constant-current conditions, therefore, the greater the voltage required to attain the desired current level. We expect, furthermore, that the time to attainment of steady state flux under iontophoresis will be inversely proportional to sample thickness. Another factor, important in the selection of a suitable animal model, is the sensitivity of the skin to current-induced barrier damage. This undesirable possibility may be exaggerated in vitro because the natural regeneration processes of the skin cannot take place.

An elegant compromise to the in vitro-versus-in vivo dilemma is the recently characterized "isolated perfused porcine skin flap" (50,51). This ex vivo technique maintains the skin in a viable biochemical state for several hours and permits sophisticated experimentation in drug delivery and percutaneous pharmacokinetics. The use of the procedure to study iontophoresis has now been described for several molecules (52,53).

IV. FACTORS AFFECTING IONTOPHORETIC DELIVERY

A. Current

The steady state flux J_i of an ion i across a membrane under the influence of an applied electrical potential (E) is described by the Nernst–Planck equation (Eq. 1) (54,55). The flux is the sum of two contributions: (a) a passive transport term $[-D_i(\delta c_i/\delta x)]$, and (b) an electrorepulsive term resulting from the applied field $[-D_i (C_i Z_i F/RT) (\delta E/\delta x)]$ where D_i = diffusivity of i, C_i = concentration of i, Z_i = charge, F = Faraday's constant, R = gas constant, and T = absolute temperature.

$$J_i = -D_i \{ (\delta C_i/\delta x) + ((C_i Z_i F)/(RT))\cdot[\delta E/\delta x] \} \qquad [1]$$

The Nernst–Planck equation, combined with the Goldman approximation (56), has been used to predict iontophoretic enhancement ratios i.e., the steady state flux in presence of an applied field divided by the passive steady state flux (28,33,54,55). Masada et al. (33) have used Eq. 1 to model their experimental data. In their studies, a four-electrode potentiostat system was used to maintain a voltage drop across hairless mouse skin; iontophoretic enhancement ratios were measured for several charged permeants at various potentials. They found that, at and below 0.25 V, the experimental and predicted ratios were in close agreement. Above 0.25 V, the measured ratios diverged appreciably from the theoretical predictions; the differences were attributed to the fact that, at these higher voltages, changes in skin resistance were induced leading to increases in current (i.e., ion) flow.

The Nernst–Planck equation does not include a term to describe convective flow and, on this basis alone, therefore, one can expect discrepancies between theory and experiment to occur. Burnette and Marrero (17) included the contribution of convective flow into the Nernst–Planck equation and then showed that the flux of neutral and charged molecules was proportional to the current density. Pikal and Shah (22–24) and Srinivasan and Higuchi (57) have also incorporated this flow term into their analyses and have then been able to predict iontophoretic enhancement ratios.

The iontophoretic current (I) is carried across the membrane by a number of ions. From Faraday's law, 1 mol of any charged species (of unit charge) carries 9.65×10^4 Coulomb (Eq. 2):

$$I = \Sigma Z_i F J_i \qquad [2]$$

The flux of an ion i (J_i), at current I, is a function of its transport number, t_i (Eq. 3):

$$J_i = t_i/(Z_i F) \qquad [3]$$

Although it has been stated that current densities less than 0.5 mA/cm^2 are well-tolerated in humans (58), several studies have suggested that iontophoresis results in effects on the skin that are not fully reversible (18,24,28,32,33,59). These findings are consistent with the observation that application of an iontophoretic current causes a rapid reduction in the resistance of the skin (59). The resistance eventually plateaus at a relatively constant level, well below the initial resistance (18,23). Pikal and Shah (24) demonstrated that the passive flux of glucose across the skin after the application of a current of 3.2 mA/cm^2 for 3 hr was ten times greater than that before current application. Although this observation may be partly explained by a reservoir effect and slow desorption subsequent to current termination (13), an iontophoretically induced modification of skin barrier function is a probable contributor to the phenomenon (18).

The precise physiological changes that are induced in the skin by iontophoresis are not defined. One possible scenario is that the concentration of current flow through appendageal "shunts," or other skin imperfections, results in significant local heating owing to the resulting high-current densities. This heating may disorder the adjacent intercellular SC lipids with a concomitant increase in overall skin permeability (60,61) as the passive contribution to the flux becomes much more important. A recently published paper (62) reported that iontophoresis induced epidermal alterations in pigs in vivo. However, by 6 days posttreatment, the skin had recovered to its normal state. Parenthetically, one might add that the electrical treatment of damaged skin accelerates the wound-healing process (63). Concerns over the potentially damaging effects of electric current on the skin have led many investigators to use pulsed DC iontophoresis for drug delivery (29,31,41,46,64,65). The rationale for this approach is that the skin can be electrically characterized as a resistor and a capacitor in parallel (66). Thus, one can expect polarization of the skin to be induced by an applied electric field and, therefore, a resulting opposition to the flux of drug ions across the skin. Pulsed current, with appropriate depolarizing frequencies, has consequently been employed to reduce the extent of this problem.

B. Electrolyte Composition

1. Buffer Components

Electrolytes used in iontophoresis typically include a buffer to maintain pH in the event of electrolysis of water during current passage. Buffers are usually salt solutions containing small inorganic ions. The presence of such salts introduces a competitive current carrier into the drug reservoir. Consequently, the efficiency of drug transport is likely to be reduced. The problem can be circumvented in certain cases. For example, Burnette and Ongpipattanakul (25) employed HEPES buffer in their iontophoresis experiments: the principal buffering ion is a large zwitterionic molecule, with pK_a = 7.4. It can be usefully employed, therefore, at physiological pH with relatively small effect on the transport number of the drug.

2. Ionic Strength

Obviously, in iontophoresis, the applied drug solution must contain a reasonable concentration of electrolyte so that the current can be efficiently conducted. If the drug is neutral, the presence of electrolyte is essential for the electroosmotic effect to be operable. Furthermore, the operation of reversible electrodes such as Ag/AgCl demands the presence of aqueous chloride ions in the surrounding anode medium. However, it is well-recognized that the addition of electrolyte to the drug solution will, almost inevitably, cause the transport number of the permeant to decrease. In particular, the Na^+ and Cl^- ions that compose saline are small, very mobile, and highly competitive charge carriers. Several studies have illustrated the foregoing points with a variety of drug species, including benzoic acid (32), the divalent peptide arginine-vasopressin (41), the monovalent cation verapamil (31), and the monovalent anion butyrate (27). In the latter example, the replacement of NaCl as the electrolyte with salt solutions containing multivalent ions resulted in more efficient butyrate transport, reflecting the alteration in electrolyte ion transport number.

For neutral molecules, the effect of ionic strength is more complicated because convective flow plays the major role. Pikal et al. (23) have recently shown that the flux of water across hairless mouse skin decreases with increasing ionic strength of the electrolyte. A similar inverse dependence, at high-ionic strength, was also seen with glucose (24). Wearley and Chien (29), on the other hand, showed that increasing the ionic strength of the electrolyte increased the anodal iontophoresis zidovudine (azidothymidine; AZT) across hairless rat skin, but that eventually this augmentation leveled off at the highest salt concentrations used. There is evidence that molecules flow through porous pathways during iontophoresis (14–18). When an electric field is established across a membrane containing pores, a diffuse double layer is established at the surface of the pore. The thickness of this double layer is directly proportional to the zeta potential. As the ionic strength of the electrolyte is increased the thickness of the double layer and, hence, the zeta potential, decreases. These changes, in turn, would be expected to lower the electroosmotic flow of water (29). From the standpoint of iontophoretic efficiency, therefore, it would appear that it is desirable to reduce, as much as possible, the ionic strength of the electrolyte. However, certain practicalities dictate that the electrolyte level must remain finite. For example, as stated earlier, the effective function of Ag/AgCl electrodes requires a supply of aqueous chloride ions. If these are not available, then the electrodes themselves begin to break down in the attempt to mobilize Cl^- into solution. This process results, typically, in precipitation of insoluble silver hydroxy species (since Ag^+ must also be mobilized) and poisoning of the system. A further drawback of low electrolyte levels can be illustrated by considering the delivery of a cationic drug (D^+) from a donor solution containing only a modest amount of NaCl. If a constant current is passed, the charge from the anode compartment will initially be carried by Na^+ (which is likely to have a higher transport number than D^+). With increasing time, though, as Na^+ depletes significantly, more and more current will be carried by D^+ (67). It follows that the flux of D^+ will increase progressively with time (as long as the supply of drug is relatively large), and that the delivery control, which is often expressed as one of the major advantages of iontophoresis, is lost. This phenomenon was observed during the iontophoresis of lysine from a solution at pH 7.4, in which the initial concentration of Na^+ was 147 mM (Fig. 7) (68).

3. pH

In addition to the composition of the electrolyte, the maintenance and selection of the vehicle pH is important. For weak acids and bases, pH control is required to maintain the species in an ionic form. Thus, in the iontophoresis of lidocaine, for example, it was shown that decreasing the vehicle pH, which increased the percentage ionized form of the drug, caused the flux to rise concomitantly (69). On the other hand, the opposite effect has been observed for the tripeptide thyrotropin (TRH) (17). For this drug, iontophoretic delivery of the neutral form, from a donor solution at pH 8, was higher than that of the cationic species at pH 4. The results were explained in terms of electroosmotic flow and the charge of the skin. At pH 8, skin carries a net negative charge; therefore, as the pH is lowered the charge on the skin is progressively neutralized. The impact on TRH flux is as follows: At high pH, because the peptide is un-ionized, electroosmosis is the

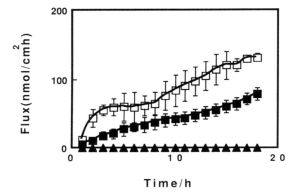

Figure 7 Iontophoretic flux of lysine across hairless mouse skin in vitro. (a) Passively (closed triangles), (b) from the anode at pH 4.0 (closed squares), and (c) from the anode at pH 7.4 (open squares). Each data point represents the mean (±SD) of four determinations. Electrode chamber contained 10 mM lysine in HEPES-buffered saline. Iontophoresis was performed at 0.36 mA/cm². (From Ref. 68)

dominant effect, owing to the high flux of Na⁺ present in the electrolyte. At low pH, electroosmosis is significantly attenuated (because the negative charge density on the skin has been reduced) and TRH moves under the influence of electrorepulsion. The relatively low transport number of TRH⁺, however, makes this an inefficient process. A parallel observation has recently been made with the cationic amino acid lysine (68) (see Fig. 7).

C. Physicochemical Properties of the Permeant

1. Charge

A systematic investigation of the effect of permeant charge on iontophoretic flux has not been undertaken. The difficulty with such a study is to isolate the charge variable from other important parameters, such as molecular weight, pK_a, and lipophilicity.

Phipps et al. (36) have compared the iontophoretic fluxes of Na⁺ and Mg²⁺, and of K⁺ and Ca²⁺, across excised pig skin. The delivery of the divalent ions was approximately half that of the monovalent species, an observation attributed this to the stronger binding of divalent cations to fixed negative sites in the skin. Similarly, Burnette and Ongpipattanakul (25) demonstrated that the replacement of NaCl by CaCl₂ as the electrolyte in an iontophoretic experiments resulted in the increased cathodal iontophoresis of Cl⁻ (owing to the strong binding of Ca^{2+} to the negative skin sites, and alteration of the membrane's permselectivity). In addition, there was an increase in electroosmotic flow from cathode to anode.

The iontophoretic flux of an anion is expected to be less than that of a similarly sized cation at, for example, pH 7.4, because the flow of the anion is counter to the electroosmotic flow of water (20). If the anion is so large that its transport number approaches zero, then it will remain within the donor chamber. In such a case, one possible method to induce the permeation of the anion is to place it into the anode chamber and to rely upon its convection by electroosmotic flow (70). Such an approach requires that the anion and electrode be separated physically by (for example) a salt bridge, so that the putative permeant cannot undergo electrochemical degradation.

2. Lipophilicity

Del Terzo et al. (27) used series of n-alkanols and n-alkanoic acids to investigate the effect of lipophilicity on iontophoretic enhancement. Not unexpectedly, given that iontophoresis is an approach targeted at the augmented delivery of polar compounds, the enhancement of both chemical classes decreased as permeant lipophilicity increased.

Recently, the dependence of iontophoretic delivery upon penetrant lipophilicity was also examined using (neutral) zwitterionic amino acids, and a series of "blocked" (and, again, neutral) tripeptides (71). Although the overall trend was diminishing enhancement with increasing lipophilicity, the dependence was very weak (i.e., a 4-log unit increase in lipophilicity resulted in only an order of magnitude decrease in normalized flux; Fig. 8).

3. Molecular Size

Recent reports that insulin can be delivered across skin by iontophoresis (45,64,65) have implied that the technique is applicable to relatively large molecules [relative molecular mass (M_r) insulin is ~6000 Da, and the protein frequently exists in solution in a multimeric form; 42].

A major driving force for the iontophoretic delivery of charged molecules is electrorepulsion. Because it appears that iontophoretic transport follows a porous pathway, one expects that the degree of enhancement will be penetrant size- dependent, and that, as size increases, the flux will diminish (until, ultimately, very large species will be reflected away from the skin surface; 24). The predicted inverse relation between M_r and ionophoretic flux has been shown for the series of n-alkanoic acids and n-alkanols (27), and for a collection of negatively charged amino acids, N-acetylated derivatives, and tripeptides (Fig. 9) (71).

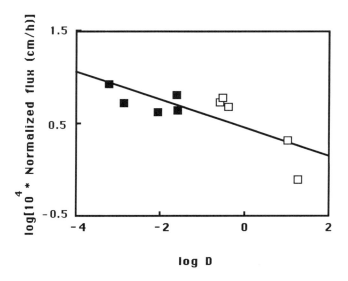

Figure 8 Normalized flux (relative to donor compartment concentration) after 12 hr of anodal iontophoresis (a) for zwitterionic amino acids (closed squares) and (b) neutral tripeptides (open squares), plotted as a function of octanol/aqueous electrolyte distribution coefficient (D). Each data point is the mean of six determinations. (From Ref. 71)

V. FUTURE DEVELOPMENTS

A. Peptide Delivery

Recent advances in genetic engineering have enabled the large-scale production of therapeutically active peptides and proteins. These molecules are particularly difficult to administer by the oral route because of their susceptibility to degradation in the gastrointestinal tract and extensive hepatic metabolism. Intravenous administration is widely used, therefore. However, this approach is clearly undesirable for long-term therapy, particularly if the peptide or protein has a short biological half-life.

Under ideal circumstances, the drawbacks associated with intravenous or oral administration can be overcome with transdermal delivery. The major difficulty with passive peptide permeation across the skin is that their intrinsic hydrophilicity considerably restricts their transport through the lipophilic stratum corneum. Nevertheless, a recent study has shown that a peptide, containing 13-amino acid residues, was able to passively penetrate split-thickness human skin (72). Furthermore, chemical penetration enhancers have been used to

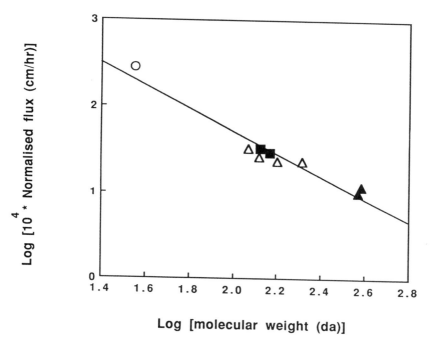

Figure 9 Normalized (steady state) flux, relative to donor compartment concentration, during cathodal iontophoresis for (a) anionic tripeptides (closed triangles), (b) anionic amino acids (closed squares), (c) negatively charged *N*-acetylated amino acid derivatives (open triangles), and (d) chloride ion (open circle) (25) plotted as a function of molecular weight. Each data point is the mean of six determinations. (From Ref. 71)

enhance passive flux: for example, dimethyl sulfoxide (DMSO) to increase insulin delivery (73), and laurocapram (Azone) to augment the flux of both vasopressin (74) and the neuropeptide, DEYE (75).

However, it is iontophoresis that offers the greatest hope for the effective delivery of peptides and proteins across the skin (76,77). For small peptides (e.g., TRH; 17), the potential of the technique looks very promising. For larger species, though, it is not yet possible to predict the likelihood of success. The uncertainty here may be illustrated by the efforts underway to deliver insulin by iontophoresis. Insulin is both charged and large, containing 51-amino acid residues; in addition, it forms aggregate structures in solution. These properties make the protein a major challenge for delivery by the transdermal route. Stephen et al. (42), however, were able to successfully deliver a strongly ionized, monomeric form of insulin to a single pig in vivo using iontophoresis. This observation prompted many investigators to pursue the iontophoretic approach. In an initial attempt, for example, Kari demonstrated that regular insulin could be delivered to rabbits in vivo, but *only* after prior disruption or removal of the stratum corneum (44). It was not until the work of Siddiqui et al. (64) that regular insulin was transported across intact skin by constant current iontophoresis. In these experiments, the pH of the donor solution was maintained below the isoelectric point of insulin; insulin cations were created as a result, and aggregation was suppressed. Meyer et al. (45) have also administered human insulin successfully to diabetic rabbits using low current densities, and application of the protein incorporated into patches containing urea. More recently, iontophoretic insulin delivery has been performed using pulsed-current iontophoresis (65). This approach prolonged the reduction of glucose blood levels in the animal model, when compared with the use of continuous direct current. Pulsing at higher frequencies was particularly effective. Parenthetically, it should be noted that pulsed-current iontophoresis has also been used to deliver arginine-vasopressin, which contains nine-amino acid residues (41,78). A more general point is that it seems reasonable to expect that certain peptidic species, especially those required in a noncontinuous fashion for optimal therapy (79,80), will benefit from the flexibility which can be programmed into the current delivery pattern by straightforward circuitry construction.

Further examples of successful peptide iontophoresis have been reported recently for the decapeptides gonadotropin-releasing hormone (GnRH) and two of its analogues (79). Although GnRH was metabolized in the skin during iontophoresis, the analogues could be delivered at rates that would be sufficient to produce therapeutic plasma levels. Meyer et al. (47) also demonstrated that leuprolide, a nine-amino acid polypeptide, could be delivered to human volunteers using low-current density iontophoresis, and that elevated peptide plasma levels could be achieved without cutaneous injury.

One of the advantages of transdermal delivery of peptides is that the skin may have a limited capacity to perform enzymatic degradation (81). However, aminopeptidases are present in dermal tissue (82), and molecules, such as gonadotropin (79), have been metabolized during iontophoresis. Iontophoresis may be useful in that it reduces the residence time of the peptide in the skin, and, therefore, reduces the exposure of the peptide to the enzymes. Although this hypothesis has not been fully tested, it appears from studies with insulin, and with a series of tripeptides (71), that peptidase activity in the skin is relatively low.

Much research continues in this area, and new information appears regularly. With our growing understanding of the mechanism of iontophoresis, the development and optimization of the technique to address relevant problems will become a reality.

B. Noninvasive Sampling of Biological Fluids

There are multiple situations in which the provision of optimal health care requires information about the level of one or more substances in the systemic circulation. Typically, then, a blood sample is drawn in a procedure that is often traumatic for the patient, and sometimes potentially hazardous to the sampler. Therefore, there is interest in the development of noninvasive procedures for sampling biological fluids. Recently, Peck et al. (83) showed that the outward, passive, transdermal migration of materials present in the plasma could be used for this purpose. Adsorbent collection devices left on the skin for several hours were used to obtain the samples. Although feasible, the approach is limited by the inherent variability in skin permeability, which adds significantly to the "noise" in the results, and by the prolonged collection period necessary. These difficulties may be circumvented by iontophoresis. Glikfeld et al. (84) have demonstrated that because of the symmetric nature of the iontophoretic procedure, and the fact that ions are moving from and to both electrodes on the skin surface, it is possible to pull various substances from beneath the skin to the surface. The idea was illustrated using clonidine and theophylline, and the amounts extracted were

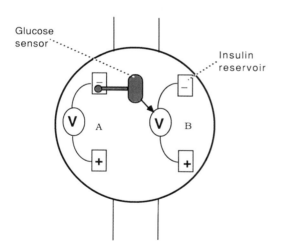

Figure 10 Hypothetical feedback system including glucose sensor and insulin delivery unit. The system (A) continuously samples glucose iontophoretically at the cathode. Within the cathode there is a glucose sensor that sends a message to unit (B) as soon as the glucose level reaches a certain preprogrammed value. This, in turn, starts the iontophoretic delivery of insulin. When the glucose level reverts back to "normal" the delivery of insulin is curtailed.

linearly correlated with the perfusing subdermal concentrations. That electro-osmosis was an important contributor to the observed findings was confirmed using glucose as the extracted species. This has raised the intriguing possibility of a novel noninvasive glucose-sensing approach to replace the currently used, and poorly tolerated, needle-stick. In the 21st century crystal ball, the optimist may now envisage, perhaps, a feedback loop system involving both the iontophoretic sensing of a diabetic's glucose level, and the subsequently controlled, ionto-phoretic input of the appropriate insulin dose (Fig. 10).

C. Local Topical Treatment

Although one typically thinks of iontophoresis as a technique to increase the systemic absorption of a topically applied compound, it can also be effective in promoting the concentration of drugs within the skin. Keister and Kasting (55) demonstrated theoretically that the steady state distribution profile of a drug iontophoresed into the skin is quite different from that achieved by passive diffusion (Fig. 11). The predicted concentration profile in the stratum corneum has been observed experimentally after short periods of iontophoresis (85).

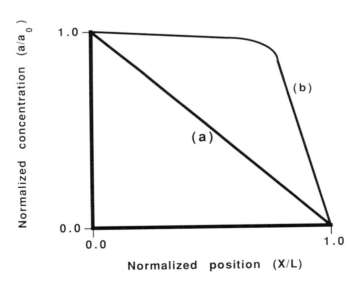

Figure 11 Theoretical normalized concentration gradient of a molecule, within a membrane of width L, following (a) passive diffusion and (b) application of an electric field. (a represents the activity of the molecule within the membrane at depth X. a_0 is the activity within the donor phase.)

In terms of therapeutic agents, iontophoresis has increased the penetration of idoxuridine, thymidine, and 9-β-D-arabinofluranosyladenine into mouse skin (26). Reservoir effects have also been demonstrated, following iontophoresis, for prednisolone in human skin (86), and verapamil in the fuzzy rat (13,85). In another study, Glass et al. (43) demonstrated that iontophoresis could be employed to increase the total amount of dexamethasone in the skin of rhesus monkey in vivo. These findings indicated, furthermore, that the drug permeated to the subcutaneous tissue in quantities significantly greater than those achieved in control (i.e., passive transport) experiments.

It follows that, in addition to the potential of iontophoresis to provide a viable administration route for the new drugs of the biotechnology revolution, the technique may also radically improve the bioavailability and efficacy of dermally active and of topically applied drugs.

ACKNOWLEDGMENTS

Supported in part by a grant from the US National Institutes of Health (HD-27839). We thank our colleagues in California and Valbonne for their constructive advice and suggestions.

REFERENCES

1. Guy, R. H. and Hadgraft, J. *J. Controlled Release 4*:237 (1987).
2. Walters, K. A. In *Transdermal Drug Delivery—Developmental Issues and Research Initiatives*. Hadgraft, J. and Guy, R. H. (eds.). Marcel Dekker, New York, p. 197 (1989).
3. Cooper, E. R. In *Solution Behavior of Surfactants*, Vol. 1. Mittal, K. L. and Fendler, E. J. (eds.). Plenum Press, New York, p. 1505 (1982).
4. Hadgraft, J., Green, P. G., and Wotton, P. K. In *Percutaneous Absorption*, 2nd ed. Bronaugh, R. L. and Maibach, H. I. (eds.). Marcel Dekker, New York, p. 555 (1989).
5. Hadgraft, J., Walters, K. A., and Wotton, P. K. *Int. J. Pharm. 32*:257 (1986).
6. Green, P. G., Guy, R. H., and Hadgraft, J. *Int. J. Pharm. 48*:103 (1988).
7. Green, P. G., Hadgraft, J., and Ridout, G. *Pharm. Res. 6*:628 (1989).
8. Neubert, R. *Pharm. Res. 6*:743 (1989).
9. Leduc, S. *Ann. Electrobiol. 3*:545 (1900).
10. Gibson, L. E. and Cooke, R. E. *Pediatrics 23*:545 (1959).
11. Grice, K., Sattar, H., and Baker, H. *Br. J. Dermatol. 86*:72 (1972).
12. Levit, F. *Cutis 26*:192 (1980).
13. Wearley, L., Liu, J.-C., and Chien, Y. W. *J. Controlled Release 9*:231 (1989).
14. Abramson, H. A. and Gorin, H. H. *J. Phys. Chem. 44*:1094 (1940).
15. Abramson, H. A. and Engel, M. G. *Arch. Dermatol. Syphilol. 44*:190 (1940).
16. Grimnes, S. *Acta Dermatol. Venereol. 64*:93 (1984).
17. Burnette, R. R. and Marrero, D. *J. Pharm. Sci. 75*:738 (1986).
18. Burnette, R. R. and Ongpipattanakul, B. *J. Pharm. Sci. 77*:132 (1988).

19. Rosendal, T. *Acta Physiol. Scand.* 5:130 (1942-43).
20. Burnette, R. R. In *Transdermal Drug Delivery—Developmental Issues and Research Initiatives.* Hadgraft, J. and Guy, R. H. (eds.). Marcel Dekker, New York, p. 247 (1989).
21. Barry, P. H., Diamond, J. M., and Wright, E. M. *J. Membr. Biol.* 4:358 (1971).
22. Pikal, M. J. *Pharm. Res.* 7:118 (1990).
23. Pikal, M. J. and Shah, S. *Pharm. Res.* 7:213 (1990).
24. Pikal, M. J. and Shah, S. *Pharm. Res.* 7:222 (1990).
25. Burnette, R. R. and Ongpipattanakul, B. *J. Pharm. Sci.* 76:765 (1987).
26. Gangarosa, L. P., Park, N. H., Wiggins, C. A., and Hill, J. M. *J. Pharmacol. Exp. Ther.* 212:377 (1980).
27. Del Terzo, S., Behl, C. R., and Nash, R. A. *Pharm. Res.* 6:85 (1989).
28. Srinivasan, V., Higuchi, W. I., and Su, M. W. *J. Controlled Release* 10:157 (1989).
29. Wearley, L. and Chien, Y. W. *Pharm. Res.* 7:34 (1990).
30. Kasting, G. B. and Bowman, L. A. *Pharm. Res.* 7:113 (1990).
31. Wearley, L., Liu, J.-C., and Chien, Y. W. *J. Controlled Release* 8:237 (1989).
32. Harper Bellantone, N., Rim, S., Francoeur, M. L., and Rasadi, B. *Int. J. Pharm.* 30:63 (1986).
33. Masada, T., Higuchi, W. I., Srinivasan, V., Rohr, U., Fox, J., Behl, C., and Pons, S. *Int. J. Pharm.* 49:57 (1989).
34. Glikfeld, P., Cullander, C., Hinz, R. S., and Guy, R. H. *Pharm. Res.* 5:443 (1988).
35. Unterecker, D. F. and Phipps, J. B. European Patent Application 0182520 (1985).
36. Phipps, J. B., Padmanabhan, R. V., and Lattin, G. A. *J. Pharm. Sci.* 78:365 (1989).
37. Sanderson, J. E., Del Riel, S., and Dixon, R. *J. Pharm. Sci.* 78:361 (1989).
38. Sanderson, J. E., Caldwell, R. W., Hsaio, J., Dixon, R., and Tuttle, R. R. *J. Pharm. Sci.* 76:215 (1987).
39. Schaefer, H., Duteil, L., and Juhlin, L. UK Patent Application 2206493A (1989).
40. Behl, C. R., Kumar, S., Malick, A. W., Del Terzo, S., Higuchi, W. I., and Srinivasan, V. In *Percutaneous Absorption*, 2nd ed. Bronaugh, R. L. and Maibach, H. I. (eds.). Marcel Dekker, New York, p. 255 (1989).
41. Lelawongs, P., Lui, J. C., Siddiqui, O., and Chien, Y. W. *Int. J. Pharm.* 56:13 (1989).
42. Stephen, R. L., Petelenz, T. J., and Jacobson, S. C. *Biomed. Biochim. Acta* 43:553 (1984).
43. Glass, J. M., Stephen, R. L., and Jacobson, S. C. *Int. J. Dermatol.* 19:519 (1980).
44. Kari, B. *Diabetes* 35:217 (1986).
45. Meyer, B. R., Katzeff, H. L., Eschbach, J. C., Trimmer, J., Zacharias, S. B., Rosen, S., and Sibalis, D. *Am. J. Med. Sci.* 297:321 (1989).
46. Okabe, K., Yamaguchi, H., and Kawai, Y. *J. Controlled Release* 4:79 (1986).
47. Meyer, B. R., Kreis, W., Eschbach, J., O'Mara, V., Rosen, S., and Sibalis, D. *Clin. Pharmacol. Ther.* 44:607 (1988).
48. Kasting, G. B. and Bowman, L. A. *Pharm. Res.* 7:1141 (1990).
49. Potts, R. O. and Francoeur, M. L. *J. Invest. Dermatol.* 96:495 (1991).
50. Williams, P. L. and Riviere, J. E. *J. Pharm. Sci.* 78:1 (1989).
51. Williams, P. L., Carver, M. P., and Riviere, J. E. *J. Pharm. Sci.* 79:305 (1990).
52. Sage, B. and Riviere, J. E. *Proc. Int. Symp. Controlled Release Bioact. Mater.* 16:49 (1989).

53. Riviere, J. E., Sage, B., and Monteiro-Riviere, N. A. *J. Toxicol. Cutan.-Ocular Toxicol.* 9:493 (1990).
54. Kasting, G. B., Merritt, E. W., and Keister, J. C. *J. Membr. Sci.* 35:137 (1988).
55. Keister, J. C. and Kasting, G. B. *J. Membr. Sci.* 29:155 (1986).
56. Goldman, D. E. *J. Gen. Physiol.* 26:37 (1943).
57. Srinivasan, V. and Higuchi, W. I. *Int. J. Pharm.* 60:133 (1990).
58. Abramson, H. A. *J. Allergy* 12:169 (1941).
59. Burnette, R. R. and Bagniefski, T. M. *J. Pharm. Sci.* 77:492 (1988).
60. Golden, G. M., McKie, J. E., and Potts, R. O. *J. Pharm. Sci.* 76:25 (1986).
61. Golden, G. M., Guzek, D. B., Kennedy, A. H., McKie, J. E., and Potts, R. O. *Biochemistry* 26:2382 (1986).
62. Monteiro-Riviere, N. A. *Fundam. Appl. Toxicol.* 15:174 (1990).
63. Weiss, D. S., Kirsner, R., and Eaglstein, W. H. *Arch. Dermatol.* 126:222 (1990).
64. Siddiqui, O., Sun, Y., Liu, J.-C., and Chien, Y. W. *J. Pharm. Sci.* 76:341 (1987).
65. Liu, J.-C., Sun, Y., Siddiqui, O., Chien, Y. W., Shi, W.-M., and Li, J. *Int. J. Pharm.* 44:197 (1988).
66. Yamamoto, T. and Yamamoto, Y. *Med. Biol. Eng. Comp.* 14:151 (1976).
67. Phipps, J. B., Sunram, J. M., and Padmanabhan, R. V. *Proc. Int. Symp. Controlled Release Bioact. Mater.* 16:50 (1989).
68. Green, P. G., Hinz, R. S., Cullander, C., Yamane, G., and Guy, R. H. *Pharm. Res.* 8:1113 (1991).
69. Siddiqui, O., Roberts, M. S., and Polack, A. E. *J. Pharm. Pharmacol.* 37:732 (1985).
70. MacLaughlin, S. and Poo, M.-M. *Biophys. J.* 34:85 (1981).
71. Green, P. G., Hinz, R. S., Kim, A., Szoka, F. C., and Guy, R. H. *Pharm. Res.* 8:1121 (1991).
72. Dawson, B. V., Hadley, M. E., Levine, N., Kreutzfeld, K. L., Don, S., Eytan, T., and Hruby, V. J. *J. Invest. Dermatol.* 94:432 (1990).
73. Kazim, M., Webber, C., Strausberg, L., Laforet, G., Nicholson, J., and Reemksma, J. *Diabetes* 33:181A (1984).
74. Benarjee, P. S. and Ritschel, W. A. *Int. J. Pharm.* 49:199 (1989).
75. Boddé, H. E., Verhoef, J. C., and Ponec, M. *Biochem. Soc. Trans.* 17:943 (1989).
76. Sibalis, D. and Rosen, S. European Patent Application 0278474 (1988).
77. Chien, Y. W., Siddiqui, O., Shi, W.-M., Lelawongs, P., and Liu, J.-C. *J. Pharm. Sci.* 78:376 (1989).
78. Lelawongs, P., Liu, J.-C., and Chien, Y. W. *Int. J. Pharm.* 61:179 (1990).
79. Miller, L. L., Kolaskie, C. J., Smith, G. A., and Rivier, J. *J. Pharm. Sci.* 79:490 (1990).
80. Koch, B. and Lutz-Bucher, B. *Endocrinology* 116:671 (1985).
81. Pannatier, P. J., Testa, B., and Etter, J. C. *Drug Metab. Rev.* 8:319 (1978).
82. Zhou, X. H. and Li Wan Po, A. *Int. J. Pharm.* 62:259 (1990).
83. Peck, C. C., Conner, D. P., Bolden, B. J., Almirez, R. G., Rowland, L. M., Kwiatkowski, T. E., McKelvin, B. A., and Bradley, C. R. In *Skin Pharmacokinetics.* Shroot, B. and Schaefer, H. (eds.). S. Karger, Basel, p. 201 (1987).
84. Glikfeld, P., Hinz, R. S., and Guy, R. H. *Pharm. Res.* 6:988 (1989).
85. Wearley, L. and Chien, Y. W. *Int. J. Pharm.* 59:87 (1990).
86. James, M. P., Graham, R. M., and English, J. *Clin. Exp. Dermatol.* 11:54 (1986).

15

Technological Aspects of Penetration Enhancers in Transdermal Systems

Thomas Hille

Lohmann Therapie Systeme GmbH & Co., Neuwied, Germany

The advantages of the transdermal application of drugs is countered by the limitation of the amount of drug that can be absorbed by the skin. Therefore, special attention must be paid to such components that enhance the ability of the human skin to absorb drugs. These components are the *enhancers*. Thus, it is not surprising that several recent reports on the enhancement of drug absorption by the skin have been published reflecting an increased interest in transdermal application. Representative examples of enhancers that have been formulated into topical systems include:

1. Hydrocarbons
2. Alcohols (e.g., ethanol, undecanol, propanediol, benzyl alcohol)
3. Ketones and their derivatives (e.g., dioxolan derivatives, cyclic ketones; 1)
4. Ethers [e.g., ethoxylated compounds (polysorbates and others)]
5. Carboxylic acids (e.g., oleic acid, ricinoleic acid, capric acid, lauric acid)
6. Esters of carboxylic acids and sulfonic acids, especially when isopropanol is the alcoholic compound (e.g., isopropyl myristate, -palmitate, -oleate)
7. Dimethyl sulfoxide and its derivatives
8. Amides (a) urea, dimethylformamide, (b) lactams (e.g., laurocapram; Azone)

There have been many attempts to describe the mechanisms of action of enhancers, and this aspect will not be discussed further in this chapter. The requirements that enhances have to meet and the resulting technological problems of incorporating these into matrix systems will be identified.

Many studies in the past have assessed enhancer activity as a result of placing the pure enhancer or solutions of it onto the skin surface. This may not be relevant to the incorporation of an enhancer into a transdermal system that must be designed such that both the active drug and enhancer are released into the skin. The first step in development will be to ensure the correct release properties of the polymeric matrix.

It is necessary to distinguish between formulation components that are genuine enhancers and those that modify the properties of the polymeric matrix into which they are incorporated. Materials that act as plasticizers or "softeners" in the polymer will speed drug release from the device, but not necessarily act as skin-enhancing agents. There may be some compounds that will have both properties.

It should be emphasized that an enhancer has to increase the penetration of a drug into the human skin in vivo. By comparison, softeners are additives to polymers that improve the softness, flexibility, extensibility, and possibly even the adhesiveness of polymers (2). An ideal softener should not migrate out of the polymer matrix. It is obvious, however, that an ingredient not being released from the polymer matrix does not penetrate into the human skin. To optimize the physical properties of transdermal systems, it is necessary to incorporate softeners and to minimize the release of these into the skin. During the development phase, the properties of these ingredients are investigated in stress tests.

Although all softeners have the tendency to migrate, this is minimized by appropriate formulation. Fick's laws can be used to assess diffusion of materials from the devices, which may reach significant levels over the time course of application to the skin (1–7 days). Normally, softeners demonstrate significant diffusion tendencies only at elevated temperatures. The migration velocity rapidly increases with temperature, from 20°C to 50°C (ten times), from 20°C to 70°C (100–200 times) (3). This could be of significance in the manufacturing processes of nonhomogeneous devices or during storage at elevated temperatures.

The in vitro dissolution of the incorporated drug should be optimized. The criteria for optimum dissolution of both the drug and the enhancer must be established. It is possible that the release of the independent components are interrelated.

After having established that a softener is a suitable vehicle for a drug, which also enhances the absorption by the skin, an appropriate polymer is selected. However, after incorporation into the polymer, the enhancing activity may be lost. It is instructive to consider other polymer systems (e.g., polyvinyl chlorides and their plasticizers) that, although not used in transdermal delivery, can provide guidance for future development. According to these studies, the migration speed depends on the temperature, the concentration, and the chemical constitution, as well as on the nature of the contact component (in the transdermal field this is the human skin) (4). For the sake of completeness, it also has to be mentioned that the chemical structure of the polymer determines the migration tendency of softeners–enhancers. This is why drugs incorporated into the matrix system using the same softeners in the same concentration, which differ in only the basic polymer, do not show identical absorption rates when penetrating into excised rodent skin, even if they had identical in vitro release patterns.

During the research and developmental phase, the concentration of the enhancer, its chemical constitution, the type of polymer and, most importantly, the construction of the matrix system can be evaluated by the technologist. One should never forget, however, that a transdermal therapeutic system (TTS) is a pharmaceutical product in which

1. The drugs and adjuvants used must be nontoxic, nonirritant, and nonallergenic.
2. The system must adhere well and have good contact during the complete scheduled application time, usually 24 hr.
3. Cohesion of product components must be guaranteed.
4. After long-term storage (in extreme cases 5 years), the in vivo penetration must be the same as immediately after production.
5. The batch content of the enhancer and drug must be uniform.

Dimethyl sulfoxide and dimethylformamide are described as enhancers, but their application has limitations owing to their irritating effects. Despite the knowledge that low-molecular-weight carboxylic acids are irritant (e.g., propionic acid), patents appear in which they are proposed for use in transdermal delivery (5). On the other hand, the thesis of Paracelsus, "The dosage alone makes the poison,"must not be disregarded [the original quotation reads *"Dosis sola facit venenum"*]. This means that compounds that cause an irritation when they are applied to the human skin in undiluted form or as concentrated solution as, for example, oleic acid, sodium lauryl sulfate, and many others, should not be condemned, a priori, because irritation of the skin and other toxic effects can be suppressed by controlled release. One is well advised to have a sound knowledge of the toxicological properties of any potential enhancers.

The second point refers to the adhesiveness of transdermal delivery systems. Here, above all, urea, the traditional "sorbent material" of classic dermatology, must be examined more closely. For example, 1% urea in polyacrylate reduces the adhesiveness in such a drastic way that the required contact with the skin cannot be guaranteed over a period of 24 hr. On the other hand, the opposite effect may also be achieved by the use of enhancers (i.e., an improvement of the adhesiveness). This can be achieved, for example, by the incorporation of oleic acid. There are no scientific nor empirical rules that can be stated to help solve these different problems. It is necessary to experiment with the different components to optimize the release and adhesive characteristics. Normal experimental design and the use of simplex techniques will be of help in minimizing the number of experiments.

Occasionally, the period of wearing a TTS may be longer than 24 hr. Then the influence of enhancer can be especially important, because the general rule for adhesion may be formulated by the concise statement: "The more brittle the adhesive, the less the adhesion." Thus, with increasing migration of the enhancer–softener, the adhesiveness may be significantly reduced. Special attention must be paid to the subject of adhesion and cohesion. As explained later, the migration tendency of an enhancer depends on its concentration. The more enhancer that is incorporated, the more is its potential for release from the system. A high proportion of a liquid component will result in systems with insufficient adhesion and cohesion. To illustrate the problematic nature of the optimal quantity of the enhancer, the literature (6) describes a formulation containing simethicone (Dimethicone; a polymeric silicone elastomer), 1,2-propanediol (enhancer) and warfarin (Coumarin; drug). Rat in vivo studies in which the transdermal systems were fixed to shaved parts of the body using silicone adhesives were conducted. Although the concentration of the drug is constant at 5%, the proportion of 1,2-propanediol was varied between 0 and 70%. Systems with enhancer concentrations between 0 and 20% provided nearly identical release patterns of the drug, whereas above 20% the in vitro release rate was increased. For in vivo examinations, samples without enhancers, with 30%, and with 50% enhancer were used. It was demonstrated that with increasing propanediol concentration higher blood levels of drug were achieved. The systems with 50% and 70% propanediol are not pharmaceutically acceptable, as far as the nature of the device is concerned, which is not surprising with such a high portion of liquid. It is astonishing, however, that systems with a 30% level of liquid should be "acceptable" according to this paper. It must be stated from the outset that there is no cohesion at such high liquid levels. It is likely that lower amounts of the enhancer could have been incorporated with maintenance of both cohesion and enhancer effects.

It is worthwhile to return to the investigation performed by manufacturers of softeners. The migration tendency and extractibility of Edenol epoxy softeners with different plastics and extracting agents has been investigated (4). As the migration tendency of a softener depends on the polymer, another polymer instead of Dimethicone could be selected to achieve the same in vitro release of this propanediol with a relatively lower portion of propanediol. To achieve an enhancer release as high as possible, a polymer should be selected with which propanediol is not compatible, according to usual procedures or that can be used only as a secondary softener. Returning to the compatibilities of polar epoxy softeners in nonpolar polyvinyl chloride (PVC) polymers, a nonpolar polymer (e.g., polyisobutylene) could be selected for the polar propanediol. How these different adjuvants can be processed will be demonstrated later on.

The penultimate point of the requirements for TTS described in the foregoing is constant release and penetration after long storage periods. Transdermal systems with a multilayered design may contain an inhomogeneous content of the enhancer. In some cases, the enhancer will be incorporated into the outermost side (i.e., that presented to the skin). After contact with the skin, the enhancer penetrates into the skin, followed by the drug. It is probable that the enhancer will migrate during storage from the outer layers into the entire matrix until equilibrium is established.

Traditional production technology involves the coating of foils with adhesive solutions or dispersions and subsequent drying or the coating of melted substances. Both procedures have certain disadvantages, especially as far as enhancers are concerned. It is obvious that highly volatile substances, such as ethanol, will be removed during drying. This "removal" of an adjuvant will also create difficulties in enhancers that have high vapor pressure, as, for example, propanediol. Polyhydric alcohols are representative examples for the description of the loss of adjuvants when drying. The reason for this is, among other things, the pronounced tendency of this class of substance to form azeotropic mixtures.

Drying during production is not achieved purely by the elevated temperatures used, but by the flow of gases (i.e., air or nitrogen) onto the moist foil webs. However, owing to a large surface area, the removal of substances in a gas flow, even below their boiling point, is significant, particularly for foils covered with moist adhesives. The loss of all volatile softeners during drying can occur (with the exception of softeners that are used with PVC, i.e., phthalic acid and terephthalic ester). Loss is more significant with enhancers. Thus, not only the drug content, but also that of the enhancer must be determined after manufacturing when wet-coating is performed. These difficulties may be avoided if transdermal systems are manufactured according to the melting procedure. It must be taken into account that some drugs that are transdermally applied are liquids with a high vapor pressure (e.g., nitroglycerol, nicotine).

Coincidentally, these drugs have short biological half-lives, which provides one of the advantages of transdermal delivery. Drug application can immediately be interrupted in emergency situations by removal of the TTS. For drugs with a long half-life value, this advantage is limited.

The stability of the drug during the drying period must be considered. In addition, reactions of the enhancer must also be taken into account. For example, urea under normal conditions is chemically inert, but after melting can undergo significant reactions. Oleic acid rapidly changes color during heating; glycerol, triglycerides, and dioxan derivatives (when glycerol is the alcohol constituent) are subject to acrolein rearrangement at elevated temperature. Diesters may be subject to the Dieckmann ester condensation; in addition, ester pyrolysis cannot be excluded.

Much effort has been devoted to defining enhancers and softeners (and other adjuvants). Enhancers may have to be considered more like drugs, since they have action on a biological system, but this must be taken in the context that they are not specific pharmacological agents. [The World Health Organization defines the term *drug* as follows: "A drug is any substance or product that is used or intended to be used to modify or explore physiological systems, or pathological states for the benefit of the recipient."]

Approaches for the incorporation of enhancers can be found for systems in which the drug is in a liquid state. An example of this type is the nicotine TTS developed and patented by the firm Lohmann Therapeutical Systems (LTS). This patent avoids the difficulties caused by nicotine (thermolabile, highly volatile, incompatible with adhesive solutions) in that a liquid drug, a drug solution, or a solution consisting of drug and enhancer will be applied to a covered fabric. Second, a matrix is applied to this covered fabric. During storage, or for highly volatile substances, during manufacturing, the matrix will be saturated by the drug and the enhancer and will become a reservoir. Figure 1 shows the nicotine TTS in cross section from which controlled release of the drug and the enhancer can be effected after removal of the protective layer. This is experimentally proved in the patent specification of the Lohmann system for nicotine. A system containing 59.5 mg of nicotine was examined. The in vitro release was achieved as follows:

After removal of the protective layer, a nicotine patch, manufactured as described in the foregoing, was immersed at 37°C into 80 mL of an isotonic salt solution, and the released nicotine was quantitatively determined by high-performance liquid chromatography (HPLC) at fixed time intervals. The volume of the receptor phase was selected in such a way that sink conditions were maintained. The following measurements were achieved:

Time (hr)	Amount released (mg)	% Release
2	23.9	40.2
4	32.34	54.0
8	41.5	69.8
24	56.54	95.0

Figures 2 and 3 show the in vitro release pattern. Both diagrams illustrate that the nicotine is released in a matrix-controlled way. An enhancer incorporated by the same procedure would be subject to the same physical laws. If the quantity of the released drug is drawn against the root of time, this will result in a straight line that deviates after the release of 60% of the drug. This is a completely normal physical phenomenon.

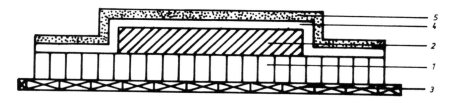

Figure 1 A cross section through the nicotine TTS. The layers are as follows: 1, matrix; 2, nonwoven foil containing nicotine; 3, release liner; 4, backing layer; 5, impermeable nonremovable metal foil.

The question must be asked: How can the release of enhancers be controlled? Initially, by the quantity of the enhancer that is applied to the textile web structure and, naturally, by the thickness of the matrix. [It is most important to emphasize that the described TTS system is not a membrane system, but a matrix system, as not only the release of nicotine, but also that of other drugs, follow the $\sqrt{t}$-law according to Higuchi.]

More importantly, however, is the design of the polymer matrix. For example, if the release of a carboxylic acid is to be controlled, it is advisable to use polyacrylate as a base polymer and as a copolymer Eudragit E 100. Experimentally, it can be shown that the release of carboxylic acids reduces as the proportion of Eudragit E 100 is increased. Release is virtually stopped if the proportion of basic polymer to acid exceeds a certain value, probably caused by salt liberation. Polyisobutylene should be used to limit the release of carboxylic acids. For vicinal alcohols (e.g., propanediol and glycerol) nonpolar polymers should be chosen if large quantities of enhancers are to be released. The release of these vicinal alcohols may be retarded by the incorporation of bivalent or trivalent metal ions. In this connection, however, attention must be paid to the increased solubility of $CaSO_4$ in glycerol compared with that in water.

Generally, however, the problem of retarding the release of the enhancer will not arise. Only carefully designed experiments will demonstrate the aforementioned requirements.

Lohmann TTS has the advantage that enhancers can be incorporated that are characterized by a high volatility (e.g., ethanol). The special characteristics of ethanol (high-migration capability and solvency for certain polymers) have to be taken into account and can be solved by selecting the correct polymer and an appropriate low loading.

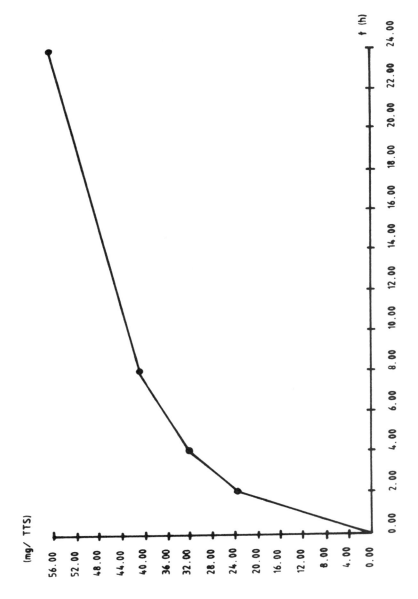

Figure 2   In vitro release of the nicotine TTS developed by LTS. Receptor phase: isotonic salt solution at 37°C.

(mg/TTS)

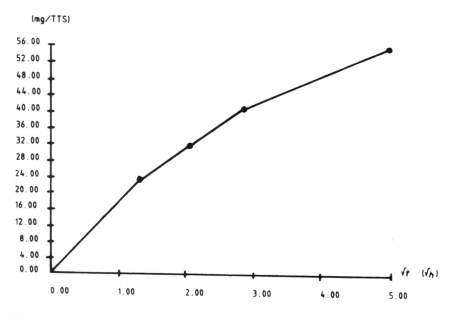

Figure 3 In vitro release plotted as a function of the square root of time for the nicotine TTS developed by LTS. Receptor phase: isotonic salt solution at 37°C.

REFERENCES

1. Hoffmann, H. R. and von Kleinsorgen, R. European patent 0 332 802 (1989).
2. *Rompps Chemie-Lexikon*, Frankh 'sche Verlagshandlung, Stuttgart, p. 3893 (1977).
3. *Rompps Chemie-Lexikon*. Frank 'sche Verlagshandlung, Stuttgart, p. 3894 (1977).
4. *Epoxy Softeners*. Manufacturing Information of the Henkel KGaA, Dusseldorf (1983).
5. Fisher, A., Levy, D., Spiegelstein, Y., Grunwald, J., Levy, A., and Kushniv, M. US Patent 4 788 063 (1988).
6. Ritschel, A. and Najak, P. M. *Arzeimittle Forschung 37*:302 (1987).
7. Hoffman, A. German patent 36 29 304 (1986).

16

Veterinary Applications of Skin Penetration Enhancers

Kenneth A. Walters

An-eX Analytical Services Ltd., Cardiff, Wales

Michael S. Roberts

University of Queensland, Queensland, Australia

I. INTRODUCTION

For the most part, this volume has been concerned with skin penetration enhancement in humans or nontarget animal models. It is becoming increasingly obvious that the mechanisms underlying the action of skin penetration enhancers involve some form of interaction with the lipids surrounding and embedding the corneocytes of the stratum corneum, the magnitude of the enhancement depending mainly on the amount and nature of this intercellular lipid. It is for this reason that some animal species, for example, the hairless mouse, appear uniquely sensitive to the action of enhancers (1). It is possible that this interspecies variation in the degree of enhancement could be exploited in the formulation of veterinary medicines, especially, but not exclusively, those designed for systemic effect by application to the skin.

There are several topical dosage forms used in veterinary medicine. These include dusting powders, suspensions, lotions, liniments, and creams (2). Of more interest in terms of skin penetration enhancement, however, are dips, sprays, and pour-on or spot-on formulations. The latter are mainly designed to delivery a systemic dose of active agent across the skin and, as such, are ideal candidates for the inclusion of enhancing agents. This chapter will outline the comparative morphology of skin from different animal species and discuss how transdermal drug delivery may be improved using penetration-enhancing agents.

II. SPECIES VARIATION IN SKIN STRUCTURE AND IMPLICATIONS FOR SKIN PENETRATION ENHANCEMENT

Most domestic animals are mammals and, as such, their skin is macroscopically separated into three layers, the stratum corneum, the viable epidermis, and the dermis. A generalized difference in structure, which is probably of little relevance to this discussion, is that the undersurface of the epidermis in large pellaged animals is smooth, whereas in pigs and humans the dermal–epidermal interface forms ridges (rete ridges). The most important differences in terms of barrier function, however, are the sebum, stratum corneum, and the presence of hairs.

A. Hair and Wool

Hair and wool can be considered to be the first absorption barrier to applied compounds in most animal species. It is possible that an enhancement effect may occur within the hair follicles. It has been estimated that there are some 2000 follicles per square centimeter in cattle (3) and up to 10,000 follicles per square centimeter in some skin regions of merino sheep (4). Accordingly, the follicular route for skin permeation may be significant, and it is likely that penetration enhancers will interact with the sebum present in the follicles and either increase or decrease the amount of applied formulation able to penetrate into the follicle, with obvious consequences for skin absorption.

Many chemicals can bind strongly to the keratin of wool, and this is also likely to occur with other animal hair. If this occurs, it would reduce the amount of applied chemicals (either active drug or enhancer) reaching the stratum corneum and, inevitably, reduce the amounts available for absorption. Although the significance of this phenomenon may be questionable in many disease states that result in hair loss, there is little doubt that it may reduce efficacy in prophylactic treatment when hair cover is normal.

Another consideration concerning the presence of hair involves the coating of the hair surface. This normally takes the form of an emulsion of sweat and sebum derived from the follicle and forms a continuous coat on wool (5). This emulsion has the capacity to absorb some applied chemicals, which are then capable of diffusing up or down the surface of the hair shaft, thereby acting to reduce the amount of active material available for absorption at the stratum corneum. The possible effects of penetration enhancers on the emulsion are unknown, but it seems likely that several types of enhancer (e.g., the surfactants) could interact with the emulsion to either enhance or reduce its capacity for absorption. It is also possible that the solvent-type penetration enhancers may dissolve the emulsion components and allow more of the active permeant to reach the skin surface.

B. Sebum

Sebum is a mixture of lipids, produced mainly in the sebaceous glands of mammalian skin, that provides a surface coat on the stratum corneum. Various studies have shown that the sebum lipids vary widely among species, both in terms of class of lipid and their aliphatic and alicyclic moieties (6). In large animals, the surface lipids appear to be predominantly produced by the sebaceous glands and are composed of varying amounts of triglycerides, phospholipids, cholesterol, cholesteryl esters, and unesterified fatty acids (7,8).

It seems likely that the presence of a film of sebum on the skin surface would act as a barrier to the migration of hydrophilic compounds to the stratum corneum, especially in the sheep in which numerous sebaceous glands produce a thick sebum layer containing desquamated stratum corneum cells (9,10). It is further likely that the presence of surfactant and solvent penetration enhancers would react to either emulsify or dissolve sebum, thereby reducing the barrier function. However, the role of sebum in the percutaneous absorption process is not yet fully understood, and it is possible that, for most drugs, it presents an extremely minor rate-limiting step.

When spreading of a formulation over the skin surface is required, however, the presence of sebum may prove disadvantageous. This is particularly significant for hydrophilic formulations that require the presence of surfactants to reduce their surface tension. Alternatively, fatty acid esters may be incorporated to improve mutual solubility between formulation and sebum (Boyle, J., personal communication). In the latter instance, it is important to select esters with a similar hydrophile–lipophile balance value to lanolin (HLB = 4.0). Examples of esters that have proved useful are 2-ethylhexyl stearate and butyl oleate.

C. Stratum Corneum

It has long been recognized that the principal barrier to percutaneous absorption is the stratum corneum. This is a coherent membrane that comprises layers of interdigitating keratinous cells embedded in a lipid matrix. The lipid matrix, which provides a tortuous, but continuous, pathway across the stratum corneum, is the main barrier to transepidermal water loss, and it is almost certainly the rate-limiting step to the inward migration of xenobiotics. Although the chemical nature of the intercellular spaces of the stratum corneum has been reasonably well established in humans, pigs, and several laboratory animals (11–13), the distribution and types of lipid present in this region of domestic animals are less clear. Those mammalian species for which the stratum corneum's intercellular regions have been studied extensively, however, show that there is not a great variation in type among different species. The lipids present are preponderantly free fatty acids, ceramides, and cholesterol, arranged in multiple lamellae. There is, however, some difference in the amount of lipid present, and this may prove important to the potential for penetration enhancement (14).

The stratum corneum's thickness in most domestic animal species is reasonably uniform, at approximately 30 μm (Table 1). Although the structure of the stratum corneum also shows reasonable consistency, there is some deviation in sheep. In the latter species, the distal layers of the stratum corneum separate from the basal layer in a disorganized manner (10) and become embedded in the sebum layer.

III. SPECIES VARIATION IN SKIN PERMEABILITY

The literature contains many references pertaining to species variation in skin permeability. Although most reports are concerned with defining a suitable animal model as a substitute for human skin, the work is pertinent to (a) the prediction of the likely penetration of undesirable compounds through the skin from both the viewpoints of veterinary toxicology and potential residues in the subsequent consumption of meat products by humans, and (b) the definition of the baseline epidermal permeabilities for therapeutic application. In general, no relation exists between the indices for toxicity, such as the median lethal dose (LD_{50}) and percutaneous penetration, as shown for organophosphorus compounds (15). The processes of percutaneous penetration and the disposition of solutes in the body, therefore, need to be defined separately and integrated.

We will briefly examine interspecies differences in solute disposition and then will consider the differences in skin permeability in more detail. The two major pharmacokinetic parameters defining the disposition of a solute in the body after input are the solute's clearance and the volume of distribution. Both of these

Table 1 Acetone-Extracted Skin Surface Lipids and Stratum Corneum Thickness for Several Species

Species	Lipids ($\mu g/cm^2$)	Stratum corneum thickness (μm)
Hairless mouse	212.4[a]	8.8[a]
Hairless rat	273.3[a]	15.4[a]
Guinea pig	224.7[a]	18.6[a]
Dog	NR	19.9[a]
Pig	130.0[a]	17.5[a]
Human	60.5[a]	18.2[a]
Sheep	NR	31.4[b]
Cattle	NR	30.9[b]

Source: [a]Ref. 14; [b]Ref. 29.

parameters can be directly related to the body weight of the species, as shown in Figure 1 for antipyrine (16). Such correlations apply to a range of other compounds. In the context of veterinary skin therapeutics, the steady state blood concentration is defined by the constant dermal rate of absorption (the flux, which is a function of the area of application and the concentration of applied permeant) divided by the clearance (53).

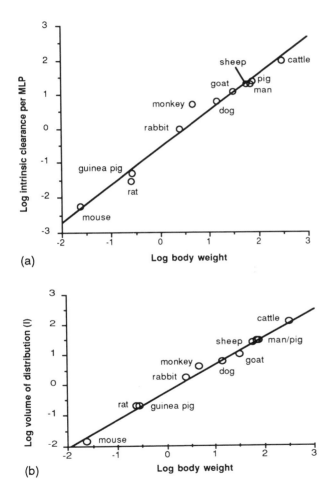

(a)

(b)

Figure 1 Allometric relation between (a) clearance per maximum life span potential (MLP) and (b) volume of distribution for antipyrine as a function of body weight for a variety of animal species. (Data from Ref. 16)

The skin permeability of different species reflect evolutionary development in particular ecological settings. Laboratory animals, such as rats, mice, and rabbits, lack sweat glands, but have more hair follicles than human skin. Larger animals appear to share more anatomical features with humans; therefore, it is not unusual that the weanling pig and rhesus monkey (17,18) may be preferable to the hairless mouse. The differing effects of hydration on hairless mouse and human skin (see Chap. 1) is of particular concern. Nevertheless, if skin permeability were related to the body size and physiological life time, the species dependence in skin permeability may be expected to be in the following order: mouse > rat > guinea pig > rabbit > monkey > dog > goat > sheep > pig > cattle > human. It should be noted that the pig body weight is very similar to that of the human (see Fig. 1). The stratum corneum thickness increases with animal size whereas the lipid content decreases with size. As shown later in Table 3, the permeability of many un-ionized solutes through the skin is lower for the larger species. The transport of ionized solutes is probably more through the shunt pathways (sweat ducts, follicles) and related to both their density and size. In reality, the permeability of the skin to ionized and un-ionized solutes show marked species variation in terms of their relative differences.

One of the earlier studies examining the transport of ionized solutes is that of Norgaard (19), who reported that the skin permeability for cobalt ions was rabbit > guinea pig > human. Tregear (20) ranks the species permeabilities as rabbit > rat > guinea pig > humans, whereas that given by McCreesh (15), for two ill-defined organophosphorous solutes was rabbit, rat > guinea pig > cat, goat, monkey > dog > pig. More recently, Scott et al. (21) reported the permeability coefficients of the dicationic herbicide paraquat in a range of species. The observed permeabilities for paraquat relative to water are shown in Table 2. Two features of paraquat permeability are readily apparent: (a) human skin is much less permeable to paraquat than any other species examined, and (b) the hairless mouse is particularly susceptible to paraquat penetration. Given that the skins of most of the laboratory species studied lack sweat glands, but do contain more hair follicles than humans, the different permeability coefficients probably reflect differences in follicular transport for the ionized compound. Unfortunately, data on the penetration of ions through larger species appear to be lacking, precluding a complete analysis.

The permeability coefficients for water (see Table 2) in each of the species studied varied by, at the most, fivefold. Durrheim et al. (22) and Huq et al. (23) reported that the permeability of alcohols and phenols through hairless mouse and human skin was similar. The aqueous concentration of phenol required to damage the human epidermis or rat and hairless mouse skin is also similar, at about 2%. However, as discussed elsewhere in this book (see Chap. 1) the effects of hydration on the permeability of hairless mouse and human skin differ markedly.

Table 2 In Vitro Absorption of Water and Paraquat Through Human and Animal Skins

Species	Permeability constant (cm/hr × 10^5)		Ratio paraquat/water
	Water	Paraquat	
Human	93	0.7	0.007
Rat	103	26.7	0.26
Hairless rat	103	35.5	0.34
Nude rat	152	35.3	0.23
Mouse	144	97.2	0.68
Hairless mouse	350	1066	3.05
Rabbit	253	79.9	0.32
Guinea pig	442	196	0.44

Source: Ref. 21.

Table 3 Relative In Vivo Absorption of Several Chemicals Through Human and Animal Skin

Penetrant	% Dose absorbed				
	Human	Pig	Monkey	Rabbit	Rat
Acetylcysteine	2.4[a]	6.0[a]	NR	2.0[a]	3.5[a]
Butter yellow	21.6[a]	41.9[a]	NR	100.0[a]	48.2[a]
Caffeine	47.6[a]	32.4[a]	NR	69.2[a]	53.1[a]
Cortisone	3.4[a]	4.1[a]	NR	30.3[a]	24.7[a]
DDT	10.4[b]	43.4[c]	1.5[c]	46.3[c]	NR
Haloprogin	11.0[a]	19.7[a]	NR	113.0a	95.8[a]
Lindane	9.3[b]	37.6[c]	16.0[c]	51.2[c]	NR
Malathion	8.2[b]	15.5[c]	19.3[c]	64.6[c]	NR
Parathion	9.7[b]	14.5[c]	30.3[c]	97.5[c]	NR
Testosterone	13.2[a]	29.4[a]	NR	69.6[a]	47.4[a]

NR, Not reported.
Source: [a]Ref. 50; [b]Ref. 51; [c]Ref. 52.

Table 3 summarizes some of the in vivo data reported on the percutaneous penetration of several un-ionized solutes through the skin of various species. In general, the magnitude of difference in skin permeability between the species is less than fivefold (cf. water in Table 2), with a rank order of rabbit > rat > pig > monkey > human. More recently, Moody et al. (24) suggested that animal models for phenoxy herbicide dermal absorption may be useful in predicting human dermal absorption. The dermal absorption of the insecticide lindane has been shown to be similar in rats and rhesus monkeys (25).

Sato et al. (14) have investigated the species difference in the percutaneous absorption of nicorandil, using hairless rat, guinea pig, hairless mouse, dog, pig, and human, and have attempted to relate this to the amount of surface lipid in these species. As part of this study the influence of the penetration enhancers laurocapram (Azone) and isopropyl myristate on nicorandil permeation was also investigated. The amounts of skin lipids extracted by acetone are shown in Table 1. Quite clearly there was a distinction between the extraction data obtained using hairless rat, hairless mouse, and guinea pig and that obtained for the other three species, and this was also true for the permeability studies (Fig. 2). Both

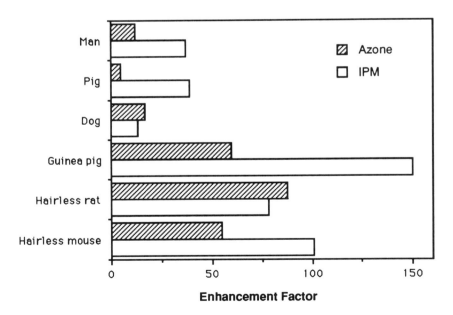

Figure 2   Effect of isopropyl myristate (IPM) and laurocapram (Azone) on the permeation of nicorandil through skin from different species. (Data from Ref. 14)

permeation and permeation enhancement of nicorandil was much greater through the skin of the hairless rat, hairless mouse, and guinea pig. These data reflect the significance of stratum corneum lipids for the permeation and penetration enhancement process. Similarly, Roberts and Mueller (26) have compared the in vitro flux of glyceryl trinitrate across hairless mouse, pig (Yucatan) and human skin and concluded that the mouse skin was an unacceptable model for the prediction of human skin permeation behavior.

A further study demonstrating the marked species differences in the response to penetration enhancement evaluated the influence of Azone on the permeation of verapamil hydrochloride across rat, hairless mouse, and human skin (27). Once again, the enhancer was much more effective on hairless mouse skin than on the other species evaluated. In addition, acetone has increased the permeability of fluorouracil by 16-fold in hairless mouse skin, but had no effect on human skin (28).

Currently, the limited literature on skin penetration in various laboratory animal species and humans does not allow the magnitude of any enhancement effect in any given species to be predicted from the data obtained in another species. Our initial generalizations, however, apply. First, the hairless mouse appears uniquely sensitive to the effect of enhancers. This is not surprising considering the amount of lipid, approximately 20% by weight, present in the stratum corneum of this species. Second, it is apparent that small, pellaged animals, for example, rat, guinea pig, and rabbit, are also relatively sensitive to the effects of penetration enhancers. Third, the skin of the domestic pig shows a response similar to human skin when exposed to penetration enhancers.

IV. SKIN PERMEABILITY IN LARGE DOMESTIC ANIMALS

The literature on the skin permeability of larger domestic animals (sheep, cattle, and horses) is sparse, with the relevant studies emphasizing therapeutic applications.

The early data on cattle and sheep skin permeability have been comprehensively reviewed by Pitman and Rostas (29). This review and the references therein give a full account of many of the veterinary therapeutic agents administered to the skin, often for systemic effect. The conclusion was that more information on the permeation characteristics of large animal skin was necessary to make more effective formulations. Several factors, of little significance to human skin permeability characteristics, can create considerable variability in the barrier function of the skin of domestic animals. For example, the temperature of sheep and cattle skin can be influenced by ambient conditions, such as radiation, leading to a significant difference in the surface temperature between black-haired and white-haired regions.

The animals' sensitivity to ambient temperature can result in seasonal variations in skin permeation rates (30). This, coupled with climate-induced alterations in sebum output, requires that any investigations into systemic drug delivery by the topical route should be normalized in terms of seasonal influences. A further complicating factor that renders prediction of effects or extrapolation of data virtually impossible is that there is considerable variability in skin morphology among breeds. Within cattle, for example, there is variability in total skin thickness and in the thickness of the various layers. This, coupled with differences in the densities of hair follicles, which are further affected by body weight, age, and sex, can lead to significant differences in skin permeability properties both inter- and intrabreed. This results in a paradox in which the formulator is required to select whether to base development activities on the least-permeable skin, and risk overdose in those breeds with a less-resistant barrier, or on the most-permeable skin, and risk underdosing the more penetration-resistant skin types.

The permeation of the anthelmintic levamisole across cattle and human skin in vitro has been determined by Pitman and Rostas (31). The formulations used in this investigation included an aqueous borate-buffered solution (pH 8.9) containing 0.85% levamisole, and an organic solvent, made up of nonaromatic hydrocarbons (15%), polyoxypropylene 15-stearyl ether (12%), and ethoxyethanol (73%), containing 10% levamisole. Interestingly, levamisole penetrated human skin from the aqueous solution at a higher rate than from the organic solvent. This is in marked contrast with cattle skin. Indeed, cattle skin appeared to be more than 400-fold more permeable than human skin using this solvent system. The data indicated that the major route for levamisole across cattle skin was through the appendages (hair follicles, and such), but, as the authors pointed out, this would not account solely for the much greater permeation rate across this tissue than across human tissue. The authors suggested that penetration through the appendages may be facilitated by the emulsified sebum, contained therein, which provided a good partitioning medium for the drug. It may be, however, that the organic solvent was removing or solubilizing the sebum and effectively acting as a penetration enhancer. Subsequent data (32) did suggest that permeability coefficients from the aqueous buffer solution across cattle skin were of a magnitude similar to those obtained with the organic solvent. It is difficult, however, to accurately compare the two sets of data, since in the former case skin was harvested in early fall and, in the latter case, in early spring. Although there is evidence to show that the cattle skin permeability to levamisole is substantially higher in midsummer than in midwinter (30) there was no indication of differences between spring and fall.

Some of the data presented by Pitman et al. (30) allow an initial evaluation of vehicle effects on the skin permeation of levamisole using individual breeds of cattle. These data are given in Table 4. One obvious observation was that the permeation of the undissociated species of levamisole (pH 8.9 buffer) was considerably higher than the cation (pH 6.0 buffer) and that this appeared to be a partitioning phenomenon. Another observation is that the permeation of the active

Table 4 Penetration of Levamisole Through Cattle Skin

Vehicle[b]	Permeability $(k_p r \times 10^6)$ cm^2/min	Diffusion coefficient $(D \times 10^6)$ cm^2/min	Partition coefficient
A	1.90	10.5	0.20
B	1.75	10.5	0.18
C	0.70	17.0	0.06
pH 8.9 aq soln	10.75	12.5	0.95
pH 6.0 aq soln	0.35	11.5	0.05
80% DMSO	1.60	86.0	0.02
Toluene	13.10	188.0	0.07

[a]$k_p r$ = product of permeability coefficient (k_p) and skin thickness (r).

[b]Vehicle A:	Levamisole	10%
	Polyoxypropylene-15-stearyl ether	12%
	Nonaromatic hydrocarbons	15%
	2-Ethoxyethanol	63%
Vehicle B:	Levamisole	10%
	Sorbitan sesquioleate	10%
	Nonaromatic hydrocarbons	20%
	2-Ethoxyethanol	60%
Vehicle C:	Levamisole	10%
	Spindle oil	10%
	Isopropanol	80%

species was considerably lower from 80% dimethyl sulfoxide (DMSO) than that from the aqueous solution of undissociated drug. Once again this appeared to be the result of unfavorable partitioning tendencies, but it can be further summarized that the activity of DMSO in cattle skin is unlike that of other species examined using this aprotic solvent. Both DMSO and toluene showed a significant increase in diffusivity within the stratum corneum, which was brought about by a marked reduction in lag time. These solvents, along with several other organic solvents, such as ether and ethanol, have been shown to be capable of removing several layers of stratum corneum cells and may prove useful as penetration enhancers, although they also increase the risk of infection (29).

A final observation on the data given in Table 4 is that the delivery of levamisole across the skin from formulation prototypes was less than that from simple aqueous solutions. Here again, the data suggested unfavorable partitioning characteristics, although there was some indication that the principle solvent, 2-ethoxyethanol, may possess some enhancement potential. It would be interesting to formulate a series of emulsions of varying aqueous proportions using these solvent-based formulations and to determine the effect on skin permeation rates. The presence of water should shift the partitioning tendency in favor of the skin.

Needless to say, the many variables in the permeability properties of the skin of large domestic animals render the empirical approach to formulation design virtually useless. It would appear that to investigate the feasibility of penetration enhancement a much greater knowledge of the properties of the skin of individual species and breeds is required. There are, however, several logical shortcuts that can be made in the formulation of pour-on and spot-on products, and these will be outlined in the following section.

V. FORMULATION ASPECTS: DEVELOPMENT AND EVALUATION

In many respects, skin penetration enhancers may provide advantageous effects on drug delivery, with beneficial consequences to the efficacy of pharmaceutical formulations. This is true not only for those formulations designed for dermatological use, but also for products designed for systemic drug availability by the dermal route. These formulations include spot-on and pour-on systems in which the basic formulation ingredients are often similar. The first pour-on application of an insecticide was reported in 1957 when poultry infested with the poultry body louse *Menacanthus stramineus* and sheep infested with the body louse *Damalinia ovis* were successfully treated by the application of a systemic insecticide, aldrin, to a small area of the skin (33,34). The pour-on method was also used for the control of the cattle grub, *Hypoderma* spp., with the organophosphate compound ruelene (35) and revolutionized lice control on cattle (36–39).

Subsequently, the application of synthetic pyrethroids, deltamethrin (40,41), cypermethrin (42), and alphacypermethrin (43) by pour-on formulations became widely used in the control of *D. ovis*. Here, a highly concentrated formulation of the active agent is deposited in a band along the animal's back. The insecticide is then able to spread through the fleece, most likely by diffusion within the emulsion layer on the wool and skin surface. The concentration of active agents, therefore, decreases with distance from the application site (40; Johnson et al., unpublished data). This is in contrast with the action of organophosphorus compounds, which are believed to be systemically absorbed following application to the skin, distributed in the blood stream, and excreted into the skin, thereby, reaching all areas containing sebaceous glands.

By using autoradiography, Jenkinson et al. (44) found that [14C]cypermethrin, applied as a pour-on formulation, spread radially across the skin within the stratum corneum at a rate that exceeded 11 cm/hr. This spread was accompanied by some dermal infiltration, which was most marked at the site of application. With a similar technique, Johnson and Dixon (unpublished data) found radiolabeled cypermethrin on wool fibers both above the surface and in the follicles, extending into the dermis. Darwish et al. (unpublished data) obtained data indicating that the synthetic pyrethroid, deltamethrin, achieved higher levels on the wool compared with skin, following pour-on application.

For both pour-on and spot-on products, there are some general factors that are essential considerations for the formulator. In the first instance, it is necessary to develop physically, chemically, and microbiologically stable preparations. Second, the developed formulations should be evaluated and optimized for drug delivery characteristics. Because of the diverse nature of domestic animal skin, this latter aspect can be realistically determined only by using skin from the target animal species either in vitro or in vivo. In the early stages of development, during which the number of formulation prototypes is relatively large, it is more rational to determine a rank order of skin permeation in vitro using laboratory animals. The advantages of this approach are based on the ability to control several parameters, such as area of application, amount applied, temperature, and receptor medium conditions. Here, the only variable is the formulation and a greater confidence in the validity of the data can be achieved.

The marked influence that formulation, components can display on drug delivery characteristics is shown in Figure 3. The peak blood levels of levamisole in heifers from two marketed pour-on preparations containing 20% active agent were 0.73 ± 0.25 µg/mL and 0.38 ± 0.18 µg/mL at 2 and 5 hr, respectively. At 24 hr after application, the concentrations of levamisole remaining were 0.05 ± 0.02 µg/mL and 0.12 ± 0.05 µg/mL respectively [Forster, M., Vibrac (Australia) Pty Ltd, personal communication]. These data illustrate the importance of bioequivalence studies in the evaluation of pour-on products.

Another important consideration for development is that the formulation should minimize the risk of irritant or sensitization reactions following application. It is possible to predict, with some certainty, the potential toxic effects of individual formulation excipients and active drugs using various in vitro methods. However, skin permeation characteristics of the individual components may be modified following mixing and processing of the formulation and, consequently, it is essential to determine skin permeation and toxicity of the final formulation.

Two basic varieties of pour- or spot-on formulations have been described in the literature; organic solvent-based and aqueous suspensions. Because most active agents are pyrethroid or organophosphorus compounds (Table 5), the majority of these formulations comprise nonaqueous solvent mixtures in which the drug is dissolved. Typical solvents used in this type of formulation are shown in Table 6. Although some of these solvents are inactive for skin penetration enhancement when applied as a single solvent solution of the active drug (e.g., mineral and vegetable oils, dimethylisosorbide and propylene glycol), there is evidence of

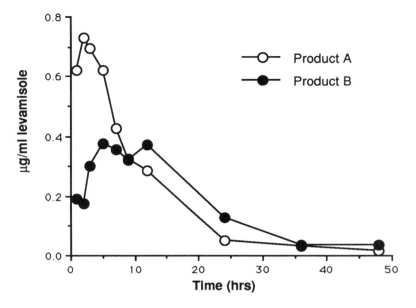

Figure 3 Comparative bioavailability of levamisole from two marketed pour-on products. [Data courtesy of Dr. Michael Forster, Vibrac (Australia) Pty. Ltd.]

synergism when binary solvent mixtures are used (45). Therefore, it is likely that mixtures of solvents, such as dimethylacetamide and butoxyethanol, with a glycol, such as ethylene glycol monoethyl ether, may prove more useful in transdermal drug delivery than either solvent alone.

An optimal formulation may be derived theoretically using solubility parameters (46). The *solubility parameter* can be defined as the sum of all the intermolecular attractive forces that are related to the extent of mutual solubility between chemical species. Lists of the solubility parameters of several formulation excipients are available (e.g., 47,48). From these values, it may be feasible to predict a drug and solvent mixture with a solubility parameter close to that of skin. Because of the mutual solubility, thereby obtained, penetration of the formulation into the skin should be comparatively rapid.

Penetration enhancers should facilitate faster penetration than can be provided by an optimal drug availability alone. Since many penetration enhancers are readily soluble in organic solvents, their addition to a formulation should be possible, providing the solubility parameter of the vehicle is maintained close to that of the skin. In addition, owing to potential hydrolytic or oxidative breakdown, drug instability must be minimized.

Table 5 Veterinary Antiparasitic Drugs[a]

Compound name	Molecular weight	Melting point (°C)	Log P (estimated)[b]	Log P (measured)[b]
Levamisole	204.31	60–61.5		
Crufomate	291.71	60–60.5	3.33	3.42
Coumaphos	362.78	91	3.98	
Trichlorfon	257.45	83–84	0.30	0.51
Phosmet	317.32	71.9	2.51	2.78
Chlorpyrifos	350.57	41–42	4.69	4.96
Chlorfenvinphos	359.56	Liquid (BP 167)	3.27	3.82
Dioxathion	456.54	−20	2.99	
Crotoxyphos	314.28	Liquid (BP 135)	2.04	3.30
Methidathion	302.31	39–40		2.42
Temephos	466.46	30–30.5	5.77	5.96
Fenthion	278.34	Liquid (BP 87)	3.86	4.09
Dichlofenthion	315.17	Liquid (BP 164)	5.06	5.14
Bromophos	365.98	53–54	5.00	4.88

Source: [a]Ref. 29; [b]Medchem Version 3.54, Daylight Chemical Information Systems Inc. (1989).

Table 6 Some Solvents and Spreading Agents Used in Pour-on and Spot-on Formulations

Glycols
  Polyethylene glycols (200–400)
  Propylene glycol
  Butyl diglycol
Glycol ethers
  Ethylene glycol monoethylether
  Butoxyethanol
  Butoxyethoxyethanol
  Methoxyenthanol
Amides
  Dimethylacetamide
  Dimethylformamide

Alcohols
  Ethanol
  Isopropanol
Hydrocarbon oils
  Mineral oil
  Vegetable oil
  Corn oil
Miscellaneous
  Dimethylsulfoxide
  Dimethylisosorbide
Spreading agents
  Polypropylene glycol-2-myristyl ether
  Polysorbate 80
  Butyl oleate
  2-Ethylhexyl stearate

The use of a simple organic solvent solution of active ingredients may not always be feasible. A water-soluble active agent or a combination of a water-soluble active and a water-insoluble active may require the use of aqueous suspensions or emulsions. Examples of this type of formulation are disclosed in UK Patent GB2109236B (49). A typical formulation (Table 7) would contain the active ingredient (usually micronized), a wetting agent, an antisettling agent, a viscolizer, antifreeze agent, preservative, antifoaming agent, water, and pigment (if necessary). When the active agent is a liquid the resultant formulation would be an oil-in-water emulsion. As with the organic solvent-based formulations, the incorporation of penetration enhancers into aqueous-based emulsions or suspensions would be feasible if the drug delivery characteristics were in need of improvement. For example, it may be possible to obtain both skin penetration enhancement effects and increased surface spreading using a single surface-active component, such as polyoxyethylene-2-stearyl ether (HLB = 4.9). Once again, however, there are no empirical rules to aid the formulator, and the optimization exercise should be carried out on the basis of previous experience and simplicity.

Examples of marketed pour-on and spot-on products are detailed in Table 8.

VI. CONCLUDING REMARKS

This chapter has briefly reviewed the species differences in skin permeability and considered the development of formulations to enable the transdermal delivery of

Table 7 Sample Formulation for an Aqueous Pour-on Product Containing Decamethrin

Ingredient	Function	Concentration (% w/v)
Micronized decamethrin	Active	1.01
Nonylphenol ethoxylate	Wetting agent	0.15
Fumed silicon dioxide	Antisettling agent	0.50
Xantham gum	Viscolizer	0.40
Propylene glycol	Antifreeze	6.00
Formaldehyde	Preservative	0.10
Silicone oil	Antifoaming agent	0.01
Pigment	Coloring agent	qs
Water		to 100

Source: Ref. 49.

Table 8 Marketed Pour-on and Spot-on Formulations

Product	Manufacturer	Active ingredient	Concentration (%)
Co-Ral	Cutter	Coumaphos	4
Neguvon	Cutter	Trichlorfon	8
Tiguvon	Cutter/Bayer	Fenthion	3/2
Ruelene	Dow Chemical	Crufomate	5, 8.3, 9.4
Citarin-L	Bayer	Levamisole	10
Spotton	Chemagro	Fenthion	20
Porect	Beechams	Phosmet	20
Ridect	Beechams	Permethrin	4 (80:20 *cis:trans*)
Vetrazin	Ciba-Geigy	Cryomazine	6
Coopers Spot-on	Coopers	Deltamethrin	1
Ripercol Pour-on	Janssen	Levamisole	20
Anthelpor 20	Youngs	Levamisole	20
Cypor	Youngs	Cypermethrin	2.5 (40:60 *cis:trans*)

active agents in domestic animals. Because of the diverse skin morphology and permeation characteristics exhibited by this variety of species, it is difficult to make broad generalizations on the potential usefulness of skin penetration enhancers. Despite this, it may be possible to predict the necessity for increasing the rate of skin permeation of a given drug in a given species if the required blood levels are known. However, it needs to be recognized that in those species in which the skin is more permeable, the clearance of any given solute is also likely to be higher.

Many of the excipients already in use in veterinary medicine are potential enhancers of skin penetration, and their judicious selection in the formulation of a new active agent may considerably reduce the need for multiple prototype development with obvious time and cost implications.

ACKNOWLEDGMENTS

One of us (MSR) acknowledges the support of the NH&MRC (Aust) and the Lions Kidney and Mutual Research Foundation of northern New South Wales and Queensland. Our thanks are also due to Dr. Peter Johnson for invaluable information on pour-on products.

REFERENCES

1. Bond, J. R. and Barry, B. W. Hairless mouse skin is limited as a model for assessing the effects of penetration enhancers in human skin. *J. Invest. Dermatol. 90*:810–813 (1988).
2. Pope, D. G. and Baggot, J. D. The basis for the selection of the dosage form. In *Formulation of Veterinary Dosage Forms*. Blodinger, J. (ed.). Marcel Dekker, New York, pp. 1–70 (1983).
3. Findlay, J. D. and Yang, S. H. *J. Agric. Sci. 40*:126 (1950).
4. Ryder, M. L. A survey of the follicle populations in a range of British breeds of sheep. *J. Agric. Sci. 49*:275 (1957).
5. Jenkinson, D. M. and Lloyd, D. H. The topography of the skin surface of cattle and sheep. *Br. Vet. J. 135*:376–379 (1979).
6. Lindholm, J. S., McCormick, J. M., Colton, S. W., and Downing, D. T. Variation of skin surface lipid composition among mammals. *Comp. Biochem. Physiol. 69B*:75–78 (1981).
7. Downing, D. T. and Colton, S. W. Skin surface lipids of the horse. *Lipids 15*:323–327 (1980).
8. Downing, D. T. and Lindholm, J. S. Skin surface lipids of the cow. *Comp. Biochem. Physiol. 73B*:327–330 (1982).
9. Britt, A. G., Cotton, C. L., Kellett, B. H., Pitman, I. H., and Trask, J. A. Structure of the epidermis of Australian merino sheep over a 12-month period. *Aust. J. Biol. Sci. 38*:165–174 (1985).
10. Lloyd, D. H., Dick, W. D. B., and McEwan-Jenkinson, D. The effects of some surface sampling procedures on the stratum corneum of bovine skin. *Res. Vet. Sci. 26*:250–252 (1979).
11. Gray, G. M. and White, R. J. Glycosphingolipids and ceramides in human and pig epidermis. *J. Invest. Dermatol. 70*:336–341 (1978).
12. Wertz, P. W. and Downing, D. T. Ceramides of pig epidermis: Structure determination. *J. Lipid Res. 24*:759–765 (1983).
13. Wertz, P. W. and Downing, D. T. Glucosylceramides of pig epidermis: Structure determination. *J. Lipid Res. 24*:1135–1139 (1983).
14. Sato, K., Sugibayashi, K., and Morimoto, Y. Species difference in percutaneous absorption of nicorandil. *J. Pharm. Sci. 80*:104–107 (1991).
15. McCreesh, A. H. Percutaneous toxicity. *Toxicol. Appl. Pharmacol. 7*(suppl. 2):20–26 (1965).
16. Boxenbaum, H. Interspecies scaling, allometry, physiological time, and the ground plan of pharmacokinetics. *J. Pharmacokinet. Biopharm. 10*:201–227 (1982).
17. Wester, R. C. and Noonan, P. K. Relevance of animal models for percutaneous absorption. *Int. J. Pharm. 7*:99–110 (1980).
18. Reifenrath, W. G., Chellquist, E. M., Shipwash, E. A., Jederberg, W. W., and Krueger, G. G. Percutaneous penetration in the hairless dog, weanling pig and grafted athymic nude mouse: Evaluation of models for predicting skin penetration in man. *Br. J. Dermatol. 111*(Suppl. 27):123–135 (1984).
19. Norgaard, O. Investigations with radiolabeled nickel, cobalt and sodium on the resorption through the skin in rabbits, guinea pigs and man. *Acta Derm. Venereol. 34*:440 (1957).

20. Tregear, R. T. *Physical Functions of Skin*. Academic Press, New York (1966).
21. Scott, R. C., Walker, M., and Dugard, P. H. A comparison of the in vitro permeability properties of human and some laboratory animal skins. *Int. J. Cosmet. Sci. 8*:189–194 (1986).
22. Durrheim, M., Flynn, G. L., Higuchi, W. I., and Behl, C. R. Permeation of hairless mouse skin. 1. Experimental methods and comparison with human epidermal permeation by alkanols. *J. Pharm. Sci. 69*:781–786 (1980).
23. Huq, A. S., Ho, N. F. M., Husari, N., Flynn, G. L., Jetzer, W. E., and Condie, L. Permeation of water contaminative phenols through hairless mouse skin. *Arch. Environ. Contam. Toxicol. 15*:557–566 (1986).
24. Moody, R. P., Franklin, C. A., Ritter, L., and Maibach, H. I. Dermal absorption of the phenoxy herbicides 2,4-D, 2,4-D amine, 2,4-D isooctyl and 2,4,5-T in rabbits, rats, rhesus monkeys and humans: A cross-species comparison. *J. Toxicol. Environ. Health 29*:237–245 (1990).
25. Moody, R. P. and Ritter, L. Dermal absorption of the insecticide lindane in rats and rhesus monkeys: Effect of anatomical site. *J. Toxicol. Environ. Health 28*:161–169 (1989).
26. Roberts, M. E. and Mueller, K. R. Comparisons of in vitro nitroglycerin (TGN) flux across Yucatan pig, hairless mouse, and human skin. *Pharm. Res. 7*:673–676 (1990).
27. Agrawala, P. and Ritschel, W. A. Influence of 1-dodecylhexahydro-2 H-azepin-2-one (Azone) on the in vitro permeation of verapamil hydrochloride across rat, hairless mouse, and human cadaver skin. *J. Pharm. Sci. 77*:776–778 (1988).
28. Bond, J. R. and Barry, B. W. Damaging effect of acetone on the permeability barrier of hairless mouse skin compared with that of human skin. *Int. J. Pharm. 41*:91–93 (1988).
29. Pitman, I. H. and Rostas, S. J. Topical drug delivery to cattle and sheep. *J. Pharm. Sci. 70*:1181–1193 (1981).
30. Pitman, I. H., Rostas, S. J., and Downes, L. M. Effects of breed, season, temperature, and solvents on the permeability of frozen and reconstituted cattle skin to levamisole. *J. Pharm. Sci. 72*:218–221 (1983).
31. Pitman, I. H. and Rostas, S. J. A comparison of frozen and reconstituted cattle and human skin as barriers to drug penetration. *J. Pharm. Sci. 71*:427–430 (1982).
32. Pitman, I. H., and Downes, L. M. Cattle and sheep skin permeability: A comparison of frozen and reconstituted skin with that of fresh skin. *J. Pharm. Sci. 71*:846 (1982).
33. McCosker, P. J. Systemic effect of dieldrin on the body louse of poultry. *Nature 179*:790 (1957).
34. McCosker, P. J. and Osborne, H. G. The systemic effect of aldrin on the sheep body louse (*Damalinia ovis*). *Austr. Vet. J. 33*:330 (1957).
35. Rogoff, W. M., and Kohler, P. H. Effectiveness of ruelene applied as a localised pour-on and as a spray for cattle grub control. *J. Econ. Entomol. 53*:814 (1960).
36. Nickel, W. E. The economical importance of cattle lice in Australia: Advances in systemic control by pour-on method. *Vet. Med. Rev. 2–3*:392 (1971).
37. Neuhauser, H. Improvement of systemic cattle lice control by spot-on method. *Vet. Med. Rev. 4*:348 (1974).
38. Kettle, P. R. Pour-on lousicides for the control of *Linognathus vituli. N. Z. Vet. J. 20*:167 (1972).

39. Kettle, P. R. and Lukies, J. M. The efficacy of some pour-on insecticides for the control of long nosed suckling lice (*Linognathus vituli*) on cattle. *N. Z. Vet. J. 27*:28 (1979).
40. Kettle, P. R., Watson, A. J., and White, D. A. Evaluation of a deltamethrin formulation as a back-line treatment for the control of the sheep body louse (*Damalinia ovis*). *N. Z. J. Exp. Agric. 11*:321 (1983).
41. Bayvel, A. C. D., Kieran, P. J., and Townsend, R. B. Technical details of a new treatment for external parasites in sheep. *Wool Technol. Sheep Breeding 29*:17 (1981).
42. MacQuillan, M. J., Northam, A., and Amery, M. I. Effectiveness against sheep body louse and itch mite of a cypermethrin formulation. *Wool Technol. Sheep Breeding 31*:99 (1983).
43. Sherwood, N. S. and Page, S. W. Control of lice on sheep with long wool. *Proc. Aust. Soc. Anim. Product. 17*:334 (1988).
44. Jenkinson, D. M., Hutchison, D., Jackson, D., and McQueen, L. Route of passage of cypermethrin across the surface of sheep skin. *Res. Vet. Sci. 41*:237 (1986).
45. Walters, K. A. Penetration enhancers and their use in transdermal therapeutic systems. In *Transdermal Drug Delivery*. Hadgraft, J. and Guy, R. H. (eds.). Marcel Dekker, New York, pp. 197–246 (1989).
46. Sloan, K. B., Koch, S. A. M., Siver, K. G., and Flowers, F. P. Use of solubility parameters of drug and vehicle to predict flux through skin. *J. Invest. Dermatol. 87*:244–252 (1986).
47. Barton, A. F. M. Solubility parameters. *Chem. Rev. 75*:731–753 (1975).
48. Vaughan, C. D. Using solubility parameters in cosmetic formulations. *J. Soc. Cosmet. Chem. 36*:319–333 (1985).
49. Kieran, P. J., Townsend, R. B., Hackney, R. J., Gayst, S., and Maguire, M. J. Aqueous pour-on formulation. UK Patent GB2109236B, 1-25 (1982).
50. Bartek, M. J., LaBudde, J. A., and Maibach, H. I. Skin permeability in vivo: Comparison in rat, rabbit, pig and man. *J. Invest. Dermatol. 58*:114–123 (1972).
51. Feldmann, R. J. and Maibach, H. I. Percutaneous penetration of some pesticides and herbicides in man. *Toxicol. Appl. Pharmacol. 28*:399–404 (1974).
52. Bartek, M. J. and LaBudde, J. A. Percutaneous absorption, in vitro. In *Animal Models in Dermatology*. H. I. Maibach (ed.). Churchill-Livingstone, New York, 103–112 (1975).
53. Roberts, M. S. Structure–permeability considerations in percutaneous absorption. In *Prediction of Percutaneous Penetration 2*. Scott, R. C., Hadgraft, J., Guy, R. H., and Boddé, H. E. (eds.). IBC Press, London, pp. 210–228 (1991).

17

Hydrotropy and Penetration Enhancement

Anthony J. I. Ward

Clarkson University, Potsdam, New York

David W. Osborne

Calgon Vestal Laboratories, St. Louis, Missouri

I. INTRODUCTION

It is often true that quite different areas of endeavor involve studies of a phenomenon that is the same on the molecular level, but is referred to in each discipline in terms of a different vocabulary. Such is the case of the phenomenon known in the detergency field as hydrotropy and that known as penetration enhancement, which is of great interest in the areas of pharmaceuticals and cosmetics. In the first instance, the technology of reducing the stability of viscous lyotropic surfactant phases has been developed to prevent the deposition of detergent either onto clothes in a washing machine or onto hair for a shampoo. This compares with the emergent strategies that are currently under investigation that look at the reversible and usually transient destabilization of the lipid layers of the stratum corneum, which are considered important in the barrier to drug delivery formed by the skin.

This chapter will try to bring these two apparently disparate areas together within a framework that exists at the molecular level. Use of suitable systems to model the behavior of complex systems, such as the stratum corneum, will also be discussed.

II. BACKGROUND

A. Self-Assembly of Surfactants and Lipids

Throughout this article the terms *surfactant* and *lipid* will be used interchangeably, since the second merely refers to those of the first that are naturally occurring; for example, phospholipids are surfactants (i.e., surface-active agents that occur in nature) and are genetically referred to as lipids.

It is the dominant feature of these types of molecules that they contain portions that are both hydrophilic and hydrophobic within the same molecule (Fig. 1). This has the effect that these molecules are surface-active when placed in water, since the solvent–hydrophobe contact is reduced by adsorption of the molecules. Such tendency of surface-active molecules to self-assemble into aggregated structures, the simplest form of which is commonly known as micelles, has been the subject of intensive study for several decades. The relation between the geometric attributes of the molecules and their formulation of self-assembled structures has been successfully explained (1,2).

Essentially, there are four main conditions of self-assembly that produce different-shaped aggregates. These depend on the commonly called *packing factor, P*, as defined as

$$P = \frac{V}{lA} \qquad [1]$$

where V is the volume of the hydrophobe, l is the effective length of the hydrophobe and A is the area occupied by the headgroup in the surface of the aggregate (see Fig. 1). Consideration of the free energy relative to the shape of the aggregate (2) showed that the most probably self-assembled structures obtained (Fig. 2) are

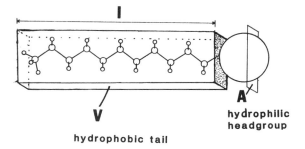

Figure 1 Representation of a surfactant molecule emphasizing the hydrophobic and hydrophilic regions. V is the volume of the hydrophobe, 1 is the effective length of the hydrophobe, and A is the area occupied by the headgroup in the surface of the aggregate.

$P < 1/2$ Spherical Micelles,

$1/3 < P < 1/2$ Rodlike micelles

$1/2 < P < 1$ Lamellar

$P > 1$ Inverse structure

It has been the lamellar structure that has attracted most attention as a potential model system for membranes, since the biomolecular lipid arrangement is similar to that found in cell walls. More recently (3–5), a similar arrangement has been suggested for the lipid component of the stratum corneum. Generally speaking, single-chained surfactants form the lamellar phase at surfactant concentrations in the range of 50–80% (w/w) when mixed with water. Double-chained surfactants of the type often found in biologically important systems have an even more marked tendency to form this bilayer arrangement. This can be seen from a consideration of P where V is twice that of a single-chain surfactant, whereas l and A are similar.

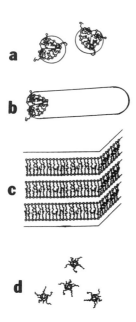

Figure 2 Most probable self-assembled structures obtained from consideration of the free energy relative to the shape of the aggregate. Spherical micelles (a), rodlike micelles (b), lamellar (c), and inverse micelles (d).

The lamellar phase of surfactants usually is prepared in the form of a stable dispersion in which domains of the layered bilayer structure are randomly distributed. In some cases, if energy is added to the system (e.g., ultrasonic irradiation), spherical structures, vesicles, or liposomes form that are made up of shells of lipid bilayers. These structures have some favorable properties in terms of amenability to certain kinds of experimental observations such as high-resolution nuclear magnetic resonance (NMR) techniques. They have been extensively studied in recent years with a view to potential drug delivery applications, even though they are intrinsically unstable systems and, ultimately, will phase-separate (unlike true lamellar dispersions, which are thermodynamically stable single phases).

B. Dynamic Structure of Lipid Bilayers

The detailed arrangements and dynamics of molecular motions of surfactant bilayers have been studied extensively. One source of confusion in the understanding of such studies has been an understanding of the term *dynamic structure*, which at first sight, presents a paradox. It may best be understood if the state of the amphipathic hydrophobes is considered in the solid state. Here, the chains are in a configuration in which the proteins are *trans* to each other, and the only motions are those of bond vibrations. If energy is supplied to this system (e.g., by heating) rotation occurs about the carbon–carbon bonds, which introduce *cis–trans* defects into the originally all-*trans* configured chain. Thus, the more rotational freedom introduced the greater the structural disorder of the chains.

As in all self-assembled surfactant systems, the restriction in the number of possible conformation is greatest for the chain segments closest to the aggregate–solution interface (i.e., those nearest the surfactant headgroup) and least for those near to and including the terminal methyl group. A profile of the amount of chain disordered across a bilayer, therefore, shows (Fig. 3) highest order near to the bilayer surface, then usually little variation along the chains until the middle of the chain is reached, followed by an approximately linear decrease toward the terminal methyl group at the center of the bilayer. The restrictions come from the interactions between the headgroups with each other and with the water and the presence of the other chains in the aggregate. This profile of order in bilayer and simple micellar systems has been theoretically predicted by molecular dynamics and statistical mechanical calculations (6).

C. Solubilizate Perturbations of Bilayers

The incorporation or solubilization of other components in such bilayer system leads to changes in the local environments depending on the location or distribution of the component throughout the system. These perturbations may lead to

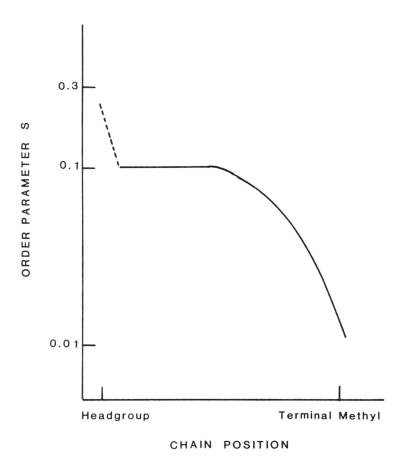

Figure 3 The typical form or order profile of hydrophobe chains observed for surfactants and lipids in lamellar phases.

increased or decreased stability of the bilayer structure, and it is these changes that form the basis of our consideration of hydrotropy or penetration enhancement.

A consideration of the possible types of interaction with the bilayers indicate the following possibilities (Fig. 4):

1. Solubilization into the bilayer interior with the maximum distribution of the solubilizate in the center of the bilayer. Such behavior would be expected for a hydrophobic solubilizate (e.g., an alkane) which has no affinity for the solvent or potential interaction with the headgroup.

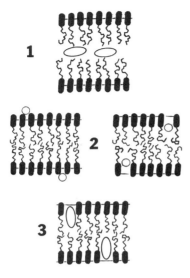

Figure 4 Possible types of interaction with bilayers. 1. Solubilization into the bilayer interior with the maximum distribution of the solubilizate in the center of the bilayer. 2. Incorporation near to, or adsorption on, the bilayer interface. 3. Interdigitation (intercalation) between the bilayer-forming molecules.

2. Incorporation near to, or adsorption on, the bilayer interface. This may occur on either side of the interface depending on the partition coefficient of the solubilizate. This would be found for molecules that have some affinity either for the surfactant headgroup, surfactant counterion (changed surfactants), or for the solvent chemicals. The interaction would potentially cause changes in the solvation of the bilayer surface and its curvature.
3. Interdigitation between the bilayer-forming molecules, as is expected for medium- to long-chained amphipathic molecules. Here is a point of attraction on the solubilizate molecule for the solvent, and a sufficiently large hydrophobic group that the molecules pack between the similar chains of the surfactant molecules, rather than distributing totally in the center of the bilayer, as in example 1.

Which one of these possibilities is found for a particular system is governed by general considerations of free energy. Interrelation of molecules between the host bilayer-forming molecules is unfavorable entropically, but leads to a generally favorable enthalpy change. On the other hand, incorporation in the most disordered region of the bilayer near the terminal methyl groups of the lipid is favorable entropically, but less favorable energetically. The effects of these differing types of solubilization on the stability of the bilayer can be judged from the ternary-phase behavior of such systems.

Such interactions have also been studied by use of NMR spectroscopy (7,8). Use has been made of the deuterium resonance in systems for which hydration changes may be used to monitor these interactions (e.g., in nonionic surfactant bilayers; 9,10). For molecules that compete with the hydration water [e.g., small-chain alcohols, such as isopropyl alcohol (IPA), or diols, such as the commonly used propylene glycol (PG)], the redistribution of water molecules from a bound site to one in which they are essentially free isotropes can be seen. Since the observed quadrupolar splitting of the water, Δv, is an average of the two types of water, that is,

$$\Delta v = F\Delta v_i = F_{\text{free}}\,\Delta v_{\text{free}} + F_{\text{bound}}\Delta v_{\text{bound}} \qquad [2]$$

where F_i and Dv_i, are the fractions and quadrupolar splittings, respectively of the water molecules in each fraction, a decrease in Δv indicates an increase in the free fraction. This is seen (Fig. 5) for samples containing a fixed amount of water as the amount of IPA or PG increased. A semiquantitative estimate of the amount of water displaced indicates that 2–3 mols of water per mole of surfactant are replaced by 1 mol of IPA or PG. A similar analysis applied to the extremely efficient hydrotrope sodium xylene sulfonate [N.B., SXS is also a strong skin irritant] shows a more complex situation (see Fig. 5). Here the decrease observed in Δv is too large to be accounted for in terms of changes in the solvation layer of the surfactant. These molecules both have moieties that are hydrophobic and that would be expected to incorporate into the bilayer interior. This is offset by the hydrophilic headgroups that will tend to hold the molecules near to the bilayer–water interface. In these cases, incorporation in the region of the bilayer near to the interface causes disruption of the amphipathic molecular packing precisely in the region where it is most sensitive. Such disruption effectively also reduces Δv_{bound} in addition to any possible solvation changes. It is the ability of these molecules to incorporate in the upper part of the bilayer that causes profound changes in the surface curvature of the aggregates, with associated decreased bilayer stability.

Molecules that locate in the center of the bilayers because of the hydrophobic nature, and that would not be expected to have any contact with the aqueous layer, do not affect the quadrupolar splitting of the water. Only with a high solubilizate content is a decrease seen, which is a result of an overall increase in the bilayer fluidity. This is seen in the example of an *n*-alkane solubilized in a bilayer formed by a nonionic surfactant and water (Fig. 6).

Solubilization of amphipathic molecules, from considerations of the molecular-packing requirements of the aggregates, should tend to increase the stability of the bilayers and, generally speaking, cause more overall order in the system. This is

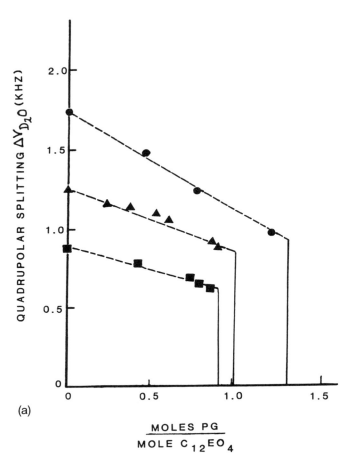

(a)

$$\dfrac{MOLES\ PG}{MOLE\ C_{12}EO_4}$$

Figure 5   Effects of additives on lamellar $C_{12}EO_4/D_2O$ liquid crystals. The vertical lines denote the phase boundary, whereas the line passing through the points was calculated using Eq. 2. (a) ●, propylene glycol (67:33 w/w $C_{12}EO_4/D_2O$); ▲, propylene glycol (60:40 w/w $C_{12}EO_4/D_2O$); ■, propylene glycol (50:50 w/w $C_{12}EO_4/D_2O$). (b) ○, isopropyl alcohol (60:40 w/w $C_{12}EO_4/D_2O$; Δ, sodium xylene sulphonate (60:40 w/w $C_{12}EO_4/D_2O$).

seen in the increase of the order parameter of the water component (Fig. 7) upon addition of propylene glycol to the system n-dodecylpentaoxyethylene glycol ether ($C_{12}EO_5$)–water, which has been used (11,12) as a model for the stratum corneum lipid fraction. Obviously, some of this increase is a result of headgroup conformation changes that allow the hydration water to more significantly

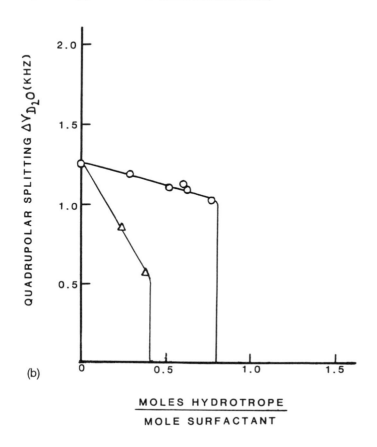

(b)

MOLES HYDROTROPE

MOLE SURFACTANT

contribute to the observed quadrupolar splitting. It is, however, still an indirect observation of what is occurring, primarily in the bilayer, that has consequences in the bilayer–solvent interfacial region.

D. Hydrotropism, Solubilization, Complexation, and Cosolvency

The mechanism of hydrotropic action that is applicable to the selection and evaluation of penetration enhancers involves destabilization of the lyotropic lamellar liquid crystalline phase. Incorporation of a hydrotrope into the bilayer system, therefore, leads to a disruption of the bilayers until the preferred aggregate structure is formed, usually either simple normal or reversed micellar. This destabilization process has been studied in detail, with particular emphasis on the

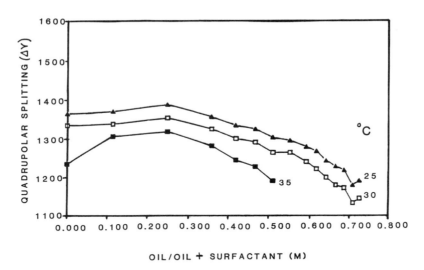

Figure 6   Variation of the quadrupolar splitting of ^2H_2O in the system $C_{12}EO_4$/water/*n*-hexadecane as a function of oil content, at different temperatures. Surfactant/water ratio of 60:40.

relation between the structure of the hydrotrope and the degree of destabilization. However, this use of hydrotropes is probably less familiar than the traditional pharmaceutical description of hydrotropy. Historically, hydrotropy has been considered synonymous with *salting-in*, in which the hydrotrope was a salt of a large organic ion. As various hydrotropes were studied with increasing ion size, the type of organic ions that were salted-in were also varied. The underlying molecular events were not necessarily clearly differentiated and hydrotropy seemed a complex phenomenon.

The hydrotropic effect can be significantly simplified by identifying the molecular events that increase the aqueous solubility of poorly soluble compounds. By briefly describing and distinguishing between these molecular events, a clear understanding of hydrotropy is possible. Of particular emphasis will be the subclass of hydrotropes most important as percutaneous penetration enhancers. To use the relation between hydrotropy and penetration enhancement, the mechanistically similar, yet molecularly distinct, phenomena of hydrotropy, solubilization, complexation, and cosolvency must be described.

The addition of an electrolyte to water usually decreases the quantity of non-electrolyte that can be dissolved. This well-known process, termed *salting-out*, has been described in terms of the electrolyte competing with the nonelectrolyte

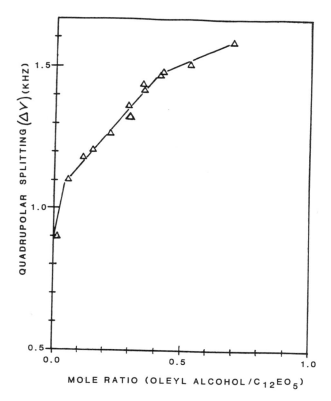

Figure 7 The effect of addition of oleyl alcohol has on the 60% $C_{12}EO_5$/D_2O host system.

for water (*hydration theory*), or the increased gap between dielectric constants of the nonelectrolyte solute and water, owing to the added electrolyte increasing the dielectric constant of water (*electrostatic theory*). Although both theories provide a sound explanation of salting-out, neither can explain the salting-in phenomenon, first described by Neuberg in 1916 (13). In this study it was noted that the aqueous solubility of nonelectrolytes could be increased by salts with large anions, such as sodium xylene sulfonate. Neuberg termed this phenomena hydrotropism and investigated the increased aqueous solubility of substances, such as benzene, benzoic acid, and aniline. This traditional hydrotropic phenomenon has been attributed to the large organic ions causing expansion of the partial molar volume of the water (*internal pressure concept*). Note, that traditional Neuberg hydrotropism concerns the increased aqueous solubility of a nonelectrolyte by addition of a salt containing a large ion. Furthermore, minimal interaction between the nonelectrolyte solute and the hydrotrope is assumed, and minimal interaction between the hydrotrope molecules with increasing hydrotrope concentration is assumed. These two assumptions must be well understood. As interactions between the solute and the hydrotrope increase, hydrotropy begins to resemble complexation. As interaction between the hydrotrope molecules increases, hydrotropy may begin to resemble solubilization.

First, consider the difference between hydrotropy and solubilization. *Solubilization* is defined by McBain and Hutchinson (14) as "a particular mode of bringing into solution substances that are otherwise insoluble in a given medium. Solubilization involves the previous presence of a colloidal (organized) solution [the] particles [of which] (organized) take up and incorporate within or upon themselves the otherwise insoluble material." Winsor (15) considered hydrotropy and solubilization to be essentially similar processes. Examples of the continuum between hydrotropy and solubilization are described by Klevens (16). In ascending an homologous series of the sodium salts of straight-chain carboxylic acids (i.e., C_1–C_{11}) a gradual change in solubilizing properties occurs. For the lower members of the series, the solubilizing properties do not become evident until 30–50% of the hydrotrope is added. For the higher members, which are surfactants (17), solubilization occurs at lower concentrations corresponding to the critical micellization concentration (CMC). However, the general character of the processes involved are essentially the same throughout the homologous series. These early experiments show that the onset of interaction (i.e., association) between the hydrotrope molecules, transforms Neuberg's traditional hydrotropic phenomenon into the familiar phenomenon of micellar solubilization. However, an exact distinction between hydrotropes and surfactants cannot be generally applied, just as an exact definition of surfactant behavior is difficult to generalize (18).

The relation between hydrotropy and *complexation* has been less firmly established in the literature; however, the concept is straightforward. If an interaction between the solute and hydrotrope occurs in simple mole ratios of the two components, then hydrotropy is essentially a process similar to complexation. James (19) showed that application of the law of mass action to a 1:1 association between a substrate S and complexing agent L to give a soluble complex SL is described by

$$\frac{[SL]}{[S]} = \frac{M_s}{M_s^0} = K_{1,1}[L] \qquad\qquad [3]$$

which is similar to that of the empirical Setschenow equation

$$\log\frac{M_s^0}{M_s} = K_s M_{salt} \qquad\qquad [4]$$

where K_s is the Setschenow constant, M_s is the solubility of the nonelectrolyte in pure water, and M_s^0 the solubility in the electrolyte solution of electrolyte concentration M_{salt}. The Setschenow equation is used to describe both salting-in (K_s negative) and salting-out (K_s positive). James (19) suggests that hydrotropy and complexation are possible extremes of the same process.

Up to this point, our description of hydrotropy has implied that the solute is a nonelectrolyte, that the solvent is water, and that the hydrotrope is a salt that dissociates upon addition to the water. For this restriction of solute, solvent, and hydrotrope, the molecular events leading to hydrotropy can be contrasted with the molecular events leading to solubilization or complexation. Increased solubility of the solute upon addition of the hydrotrope is caused by changes in solvent properties owing to solvent–hydrotrope interactions, provided that minimal solute–hydrotrope and hydrotrope–hydrotrope interactions occur. If increased aqueous solubility is predominately the result of solute–hydrotrope interactions then complexation rather than hydrotropy occurs. [For complexation the terminology would be that substrate–complexing agent interactions result in the formation of a soluble complex.] Alternatively, if increased aqueous solubility is predominately the result of hydrotrope–hydrotrope interactions, then solubilization, rather than hydrotropy occurs. [For solubilization the terminology would be that surfactant association results in solubilization.]

Not all hydrotropes are solid salts, and often in the pharmaceutical industry the solute is not a nonelectrolyte (i.e., benzene), but rather, a drug that is often a weak acid or weak base. For liquid hydrotropes, such as propyene glycol, the increased solubilization of the solute can be confused with cosolvency. For nonelectrolytes, cosolvency can be understood in terms of regular solution theory. To predict solubilities in solution in which molecular interactions are small, the following form of the regular solubility equation can be used (19).

$$-ln\, X_2 \;=\; -ln\, X_2^i + \frac{V_2 \Phi_1^2 (\delta_1 - \delta_2)^2}{RT} \qquad [5]$$

The solubility parameter of the solvent is δ_1, whereas the solubility parameter of the solute is δ_2. The addition of a cosolvent results in a change in the value of δ_1. The regular solubility of the solute (X_2) will approach the ideal solubility (X_2^i) as cosolvent is added, such that the value of δ_1 approaches the value of δ_2. The ideal solubility (X_2^i) is the maximal solubility of the solute in the solvent. Thus, solute solubility will increase upon addition of a miscible cosolvent that has a solubility parameter value closer to that of the solute than to the solubility parameter value of the solvent. Since water has a solubility parameter greater than the solutes considered, addition of an organic cosolvent will usually increase the solute solubility. It may be useful to emphasize that the second term on the right-hand side is the energy, in excess of ideal, necessary to maintain the solute in solution.

By matching the solubility parameters of solvent and solute, additional energy is not required to maintain the solute in solution. Increased solubility of drugs by cosolvents, such as ethanol, propylene glycol, and glycerin, has been extensively studied by Yalkowsky et al. (20).

With this description of *cosolvency*, it is possible to distinguish between cosolvency and hydrotropy. First, the liquid that increases aqueous solubility of the solute should be miscible or highly soluble in water for cosolvency to occur. It this criteria is met, then the solubility parameter of solvent, solute, and suspected cosolvent should be obtained from the literature (21), experiment, or calculation (22). As described by James (19), if one plots the solute solubility against solvent blend solubility parameter, then a curve similar to Figure 7 results. This is a direct result of regular solution theory as described in Eq. 5. Thus, increases in solute solubility by addition of a cosolvent should agree with Eq. 5, and a plot of solute solubility verses water–cosolvent solubility parameters should follow a form similar to Figure 8. If these conditions are not met, then cosolvency does not occur, and hydrotropy, complexation, or solubilization may be responsible for observed increases in solute solubility.

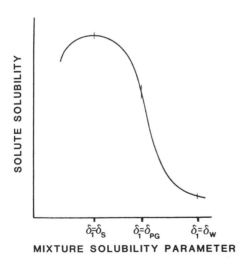

Figure 8 Variation of solubility of a solute (S) with the solubility parameter of the water–cosolvent mixture. If this idealized curve was for a mixture of propylene glycol (PG) and water (W), then the relative solubility parameters would be as marked.

III. PERTURBATION OF BILAYERS BY HYDROTROPES

The foregoing discussions are useful in providing the molecular events associated with traditional hydrotropy, but the relation between hydrotropy and skin permeability enhancement is probably not yet obvious. The work by Friberg and collaborators provides the link between hydrotropy and penetration enhancement (23–25). The same molecules that increase the solubility of nonelectrolyte solutes in water, increase the solubilization of amphipathic substances with predominantly hydrophobic properties, such as a long-chain carboxylic acid. As stated before, traditional hydrotropes function by destabilizing bilayer structures (23,24). When the short-chain hydrotrope locates at the interface, the mixture of long-chain amphipaths and short-chain hydrotropes is incompatible with the formation of bilayers (25). In simplest terms, this is an additive effect. Thus, the greater the amount of long-chain amphipath present, the greater the amount of hydrotrope required to maintain a micellar solution (i.e., destabilize the bilayer liquid crystalline structure). This explains the need for large hydrotrope concentrations (20–40%) when they are used extensively in cleaners to prevent gelation of the concentrated product and to aid in the laundry process.

An example of hydrotropy for an amphipathic system is shown in Figure 9. The comparison of the ternary system water–octanoic acid–hydrotrope with the

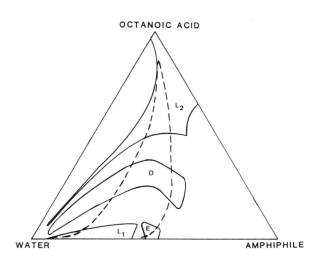

Figure 9 The difference in phase equalibria for a system of water–octanoic acid, with a surfactant as amphipath (solid line) and with a xylene sulfonate hydrotrope as amphipath (dashed line).

system water–octanoic acid–surfactant emphasizes these two dominate features of the hydrotrope system. The solubilization of the carboxylic acid begins at high concentrations of the hydrotrope, and the solubility of the carboxylic acid reaches huge values at 40–50% hydrotrope. The first feature is expected, considering that the CMC of a surfactant is increased with shorter-chain length. Since hydrotropes have shorter-chain lengths than surfactants, solubilization owing to hydrotrope interactions does not occur until high concentrations of the hydrotrope are reached. The second feature is that the solubility of the caboxylic acid is not interrupted by the formation of a lamellar liquid crystal. As seen in Figure 8, solubilization of no more than 10 wt% carboxylic acid occurs before the separation of the bilayer-structured lamellar phase. Evidently, the huge solubilities of hydrophobic carboxylic acids found in aqueous solutions of hydrotropes is due to the association aggregates of limited size not being replaced by a lamellar liquid crystal, even when greater than 70% carboxylic acid is added. This phenomenon can readily be explained in terms of the Ninham packing factors described earlier.

The dicarboxylic acid hydrotrope (Westvaco's DIACID) shown in Figure 10 would be considered a long-chain amphipath compared with the traditional sodium xylene sulfonate hydrotrope. Although the structure of this dicarboxylic acid is nontraditional for a hydrotrope, the mechanisms by which it functions is essentially the same. Phase behavior studies (26) showed that the disodium soap of the Westvaco dicarboxylic acid (NaDA) inhibited formation of the lamellar liquid crystalline phase at concentrations below the CMC of the surfactant when combined with a long-chain alcohol. Furthermore, small-angle x-ray analysis (27) showed that NaDA maintained an interfacial conformation in which both of the carboxylic acid functional groups were anchored at the interface. The resulting partial molar area of the monosoap was 52–53 $Å^2$. Thus, by curling at the interface, NaDA functions like a short-chain hydrotrope, providing a relatively short hydrophobic "tail" compared with the surface area occupied at the interface. The degree of bilayer destabilization caused by addition of NaDA was determined by monitoring the quadrupolar splitting of octanol-d17 using deuterium NMR. In

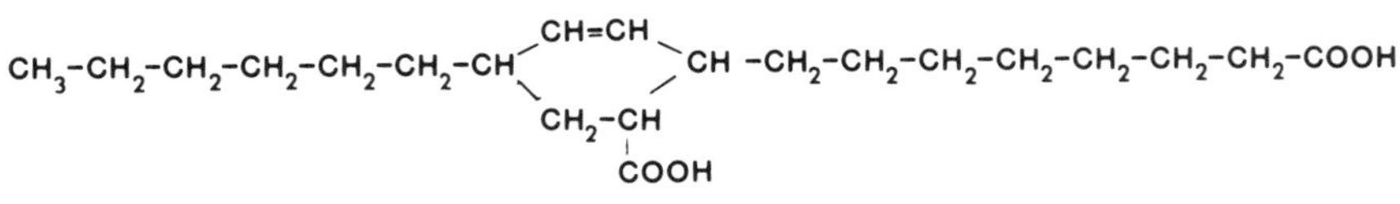

Figure 10 Chemical structure of Westvaco's DIACID, 8-(5-carboxy-4-hexyl-cyclohex-2-enyl)-octanoic acid.

that investigation the effect of NaDA addition was compared with the effect of sodium octanoate addition. Both molecules were added to a host liquid crystal of water–octanol–sodium octanoate. The study showed that addition of NaDA had a dramatic disordering effect on the methylene group adjacent to the polar head group, whereas addition of equivalent amounts of sodium octanoate had no disordering effect (25).

IV. HYDROTROPES AS PERCUTANEOUS PENETRATION ENHANCERS

It is the ability of hydrotropes to destabilize liquid crystalline phases, especially bilayer-structured liquid crystalline phases, that makes hydrotropes of interest to the researcher of percutaneous transport enhancement. The early speculation that epidermal lipids are arranged as bilayers (3,4), combined with the understanding that the stratum corneum provided the barrier function of the skin (28), led to the establishment that the barrier function of the skin can be described in terms of the integrity of the epidermal lipid bilayers (29,30). Although the effects of some enhancers, such as urea, undoubtedly stem from their interaction with the protein cells of the stratum corneum, destabilization of the bilayer-structured epidermal lipids has also been suggested as a mechanism for enhanced percutaneous absorption (31).

The dicarboxylic acid hydrotrope described earlier was previously evaluated as a potential percutaneous transport enhancer for minoxidil (32). In vitro transdermal transport results using human cadaver skin showed that the addition of 10 wt% NaDA to the water–propylene glycol–ethanol minoxidil formulation resulted in no change in drug transport. It was concluded that NaDA functions as a selective hydrotrope, destabilizing only bilayer systems that are formed from amphipaths with relatively small-sized head groups. This conclusion was based on the systematic characterization of the bilayer systems listed in Table 1. The effectiveness of NaDA as a bilayer-destabilizing molecule was compared with a nondestabilizing molecule of similar properties, sodium octanoate. Sodium octanoate (NaC_8) was selected because it presumably extends into the bilayer to approximately the same degree that NaDA does in its curled conformation. Thus, a primary difference between the interaction of these molecules at the interface is the greater bulkiness of the curled NaDA (i.e., bilayer-destabilizing hydrotrope effect). If the amount of NaC_8 required to disrupt the bilayer-structured host (as evidence by a phase transition) is compared with the amount of NaDA required to cause the same phase change, then the ratio of these amounts reflects the effectiveness of NaDA as a bilayer-disrupting molecule. A large value for the (amount NaC_8)/(amount NaDA) ratio would indicate that NaDA was an effective bilayer-disrupting molecule, whereas a ratio value of unity would indicate NaDA was no

Table 1 Comparison of the Amounts of Sodium Octanoate (NaC8) and NaDA
Required to Cause a Phase Change of the Bilayer-Structural Host

Bilayer-structured host	S_A (Å^2)	X_{NaC8}	X_{NaDA}	Host solvent/ amphipath mole ratio	$\dfrac{X_{NaC8}}{X_{NaDA}}$
Sodium octanoate/ octanol/water	25	0.080	0.011	6.9	7.4
Monocaprylin/ water	30	0.056	0.016	3.0	3.5
		0.032	0.016	5.6	2.0
Lecithin/water	53	0.079	>0.10	7.9	<0.77
Lecithin/ ethylene glycol	70	0.034	0.11	4.8	0.33
		0.034	0.066	8.6	0.52

Source: Ref. 32.

more disruptive to the bilayer system than sodium octanoate. As seen in Table 1 the effectiveness of NaDA to disorder the bilayer host decreases as the extrapolated effective surface area per amphipathic headgroup increases.

Since bilayer-structured lipids represent a primary barrier to transdermal delivery of drugs, any molecule that disorders bilayer structures should enhance the delivery of drugs. However, NaDA did not appear to function as a transdermal delivery enhancer for minoxidil when added to 10 wt% to the ethanol–propylene glycol–water vehicle. This can be understood by examining the information given in Table 1. The NaDA is effective in disordering bilayers when the interfacial surface area per amphipathic headgroup is small. For bilayers of molecules with large headgroups, such as lecithin, the curled conformation of NaDA is not bulky enough to cause disorders sufficient to destabilize (i.e., break) the lamellar phase. In essence, NaDA is a selective hydrotrope, being able to totally disrupt bilayers of small headgroup amphipaths, whereas not disrupting phospholipid bilayers. It appears that NaDA has an effective destability range of extrapolated interfacial areas of 30–32 Å^2 or less. Since epidermal lipid bilayers are characterized by moderate-sized headgroups, probably in the 34–38 Å^2 range, the epidermal lipid bilayers are not disordered by NaDA addition. Thus, NaDA addition does not enhance permeation of drugs through the skin.

The most important implication of this preliminary study is the suggestion that a selective hydrotrope could exist that would strongly disorder the epidermal lipids, while not affecting the viable cell membranes. Such a molecule would probably be a nonirritating transdermal penetration enhancer and be of considerable importance to the pharmaceutical industry.

V. PERTURBATION OF BILAYERS BY PENETRATION ENHANCERS

Although phospholipid systems are good models for most membranes, some important membranes found in the body do not have lipid components that are composed of phospholipids. In the context of this chapter, it is the lipid component of the stratum corneum that is of main importance. It has been shown (33) that as the cells migrate from the basal layers, the composition of the lipid component changes from one containing 55–60% phospholipid to less than 5% at the stratum corneum. The major components are polar (i.e., uncharged) lipids (e.g., ceramides, sterols, and fatty acids). A bilayer arrangement was indicated (3,4) by electron microscopy and later supported by small-angle x-ray diffraction (34), although it was found necessary to take into account the pH of the skin, which meant that some of the fatty acid must be in neutralized form.

Use has been made of the lamellar phase formed by $C_{12}EO_5$–water mixtures as a model system for investigating interactions with penetration enhancing agents. The rationale behind the choice of this system as a model is that the headgroups are polar and interact with the aqueous component through hydrogen-bonding. This is directly analogous to the dominant interactions found in the in vivo system. Studies of reaggregated stratum corneum, using different lamellar phases for the lipid fraction (35), have shown the preeminent importance of the bilayer lipid arrangement in the barrier function. Initial studies of PG, Azone, and oleyl alcohol (11,12) showed that PG behaved as expected from the hydrotrope studies (36) (i.e., produced a change in the hydration layer of the bilayer interface). Azone and oleyl alcohol, conversely, produced a more-ordered system.

The ternary-phase behavior of these systems showed (Fig. 11) that Azone and oleyl alcohol allowed the bilayers to incorporate a larger amount of water, relative to the two-component surfactant–water bilayers. On the other hand, PG reduced the water-holding capacity of the bilayers. Both Azone and oleyl alcohol could be incorporated up to high levels (about 20% w/w), whereas only about 5% of PG could be accommodated by the system. These observations are significant, since penetration enhancement of hydrophilic drugs is related to the water content of the skin, and the formation of a larger-volume hydrophobic interior of the bilayers is probably influential in percutaneous transport of hydrophobic drugs. Furthermore, studies (37) of the bilayer internal order, using deuterated surfactant analogues as the probe, show increases in amphipath chain order, a feature that is also associated with enhanced penetration.

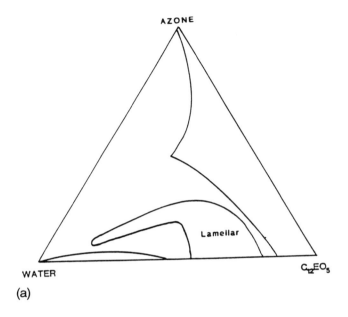

(a)

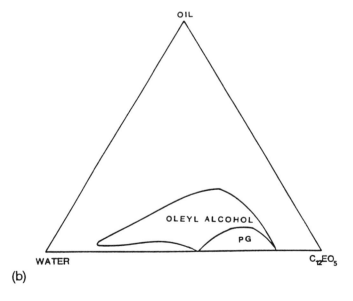

(b)

Figure 11   (a) Phase diagram at 298 K for the system $C_{12}EO_5$–Azone–water. (b) Partial phase diagrams showing the extent of the lamellar phases of the system $C_{12}EO_5$–water with oleyl alcohol and propyplene glycol at 298 K.

Another area of penetration enhancer behavior that has been investigated using this model system is that of synergism in enhancement produced by some binary mixtures of enhancing agents. Mixtures of propylene glycol with weakly amphipathic molecules, such as oleic acid and alcohol, have exhibited synergism in a number of in vitro studies (38–40) (i.e., enhanced penetration above that expected from simple addivity of the effects of the individual components). The chosen model system was studied in terms of the lamellar phase stability in the presence of such mixtures (11,12). It was observed (Fig. 12) for PG mole fractions in the mixture, X_{PG}, below 0.10 that there was no enhanced water retention capacity of the bilayers compared with the system without solubilizate. Similarly, an enhanced capacity of the bilayers to incorporate the enhancer mixture was found (Fig. 13) in the range $0.5 < X_{pg} < 0.8$, again compared with that expected from the amounts of the single components that could be solubilized. For oleyl alcohol–PG mixtures, approximately 55% (w/w) could be solubilized, compared with 26% for oleyl alcohol or 5% for PG alone. This mole fraction range corresponds to the composition range of such vehicles for which synergistic enhancement of the

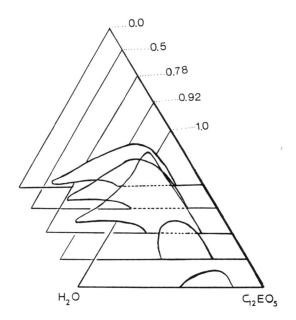

Figure 12 Partial phase diagrams of the system $C_{12}EO_5$–water with solubilized oleyl alcohol–propylene glycol of different PG mole fractions (numbers at the apex of the diagrams).

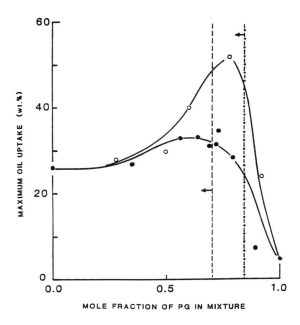

MOLE FRACTION OF PG IN MIXTURE

Figure 13 Maximum uptake of Azone–PG (closed circles) and oleyl alcohol–PG (open circles) mixtures in lamellar $C_{12}EO_5$–water (60:40 w/w) at 298 K, showing the limit of compositions at which increased water capacity is found; $\cdot - \cdot - \cdot - \cdot -$ oleyl alcohol–PG; $----$ Azone–PG.

fluxes of progesterone and glucose are observed through intact stratum corneum (41) in vitro.

Preliminary deuterium NMR and small-angle x-ray diffraction measurements of these model systems indicate (11,12) differing effects of the individual enhancing components on the dynamic structure of the bilayer lipids. With PG, competition occurs for solvation sites of the headgroups and associated disruption at the bilayer–water interface. This is balanced by structuring effects, both within the bilayer and at the bilayer–water interface, through increased hydrogen-bonding possibilities, which occur on incorporation of long-chain amphipathic molecules.

The location of the maximum distribution of an incorporated solubilizate in the bilayer system therefore, is extremely important. Molecules that can locate preponderantly in the region of the bilayer, close to the lipid headgroups, cause most disruption of the molecular packing in the bilayer. Sodium xylene sulfonate, for example, is an extremely efficient hydrotrope and, in fact, is well-known for being a skin irritant. Synergism or increased penetration enhancement is a fine balance between the competing structural influences of the vehicle components. If the balance moves to much toward too efficient bilayer disruption, the likelihood of problems of irritancy is increased.

ACKNOWLEDGMENT

The financial support of The Upjohn Company and EOLAS is gratefully acknowledged.

REFERENCES

1. Israelachvili, J. N. *Proc. Int. Sch. Phys. "Enrico Fermi" (Phys. Amphiphilas)* 90:24 (1985).
2. Ninham, B. W. and Mitchell, D. J. *J. Chem. Soc., Faraday Trans. II* 77:601 (1981).
3. Elias, P. M. and Friend, D. S. *J. Cell Biol.* 65:185 (1975).
4. Lavker, R. S. *J. Ultrastruct. Res.* 55:78 (1976).
5. Friberg, S. E., Kayali, I. H., Margosiak, M., Osborne, D. W., and Ward, A. J. I. In *Topical Drug Delivery Formulations.* Osborne, D. W. and Amann, A. H. (eds.). Marcel Dekker, New York, p. 29 (1990).
6. Gruen, D. W. R. *Prog. Colloid Polym. Sci.* 70:6 (1985).
7. Lindman, B. and Wenrerstrom, H. *Phys. Rep.* 52:1 (1979).
8. Seelig, J. *Q. Rev. Biophys.* 10:353 (1977).
9. Rendall, K. and Tiddy, G. J. T. *J. Chem. Soc., Faraday Trans. I* 80:3339 (1984).
10. Lyle, I. G. and Tiddy, G. J. T. *Chem. Phys. Lett.* 124:432 (1986).
11. Ward, A. J. I. and Tallon, R. *Drug Dev. Ind. Pharm.* 14:115–116 (1988).
12. Ward, A. J. I and Tallen, R. *Drugs Pharm. Sci.* 42:47–67 (1990).
13. Neuberg, C. *Biochem. Z.* 76:107 (1916).
14. McBain, M. E. L. and Hutchison, E. *Solubilization and Related Phenomena.* Academic Press, New York (1955).
15. Winsor, P. A. *Trans. Faraday Soc.* 44:376, 382, 287, 290 (1948).
16. Klevens, H. B. *Chem. Rev.* 47:1 (1950).
17. Ekwall, P. In *Advances in Liquid Crystals.* Vol. 1. Browne, G. H. (ed.). Academic Press, New York, p. 1 (1975).
18. Laughlin, R. G. In *Advances in Liquid Crystals,* Vol. 3. Browne, G. H. (ed.). Academic Press, New York, p. 41 (1978).
19. James, K. C. *Solubility and Related Properties.* Marcel Dekker, New York, p. 382 (1986).
20. Yalkowsky, S. H. and Roseman, T. J. In *Techniques of Solubilization of Drugs.* Yalkowsky, S. H. (ed.). Marcel Dekker, New York (1981).
21. Vaughan, C. D. *J. Soc. Cosmet. Chem.* 36:319 (1985).
22. Rheineck, A. E. and Lin, K. F. *J. Paint Technol.* 44:611 (1968).
23. Friberg, S. E. and Rydhag, L. *Tenside* 7:80 (1970).
24. Friberg, S. E. and Chiu, M. *Dispers. Sci. Technol.* 9:443 (1988–1989).

25. Friberg, S. E., Rananavare, S. B., and Osborne, D. W. *J. Colloid Interface Sci. 109*:487 (1986).
26. Cox, J. M. and Friberg, S. E. *J. Am. Oil Chem. Soc. 58*:743 (1983).
27. Flaim, T. and Friberg, S. E. *J. Colloid Interface Sci. 97*:26 (1984).
28. Scheuplein, R. J. and Bronaugh, R. L. In *Biochemistry and Physiology of the Skin*. Goldsmith, L. A. (ed.). Oxford University Press, New York, p. 1255 (1983).
29. Elias, P. M., Cooper, E. R., Kore, A., and Borwn, B. E. *J. Invest. Dermatol. 76*:297 (1981).
30. Downing, D. T. *J. Invest. Dermatol. 55*:135 (1970).
31. Cooper, E. R. In *Percutaneous Absorption*. Bronaugh, R. L. and Maibach, H. I. (eds.). Marcel Dekker, p. 515 (1985).
32. Osborne, D. W. *Colloid Surfaces 30*:13 (1988).
33. Lampe, M. A., Williams, M. L., and Elias, P. M. *J. Lipid Res. 24*:131 (1983).
34. Friberg, S. E. and Osborne, D. W. *J. Dispers. Sci. Technol. 6*:485 (1985).
35. Ward, A. J. I. and du Reau, C. *Int. J. Pharm. 74*:137 (1991).
36. Ward, A. J. I., Marie, C., Sylvia, L. A., and Phillipi, M. A. *J. Dispers. Sci. Technol. 9*:149 (1988).
37. Ward, A. J. I. and Tallon, R. Unpublished results.
38. Stoughton, R. B. and McClure, W. O. *Drug Dev. Ind. Pharm. 9*:725 (1983).
39. Hoelgaard, A. and Mollgaard, B. *J. Controlled Release 2*:111 (1985).
40. Wotton, P. K., Mollgaard, B., Hadgraft, J., and Hoelgaard, A. *Int. J. Pharm. 24*:19 (1985).
41. Tallon, R., Osborne, D. W., and Ward, A. J. I. Unpublished results.

18

Molecular Modeling of Skin Permeation Enhancement by Chemical Agents

Keith R. Brain

The Welsh School of Pharmacy, University of Wales, Cardiff, Wales

Kenneth A. Walters

An-eX Analytical Services, Ltd., Cardiff, Wales

I. INTRODUCTION

The skin penetration and permeation literature contains many suggestions concerning the mode of action of chemical permeability enhancers. There are certainly sufficient experimental data to indicate a major involvement of the intercellular lipid lamellae of the stratum corneum. The collective data, using such diverse techniques as differential-scanning calorimetry (1–4), infrared spectrometry (4,5), electron spin resonance (6), x-ray diffractometry (7–9), fluorescence spectrometry (10), and direct determination of in vitro and in vivo skin permeability (11–13) have implied that chemical skin penetration enhancement is usually a result of an increased fluidity of the hydrophobic regions of the intercellular lipid lamellar structure.

There can be little doubt that the design of skin penetration enhancers would be facilitated by a fuller understanding of their mode of action within the target tissue, and it may be possible to use the techniques of molecular modeling as part of this process. One major problem with this approach is that the exact chemical morphology of the lipid lamellae have yet to be elucidated, although several studies on model membranes give some indications.

Over the past 10 years there has been increasing use of molecular graphics and modeling programs in the determination of structure–activity relations and in drug design. Although these techniques have previously required mainframe computer power, recent developments in computing technology have resulted in the availability of effective interactive molecular graphics and modeling programs that can be run on desktop computers. This has rendered the application of these techniques accessible to a much wider spectrum of scientists. These programs, however, are only as effective as the algorithms on which they are based, and it is inevitable that these include some empirical procedures that result in approximations that may be significant. However, they allow the investigation of a number of important parameters. Structures may be built and manipulated in three dimensions; energies, partial charges, and electrostatic potentials calculated; and conformational searches and molecular fitting conducted. There have as yet been few reports on the use of these techniques in the elucidation of the mechanism of action of skin penetration enhancers. However, in this chapter, we have applied this approach to the available literature data on several types of enhancer. The molecular features of a range of related compounds are discussed in relation to both their enhancing effect and their potential interaction with the lipid components of the intercellular spaces in the stratum corneum. The model has been used to partially explain various literature observations, including the phenomenon of saturation observed with many of the enhancers studied (14–17). However, the reader is advised that the following evaluation is probably also saturated with assumptions and can be regarded as only speculative at this point.

II. STRATUM CORNEUM LIPIDS

For the purposes of this discussion the origins of the stratum corneum intercellular lipid lamellae have been considered largely irrelevant. However, in brief, the lipid sheets are believed to be derived from intracellular granules, the contents of which are secreted during cornification (18). Numerous references to the types and proportions of the intercellular lipids of the stratum corneum have illustrated considerable inter- and intraspecies variation. It is possible, however, that variable extraction procedures may be partly responsible for some of these reported differences. Nonetheless, analysis of the data does provide some general observations concerning the types and amounts of lipids present in human stratum corneum (Table 1).

It is evident that, on a molar basis, most lipid comprises cholesterol derivatives and ceramides (Fig. 1), with smaller amounts of other material, such as fatty acids and triglycerides (19,20). The percentage molar proportions of total ceramides and cholesterol (plus derivatives, with esters calculated as C_{16}) amount to about 72% of the total lipid. The precise arrangement of the various lipid components in intact stratum corneum is difficult to determine experimentally. It has been shown that the stratum corneum intercellular lipids are present in distinct structured bilayer lamellae, which provide a substantial hydrophobic barrier. The

Table 1 Composition of Human Stratum Corneum Lipids in Percentage (w/w) and Mole Percentage

Lipid	% (w/w)	mol %
Cholesterol esters	10.0	7.5[a]
Cholesterol	26.9	33.4
Cholesterol sulfate	1.9	2.0
Total cholesterol derivatives	38.8	42.9
Ceramide 1	3.2	1.6
Ceramide 2	8.9	6.6
Ceramide 3	4.9	3.5
Ceramide 4	6.1	4.2
Ceramide 5	5.7	5.0
Ceramide 6	12.3	8.6
Total ceramides	41.1	29.5
Fatty acids	9.1	17.0[a]
Others	11.1	10.6[b]

[a]Based on C_{16} alkyl chain.
[b]Based on MW of 500.
Source: Ref. 19.

fundamental stability of this lamellar structure must be dependent on both cooperative interactions between the polar headgroups and hydrophobic interactions between the alkyl chains. It is unclear whether individual components are present in distinct domains or randomly distributed. Klausner et al. (21) considered that, from a biological viewpoint, the latter would appear doubtful. Although some form of ordering would be expected to be present, it is considered most likely that this is at the micro-, rather than the macrolevel.

Most studies have only considered the importance of the ceramides, perhaps because they are relatively unusual compounds in terms of membrane components. However, these make up only approximately one-third of the total stratum corneum lipids on a molar basis, and the significance of the presence of an approximately equimolar ratio between cholesterol and total ceramides in stratum corneum has not been taken into account in most considerations of permeability modification. It has been suggested that the cohesive links between the adjacent lipid lamellae in the stratum corneum (Fig. 2) are made by the long-chain ceramide 1, which contains an ω-hydroxyacid residue; by bifunctional glucosyl ceramides; or by protein bridges. It is also theoretically possible that the

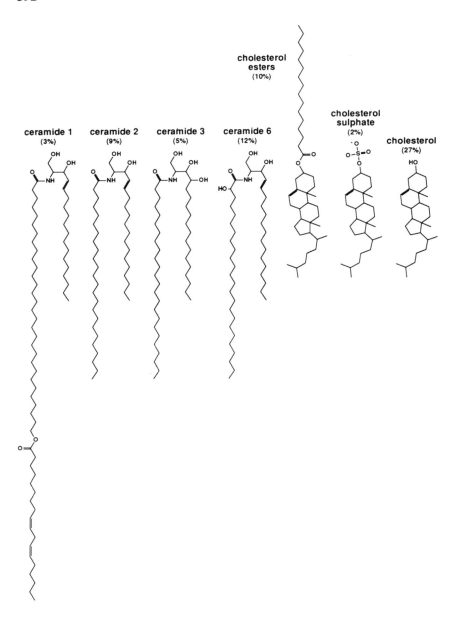

Figure 1   Major lipids of the intercellular regions of the human stratum corneum.

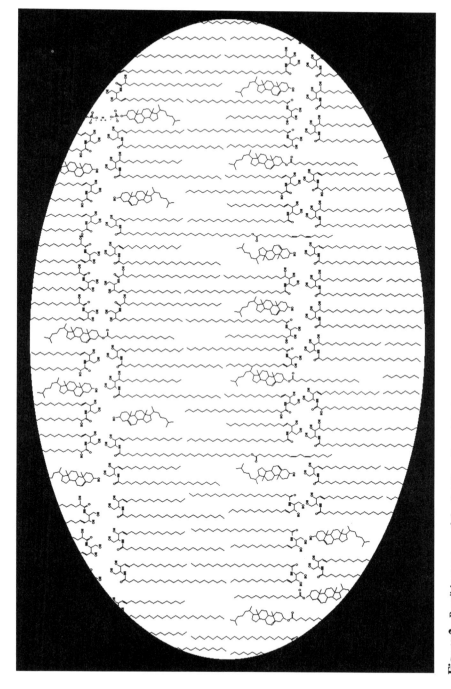

Figure 2 Possible structure of the lipid lamellae of the intercellular regions of the outer layers of the human stratum corneum.

cholesterol esters may span adjacent bilayers and that cholesterol sulfate moieties may be bridged through divalent counterions. For simplicity, this evaluation has excluded some of the other lipids that have been shown to be present in small quantities in the stratum corneum.

III. MODEL MEMBRANES

Phospholipids, such as dipalmitoylphosphatidylcholine (DPPC) and distearoyl-phosphatidylcholine (DSPC) have been used extensively for model studies on membrane structure and interactions (22–26). These lipids are readily available in pure form and have provided some useful information. However, although the alkyl chains are similar to those in skin ceramides, the structure of the polar headgroup is significantly different (Fig. 3). Some studies have been carried out using extracted skin ceramides (27–29) and these have produced results qualitatively similar to those with phospholipids. However, it is more difficult to put a precise interpretation on the skin ceramide studies owing to the heterogeneity of the systems.

Finean (23) has recently reviewed the literature on the interactions of cholesterol and phospholipids and provided strong evidence for the presence of one-to-one molar complexes (Fig. 4) involving hydrogen bonding of the 3-β-hydroxyl of cholesterol, with the glycerol oxygen at the 2 position of the phospholipid, and van der Waals bonding between the hydrocarbon structures. Two alternative packing modes were proposed, with and without cholesterol–cholesterol contact. It is probable that a similar equimolar arrangement occurs within the skin lipids.

Cholesterol has a modifying effect on the fluidity and permeability of phospholipid membranes (23,30). The presence of the rigid steroidal skeleton next to the first 10–12 carbon atoms of the alkyl chain of the phospholipid reduces the freedom of movement of those atoms. At the same, the freedom of movement of the lower part of the chain is increased owing to the increase in space produced. However, as the concentration of cholesterol increases, the area of the membrane taken up by the alkyl chains plus cholesterol exceeds that of the phospholipid headgroups, so that the chain tilt present in the pure phospholipid bilayer is abolished. At equimolar concentrations, cholesterol increases fluidity below the transition temperature (owing to pushing apart of the headgroups), but decreases fluidity above the transition temperature (owing to condensation of the alkyl chains).

The transition temperature of ceramides ($\sim$70°C) is well above normal physiological conditions, so that the ceramides will exist in the condensed state, in the absence of modifying forces. However, the headgroups of the ceramides are somewhat smaller than those of phospholipids; hence, the disruptive effect of

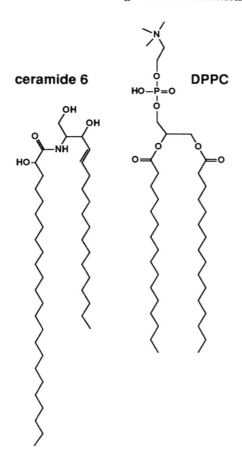

Figure 3 Comparison of the structure of ceramide 6 and that of dipalmitoylphosphatidyl-choline (DPPC).

cholesterol might be expected to be greater. Certainly, the large mole percentage of cholesterol in the stratum corneum lipids must be taken into account in any consideration of skin permeability modification. It is proposed that the 3β-hydroxyl of cholesterol is hydrogen-bonded to the headgroup of the adjacent ceramide. As cholesterol has no other functional group available for specific interaction, we suggest back-to-back pairing of cholesterol moieties held together by multiple weak interactions between the rigid skeletons (Fig. 5). The second cholesterol molecule will then hydrogen-bond with the next ceramide.

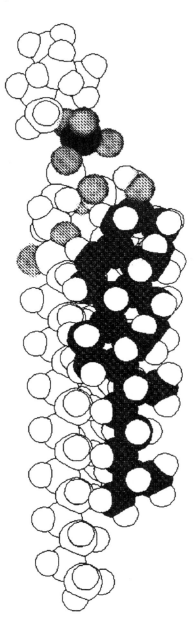

Figure 4   One-to-one molar complex of phospholipid and cholesterol as postulated by Finean (23).

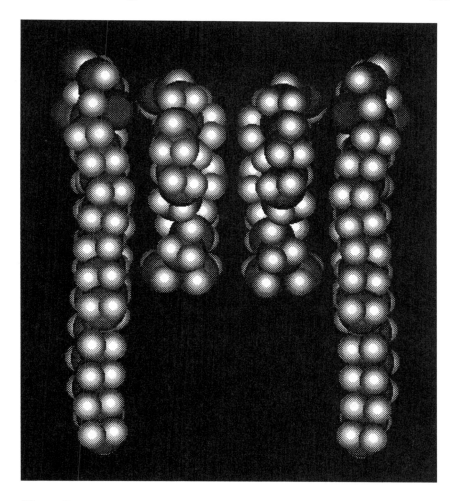

Figure 5   Possible arrangement of cholesterol and ceramides.

IV. MODELING OF ENHANCER–LIPID INTERACTIONS

The consideration of chemical enhancement here is deliberately restricted to those molecules believed to have a specific, rather than a solventlike (e.g., ethanol; 31) effect on permeation. After having established a primitive model on which to base our arguments, it is possible to speculate further and attempt to explain the potential mechanisms of chemical penetration enhancement by incorporation of these moieties into the model.

The precise configuration of a molecule depends not only on intramolecular forces, but also on interaction with the surrounding environment. It is possible to calculate optimized minimum energy configurations for enhancers, but these will not necessarily represent the molecular structure at the bilayer interface. Interactions can occur with the water of hydration and polar headgroups of the lipids. These will tend to arrange the atoms such that relatively polar groups are oriented toward the aqueous surface, or toward adjacent polar groups. It is also clear that the interactions between the nonpolar components of the molecules will be influenced by hydrophilic interactions at the polar end that alter intermolecular spacing. It is probable that different enhancers behave in different ways and also exhibit variable effects on alternative permeants.

Chemical enhancement is often considered to be largely the result of interactions in the polar headgroup region, which result in increased fluidity of the alkyl chains. Both saturated and unsaturated fatty acids and alcohols (32,33) have been established as effective enhancers. Comparison of the influence of incorporating 10% saturated alcohols on the flux of naloxone in propylene glycol through human skin (Fig. 6) showed a parabolic effect of alkyl chain length with C_{10} and C_{12} being most effective. It may be significant that the most effective alkyl chain lengths (C_{10}–C_{12}) correspond to the length of the steroid nucleus of cholesterol, suggesting that these enhancers may act by disrupting ceramide–cholesterol or cholesterol–cholesterol interaction. However, incorporation of increasing levels of unsaturation into the C_{18} derivative produced even more effective enhancement (Fig. 7). In the corresponding fatty acids a similar effect was seen, except that the C_{10}–C_{12} compounds had a higher activity than the unsaturated C_{18} derivatives (Fig. 8). There was a much greater concentration dependence of flux enhancement for lauric acid than lauryl alcohol (Fig. 9), but this could not be attributed to complexation of lauric acid with naloxone. In a similar study, Ogiso and Shintani (34) examined the effects of a series of fatty acids (C_6–C_{18}) on the flux of propranolol across rabbit skin. Once again, a parabolic relation between enhancer efficacy and enhancer alkyl chain length was observed (Fig. 10). The carboxylic acids have higher melting points than their corresponding alcohols (e.g., lauric acid, 45°C; lauryl alcohol, 25°C), but lower solubility parameters. If the enhancement by these acids and alcohols was solely due to solubility effects, then it would be predicted that the alcohols would be more effective than the acids, whereas the converse is true for alkyl chains up to C_{18}. This indicates that more specific interactions must occur. The most effective alkyl chain length corresponds to the dimensions of the cholesterol skeleton, which leads to the hypothesis that disruption of ceramide–cholesterol, or cholesterol–cholesterol, interactions is an important factor in permeability modification by these C_{10}–C_{12} compounds. Introduction of unsaturation into long alkyl chains modifies the behavior considerably and,

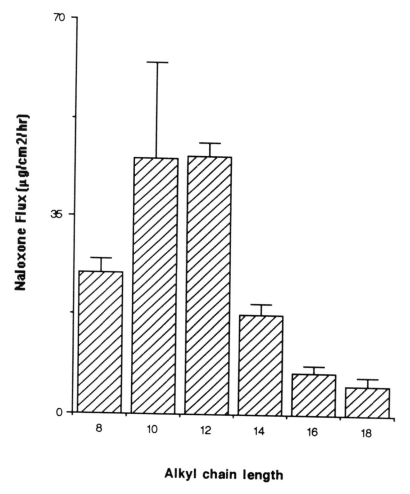

Figure 6 The influence of fatty alcohols on naloxone flux across human skin. (Data from Ref. 33)

for the C_{18} compounds, there was little difference between the corresponding acids and alcohols.

Aungst (35) further demonstrated (Fig. 11) that, for naloxone, there were no significant differences between the enhancement effects of a series of C_{16}–C_{18} cis- and trans-unsaturated fatty acids. In contrast, Cooper (32) and Golden et al. (36) have presented evidence that cis-double-bonded unsaturated fatty acids are

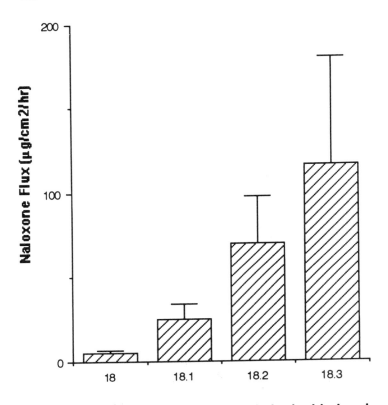

Alkyl chain length. Number of cis double bonds

Figure 7 The influence of alkyl chain unsaturation (*cis*) on the fatty alcohol induced enhancement of naloxone flux across human skin. (Data from Ref. 33)

more effective in increasing both lamellar fluidity and permeation rates than their *trans*-counterparts. Considerable differences in permeability enhancement between the isomeric C_2- and C_{16}-branched isostearic acids have been demonstrated (35). Only the latter, with the methyl group attached distally to the carboxyl was more effective than stearic acid, indicating that disruption of the packing by the out-of-plane methyl group is more effective at a deeper level.

The differential effect between saturated and unsaturated fatty acids and alcohols has been attributed to the large difference in molecular geometry between these species (Fig. 12) and the presence of distinct kinks in the alkyl chain, which could disrupt the stratum corneum lipid packing. Increasing the number of

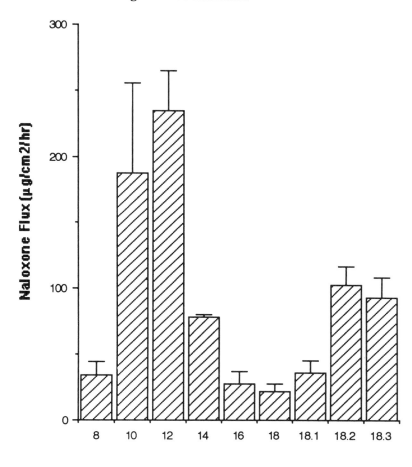

Figure 8 The influence of fatty acids on naloxone flux across human skin. (Data from Ref. 33)

cis-double bonds to two or three, with increased kinking, enhances the flux of naloxone through human skin (33).

There is some dispute over whether enhancers (and cholesterol) are distributed homogeneously or as distinct domains (37,38). There is evidence from fluorescent polarization spectroscopy of phospholipid membranes, treated with saturated and unsaturated fatty acids, to support the existence of separate lipid phases and

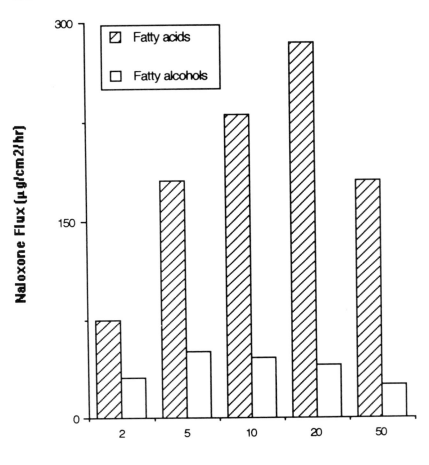

Figure 9 Concentration dependent effects of fatty acids and alcohols (C_{12}) on naloxone flux across human skin. (Data from Ref. 33)

permeable defects at phase interfaces, and differential accumulation of saturated and unsaturated fatty acids in different domains (21). Fourier transform infrared spectrometry (FTIR) evidence has been presented for the occurrence of distinct pools of perdeuterated oleic acid in porcine stratum corneum after treatment with that molecule (39). It was demonstrated that the perdeuterated oleic acid was in the liquid state, in a solid continuous lipid phase, and proposed that penetration

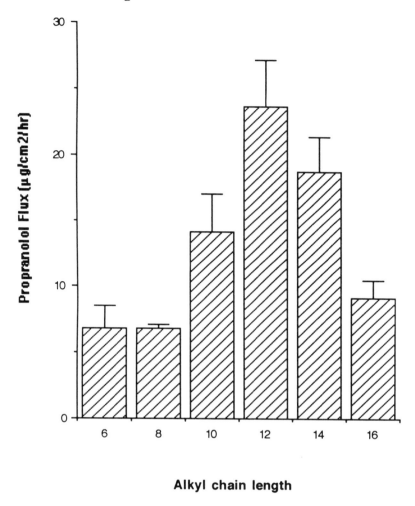

Figure 10   The influence of fatty acid chain length on the flux of propranolol across rabbit skin. (Data from Ref. 33)

enhancement resulted from the occurrence of permeable effects at the liquid–solid-phase interface. The use of perdeuterated oleic acid allowed separate resolution of the C-H and C-D stretching frequencies. However, it is possible that the ability of the normal alkyl chains of the stratum corneum lipids to pack with the perdeuterated alkyl chains was not the same as that of normal oleic acid (see, e.g., 40–42). However, neutron-scattering experiments with DPPC

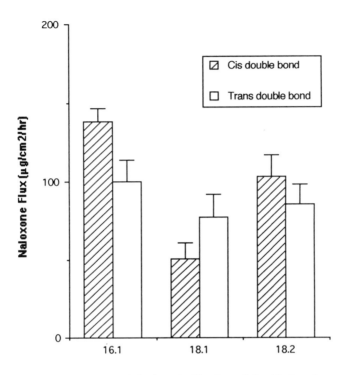

Fatty acid chain length. Number of double bonds

Figure 11 Comparison between the effects of *cis*- and *trans*-double bonds in unsaturated fatty acids on naloxone flux across human skin. (Data from Ref. 35)

liposomes containing either perdeuterated oleic acid or deuterated DPPC, both indicated that the mixtures were not homogeneous (Watkinson, A. and Hadgraft, J., personal communication). The rate of diffusion of a permeant through a liquid phase would be considerably more rapid than through a solid phase, and it is perhaps unnecessary to postulate the importance of interfacial defects. If the interfacial defect route is the most important, then increasing pool size will be disadvantageous (Fig. 13), and optimum disruption may occur at an equimolar ratio.

Several studies have compared the effectiveness of structures based on laurocapram (Azone; 1-dodecylazacycloheptan-2-one, I). The effects of variations in ring size, and incorporation of branched saturated or unsaturated alkyl chains (Fig. 14), in this series on the enhancement of the permeation of mitomycin

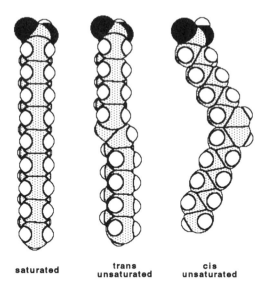

Figure 12 Molecular geometry of saturated, *trans*-unsaturated, and *cis*-unsaturated fatty acids.

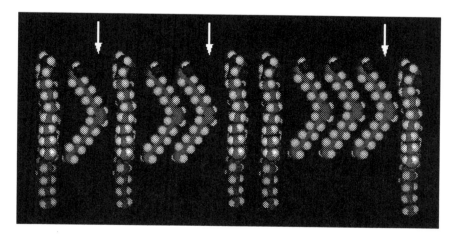

Figure 13 Influence of pool size on the frequency of interfacial defects (arrows) between ceramide and oleic acid molecules.

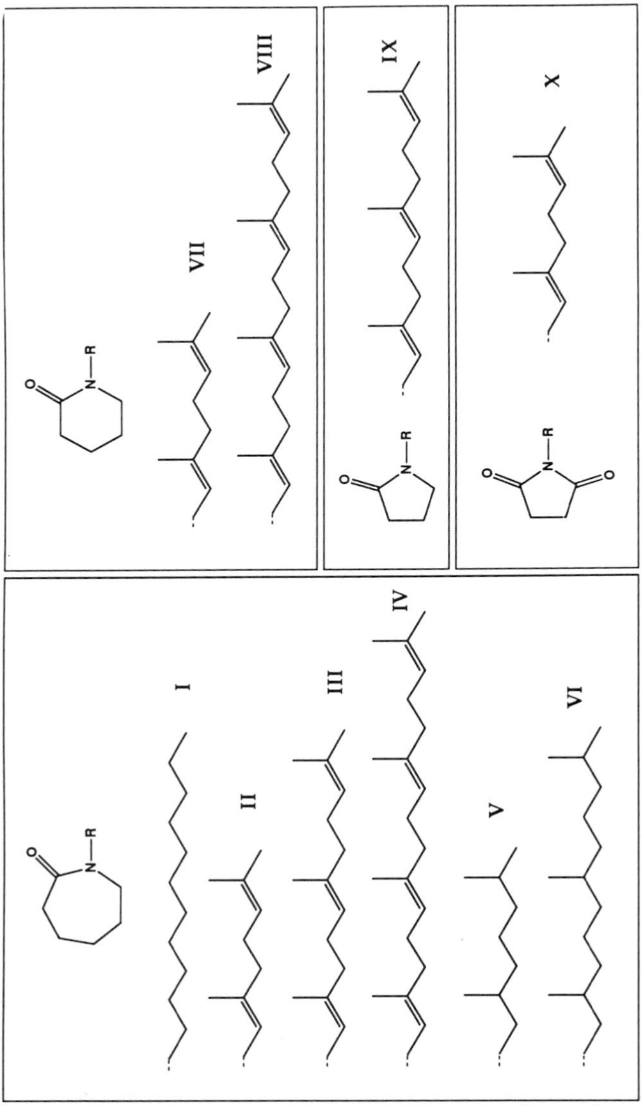

Figure 14   Azone and several analogues evaluated as skin penetration enhancers.

through hairless mouse and Wistar rat skin (43), and 6-mercaptopurine through guinea pig skin (44), have been examined. Replacement of the alkyl chain of Azone (I) with the mono-, sesqui, and diterpene geranyl (II), farnesyl (III), and geranyl-geranyl (IV) chains produced decreasing enhancement of the permeation of 6-mercaptopurine across guinea pig skin. However, there was little difference between the effect of the unsaturated mono- (II) and sequiterpene (III) derivatives and their saturated analogues (V and VI). Interpretation of this data at the molecular level is complicated because the terpene derivatives tested were actually mixtures of the 2'-*trans* and 2'-*cis*-isomers, which have considerably different molecular architectures (Fig. 15), in a 7:3 ratio. It would be predicted from the overall molecular shape that the 2'-*cis*-series would be less effective, and the corollary of that is that the 2'-*trans*-series are probably actually more active than the saturated analogues. Reduction of the ring size to five- or six-membered had little effect on the activity of the limited number of terpene derivatives examined (cf. III and IX, II and VII, and IV and VIII). However, the pentacyclic diketo-geranyl derivative (X) was much less effective than the heptacyclic-monoketo derivative (II). The same rank order of effectiveness of I, II, and III on a wider range of permeants (including acylovir, fluorouracil, and sulfanilic acid) has also been reported (45). A parabolic relation between enhancement and permeant lipophilicity was observed, with maximal effect on fluorouracil ($\log P_{oct/water} = -1$).

Hoogstraate et al. (46) have demonstrated that several linear alkyl chain analogues of Azone are less effective in enhancing the skin penetration rate of desgylcinamide arginine vasopressin (Table 2). In particular, short alkyl chains were unfavorable, and C_{10} and C_{14} alkyl chains less effective than C_{12} (Azone). Dodecyl analogues of a variety of chemical species are often most effective in terms of membrane activity (see, e.g., 47), perhaps because of interaction with cholesterol. A spoon-shaped model for the conformation of Azone was proposed by Bodde (48). Evidence for the existence of such a conformation in practice was presented by Lewis and Hadgraft (24), who examined the effect of Azone on the compressibility of DPPC monolayers, using a Langmuir trough, and determined the area per molecule in the film. They also used conformational analysis to demonstrate that the energy required to produce the spoon shape by rotation around an alkyl chain bond was small. Hoogstraate et al. (46) used computer-aided molecular modeling to demonstrate that turning the carbonyl moiety toward the interlamellar hydrophobic domain to produce a soup-spoon required only 1 kcal/mol above the minimum energy conformation.

Modeling of the electrostatic field around the headgroup of ceramides shows that electronegative and positive regions exist on opposite sides of the molecule, and it is predicted that the interaction of these charges is involved in binding the headgroups together. The spoon-shaped Azone model shows an electronegative

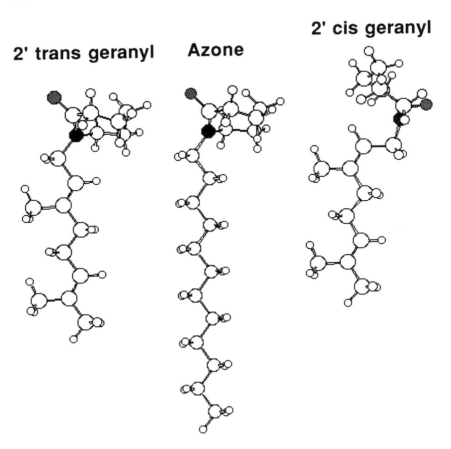

Figure 15 Molecular geometry of Azone compared with analogues containing 2'-*trans*- and 2'-*cis*-geranyl chains.

site at the carbonyl moiety, but no complementary positive site, and intercalation of Azone into the ceramide matrix will leave an unbalanced electronegative site on the ceramide, which could give rise to a permeable defect. Several novel derivatives of Azone have been examined (49) that possess either two electronegative sites or both a negative and a positive site (Fig. 16). The former is a more effective enhancer, owing to increased electrostatic repulsion, whereas the latter actually retards permeation, presumably by interacting with both adjacent ceramide molecules. The sulfur analogue of Azone is inactive. This can be explained in terms of both reduced electronegativity of the molecule and conformational

Table 2 Influence of Azone and Analogues on the Permeability Coefficients of Desglycinamide Arginine Vasopressin Through Human Stratum Corneum

Vehicle	Permeability coefficient (cm/sec $\times 10^{-11} \pm$ SD)
Control	5.3 ± 2.1
Propylene glycol	4.0 ± 0.8
C_{14} Azone analogue	13.0 ± 0.9
Azone	18.7 ± 1.9
C_{10} Azone analogue	9.9 ± 0.6
C_8 Azone analogue	5.4 ± 0.6
C_6 Azone analogue	3.8 ± 0.2

Source: Ref. 46.

analysis of the headgroup torsion, which indicates that transformation from the straight to the bent form is a much more energetic process here (Fig. 17).

Williams and Barry (50) have reported widely different enhancement ratios (3- to 380-fold) for several cyclic terpenes, using fluorouracil as the test permeant. In view of the large range of enhancement effects observed, and that the purity of the test terpenes varied from 90 to 99%, it is difficult to fully interpret the structure–activity relations. However, it is clear that the presence of an oxygen function was required for significant activity, and that the most effective compounds had bulky structures containing oxygen bridges out of the plane of the hydrocarbon ring (Fig. 18). This feature has some similarity to the F-ring structure of the spiroketal steroidal compounds, which are known to disrupt membranes (51). These bicyclic structures are quite small molecules relative to the enhancers discussed in the foregoing, and it is unclear how deeply they penetrated the bilayers. If they are restricted to the interfacial or palisade regions, they could either align themselves with the oxygen bridge projecting toward the aqueous interlamellar phase, or at right angles with the oxygen moiety, hydrogen-bonding with complementary groups on adjacent lipids. In view of the large difference in activity between cyclopentene oxide and cyclohexene oxide, the latter seems more likely. The latter comparison highlights the advantages of viewing molecular structure in three dimensions.

V. CONCLUDING REMARKS

In this consideration we have attempted to rationalize the molecular modes of action of several groups of skin penetration enhancers, based on the current state

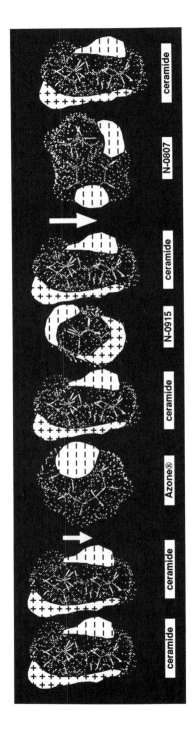

Figure 16 The electrostatic field surrounding the head groups of ceramide, Azone and analogues illustrating potential interfacial defects (arrows).

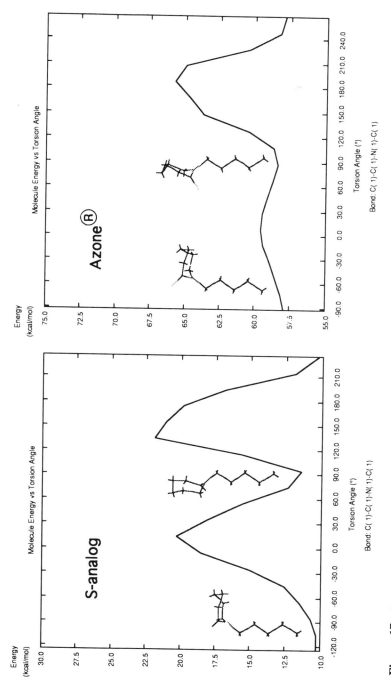

Figure 17 Comparison of the ease of rotation of the head group for Azone and its S-analogue. See text for details.

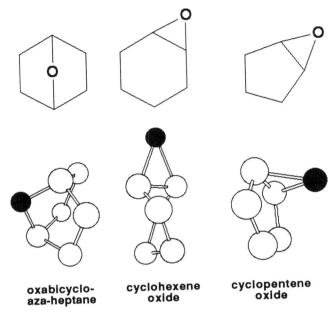

oxabicyclo- aza-heptane	**cyclohexene oxide**	**cyclopentene oxide**

Figure 18 Molecular geometry of selected cyclic terpenes. Oxabicycloaza-heptane enhancement ratio = 91.7, cyclohexene oxide enhancement ratio = 2.4, cyclopentene oxide enhancement ratio = 30.9. (Ratios from Ref. 50)

of knowledge of skin structure. However, it is important that the reader be aware that several assumptions have been made and that these must be taken into account in the assessment of the presented hypotheses. It is clear that many of the reported skin penetration enhancers possess identifiable regions in their structure that are capable of interaction with distinct regions of skin lipids. There are, however, some molecules that increase skin permeation rates, the action of which cannot be explained by the foregoing hypotheses. The latter compounds may act by alternative mechanisms, such as simple cosolvency or alteration of the thermodynamic activity of the permeant in the stratum corneum. It is also possible that some molecules may have a direct action on the keratin contained within the corneocytes. In view of the lack of information in this area, this aspect has been deliberately excluded from the foregoing discussion.

The continuing development of evermore sophisticated and sensitive physicochemical techniques is providing an improved knowledge, based on skin structure and its alteration by penetration enhancers. As more is known at the molecular level, it should be possible to use molecular graphics not only to explain empirical observations, but also to design penetration enhancers and drugs or prodrugs that act as self-enhancers. This will be useful in the optimization of human and veterinary pharmaceutical formulations for both topical and transdermal use. Similarly, it may be possible to design molecules that are capable of practical-scale retardation of penetration rates across simple or complex biological barriers, which could have a significant impact in reduction of the risks associated with deliberate or accidental exposure to xenobiotics. Therefore, the data generated from molecular modeling may be of considerable value to, and have application in, a wide range of pharmaceutical, cosmetic, and agrochemical fields.

REFERENCES

1. Goodman, M. and Barry, B. W. Differential scanning calorimetry of human stratum corneum: Effects of penetration enhancers Azone and dimethyl sulphoxide. *Anal. Proc.* 23:397–398 (1986).
2. Golden, G. M., Guzek, D. B., Harris, R. R., McKie, J. E., and Potts, R. O. Lipid thermotropic transitions in human stratum corneum. *J. Invest. Dermatol.* 86:255–259 (1986).
3. Bouwstra, J., Peschier, L., Brussee, J., and Bodde, H. Effect of *n*-alkyl azocycloheptan-2-ones including Azones on the thermal behaviour of human stratum corneum. *Int. J. Pharm.* 52:47–54 (1989).
4. Potts, R. O., Golden, G. M., Francouer, M. L., Mak, V. H. W., and Guy, R. H. Mechanism and enhancement of solute transport across the stratum corneum. *J. Controlled Release* 15:249–260 (1991).
5. Mak, V. H. W., Potts, R. O., and Guy, R. H. Percutaneous penetration enhancement in vivo measured by attenuated total reflectance infrared spectroscopy. *Pharm. Res.* 7:835–841 (1990).
6. Gay, C. L., Murphy, T. M., Hadgraft, J., Kellaway, I. W., Evans, J. C., and Rowlands, C. C. An electron spin resonance study of skin penetration enhancers. *Int. J. Pharm.* 49:39–45 (1989).
7. Wilkes, G. L., Nguyen, A. N., and Wildnauer, R. Structure–property relations of human and neonatal rat stratum corneum. I. Thermal stability of the crystalline lipid structure as studied by x-ray diffraction and differential thermal analysis. *Biochim. Biophys. Acta* 304:267–275 (1973).
8. Friberg, S. E., Goldsmith, L., Suhaimi, H., and Rhein, L. D. Surfactants and the stratum corneum lipids. *Colloids Surfaces* 30:1–12 (1988).
9. Friberg, S. and Osbourne, D. Small-angle x-ray diffraction patterns of stratum corneum and a model structure for its lipids. *J. Dispers. Sci. Technol.* 6:485–495 (1985).
10. French, E. J., Pouton, C. W., and Steele, G. Fluidization of lipid bilayers by nonionic surfactants: Structure activity studies using a fluorescent probe. In *Prediction of Percutaneous Penetration*. Scott, R. C., Guy, R. H., and Hadgraft, J. (eds.). IBC, London, pp. 308–315 (1990).
11. Ashton, P., Hadgraft, J., Brain, K. R., Miller, T. A., and Walters, K. A. Surfactant effects in topical drug delivery. *Int. J. Pharm.* 41:189–195 (1988).

12. Aungst, B. J., Blake, J. A., and Hussain, M. A. Contributions of drug solubilization, partitioning, barrier disruption, and solvent permeation to the enhancement of skin permeation of various compounds with fatty acids and amines. *Pharm. Res.* 7:712–718 (1990).

13. Walters, K. A., Walker, M., and Olejnik, O. Nonionic surfactant effects on hairless mouse skin permeability characteristics. *J. Pharm. Pharmacol.* 40:525–529 (1988).

14. Lambert, W., Higuchi, W. I., Knutson, K., and Krill, S. Dose-dependent enhancement effects of Azone on skin permeability. *Pharm. Res.* 6:798–803 (1989).

15. Hori, M., Moon, K. C., Maibach, H. I., and Guy, R. H. Lineweaver–Burk analysis of skin penetration enhancement. *J. Controlled Release* 16:263–266 (1991).

16. Hori, M., Satoh, S., Maibach, H. I., and Guy, R. H. Enhancement of propranolol hydrochloride and diazepam skin absorption in vitro: Effect of enhancer lipophilicity. *J. Pharm. Sci.* 80:32–35 (1991).

17. Schuckler, F. and Lee, G. Relating the concentration-dependent action of Azone and dodecyl-L-pyroglutamate on the structure of excised human stratum corneum to changes in drug diffusivity, partition coefficient and flux. *Int. J. Pharm.* 80:81–89 (1992).

18. Wertz, P. W. and Downing, D. T. Glycolipids in mammalian epidermis: structure and function in the water barrier. *Science* 217:1261–1262 (1982).

19. Wertz, P. W. and Downing, D. T. Stratum corneum: Biological and biochemical considerations. In *Transdermal Drug Delivery*. Hadgraft, J. and Guy, R. H. (eds.). Marcel Dekker, New York, pp. 1–22 (1989).

20. Imokawa, G., Kuno, H., and Kawai, M. Stratum corneum lipids serve as a bound-water modulator. *J. Invest. Dermatol.* 96:845–851 (1991).

21. Klausner, R. D., Kleinfeld, A. M., Hoover, R. L., and Karnovsky, M. J. Lipid domains in membranes: Evidence derived from structural perturbations induced by free fatty acids and lifetime heterogeneity analysis. *J. Biol. Chem.* 255:1286–1295 (1980).

22. Beastall, J. C., Hadgraft, J., and Washington, C. Mechanism of action of Azone as a percutaneous penetration enhancer: lipid bilayer fluidity and transition temperature effects. *Int. J. Pharm.* 43:207–213 (1988).

23. Finean, J. B. Interaction between cholesterol and phospholipid in hydrated bilayers. *Chem. Phys. Lipids* 54:147–156 (1990).

24. Lewis, D. and Hadgraft, J. Mixed monolayers of dipalmitylphosphatidylcholine with Azone or oleic acid at the air/water interface. *Int. J. Pharm.* 65:211–218 (1990).

25. French, E. J. and Pouton, C. W. Nonionic surfactants as penetration enhancers: Correlation to lipid bilayer fluidity. In *Prediction of Percutaneous Penetration*, vol. 2. Scott, R. C., Guy, R. H., Hadgraft, J., and Boddé, H. E. (eds.). IBC, London, pp. 183–200 (1991).

26. Rolland, A., Brzokewicz, A., Shroot, B., and Jamoulle, J.-C. Effect of penetration enhancers on the phase transition of multilamellar liposomes of dipalmitoyl-phosphatidylcholine. A study by differential scanning calorimetry. *Int. J. Pharm.* 76:217–224 (1991).

27. Abraham, W. and Downing, D. T. Preparation of model membranes for skin permeability studies using stratum corneum lipids. *J. Invest. Dermatol* 93:809–813 (1989).

28. Schuckler, F. and Lee, G. The influence of Azone on monomolecular films of some stratum corneum lipids. *Int. J. Pharm.* 70:173–186 (1991).

29. French, E. J. The enhancement of percutaneous absorption by nonionic surfactants. PhD Thesis, University of Bath, UK (1991).
30. Presti, F. T. The role of cholesterol in regulating membrane fluidity. In *Membrane Fluidity in Biology*, Vol. 4, *Cellular Aspects*. Academic Press, New York (1985).
31. Bommannan, D., Potts, R. O., and Guy, R. H. Examination of the effect of ethanol on human stratum corneum in vivo using infrared spectroscopy. *J. Controlled Release* 16:299–304 (1991).
32. Cooper, E. R. Increased skin permeability for lipophilic molecules. *J. Pharm. Sci.* 73:1153–1156 (1984).
33. Aungst, B. J., Rogers, N. J., and Shefter, E. Enhancement of naloxone penetration through human skin in vitro using fatty acids, fatty alcohols, surfactants, sulfoxides and amides. *Int. J. Pharm.* 33:225–234 (1986).
34. Ogiso, T. and Shintani, M. Mechanism for the enhancement effect of fatty acids on the percutaneous absorption of propranolol. *J. Pharm. Sci.* 79:1065–1071 (1990).
35. Aungst, B. J. Structure/effect studies of fatty acid isomers as skin penetration enhancers and skin irritants. *Pharm. Res.* 6:244–247 (1989).
36. Golden, G. M., McKie, J. E., and Potts, R. O. The role of stratum corneum lipid fluidity in transdermal drug flux. *J. Pharm. Sci.* 76:25–28 (1987).
37. Francoeur, M. L., Golden, G. M., and Potts, R. O. Oleic acid: Its effect on stratum corneum in relation to (trans)dermal drug delivery. *Pharm. Res.* 7:621–627 (1990).
38. Walker, M. and Hadgraft, J. Oleic acid—a membrane "fluidizer" or fluid within a membrane? *Int. J. Pharm.* 71:R1–R4 (1991).
39. Ongpipattanakul, B., Burnette, R., and Potts, R. O. Evidence that oleic acid exists as a separate phase within stratum corneum. *Pharm. Res.* 8:350–354 (1991).
40. Buckingham, A. D. and Hentschel, H. G. E. Partial miscibility of liquid mixtures of protonated and deuterated high polymers. *J. Polymer Sci. Polymer Phys. Ed. 18*: 853–861 (1980).
41. Bates, F. S., Wignall, G. D., and Koehler, W. C. Critical behavior of binary liquid mixtures of deuterated and protonated polymers. *Phys. Rev. Lett.* 55:2425–2428 (1985).
42. Dorset, D. L., Strauss, H. L., and Snyder, R. G. Chain-length dependence of the melting point difference between hydrogenated and deuterated crystalline *n*-alkanes. *J. Phys. Chem. 95*:938–940 (1991).
43. Okamoto, H., Ohyabu, M., Hashida, M., and Sezaki, H. Enhanced penetration of mitomycin C through hairless mouse and rat skin by enhancers with terpene moieties. *J. Pharm. Pharmacol. 39*:531–534 (1987).
44. Okamoto, H., Hashida, M., and Sezaki, H. Structure–activity relationship of 1-alkyl- or 1-alkenylazacycloalkanone derivatives as percutaneous penetration enhancers. *J. Pharm. Sci. 77*:418–424 (1988).
45. Okamoto, H., Hashida, M., and Sezaki, H. Effect of 1-alkyl- or 1-alkenylazacyclo-alkanone derivatives on the penetration of drugs with different lipophilicities through guinea pig skin. *J. Pharm. Sci. 80*:39–45 (1991).
46. Hoogstraate, A. J., Verhoef, J., Brussee, J., IJzerman, A. P., Spies, F., and Boddé, H. Kinetics, ultrastructural aspects and molecular modelling of transdermal peptide flux enhancement by *N*-alkylazacyclo-heptanones. *Int. J. Pharm.* 76:37–47 (1991).

47. Prottey, C. and Ferguson, T. Factors which determine the skin irritation potential of soaps and detergents. *J. Soc. Cosmet. Chem. 26*:29–46 (1975).
48. Bodde, H. E. Visualization of percutaneous transport and its enhancement. *International Symposium Present Developments and Future Challenges in Transdermal Drug Delivery*. Noordwijkerhout, The Netherlands, Nov. 8–10 (1989).
49. Williams, D. G. Mechanism of action of penetration enhancers. PhD Thesis, University of Wales (1991).
50. Williams, A. C. and Barry, B. W. Terpenes and the lipid–protein-partitioning theory of skin penetration enhancement. *Pharm. Res. 8*:17–24 (1991).
51. Brain, K. R., Hadgraft, J., and Al-Shatalebi, M. Membrane modification in activity of plant molluscicides. *Planta Med. 56*:663 (1990).

19

Skin Penetration Enhancement

Clinical Pharmacological and Regulatory Considerations

Vinod P. Shah, Carl C. Peck, and Roger L. Williams

Food and Drug Administration, Rockville, Maryland

I. INTRODUCTION

In healthy skin, the stratum corneum and viable epidermis provide an effective protective barrier to entry of exogenous substances. In diseased skin, this barrier may be breached to varying degrees. Application of a drug topically to treat dermatological disease reflects an optimum setting for drug administration. Topical drug administration results in delivery of a pharmacologically active agent directly to the site at which the pharmacological effect is intended. This opportunity is only rarely possible with other routes of administration, during which entry into the systemic circulation results in drug distribution into all organs and tissues, including both sites at which the pharmacological effect is desired and those at which it is not.

Transdermal products are intended to treat or prevent systemic disorders in locations distant from the site of topical application. Examples of such products include transdermal patches, ointments, creams, and gels for the treatment or prevention of angina (glyceryl trinitrate), hypertension (clonidine), motion sickness (scopolamine), addictive disorders (nicotine), pain (fentanyl), and estrogen deficiency (estradiol). Because the intended site(s) of action differ between a topically applied product intended for local or for systemic administration, an important difference between topical and transdermal topical and transdermal drug products is the mass transfer rate of drug within and across the skin. For topical drug products, formulations should promote drug uptake and retention by skin at the site of application. In this setting, a high flux (amount of drug transported through a unit area of skin per unit time) is not required, even though drug retained in the stratum corneum might eventually result in some systemic entry. For transdermal products, a high flux is desired so that drug can penetrate the stratum corneum to be available in sufficient amounts to the systemic circulation for therapeutic effect.

For physicochemical reasons, such as high molecular weight and polarity, most drugs are not suitable for transdermal administration. Thus, enhancement of penetration of selected drugs might significantly expand the list of drugs that could be delivered transdermally. From a regulatory standpoint, development of a drug for transdermal delivery poses several challenges to the drug development process, some of which are amplified with the addition of penetration enhancement methods. This chapter will focus on the addition of penetration enhancers to transdermal delivery systems from a clinical pharmacological and regulatory standpoint. Although methods for penetration enhancement will be reviewed briefly, more detailed information is provided in several excellent recent reviews (1–9).

II. CLINICAL PHARMACOLOGY

The application of clinical pharmacological principles to the development of a transdermal product rests on the assumption that drug effect is related to concentration of total or unbound drug in an accessible biological fluid, such as blood, plasma, or urine. A transdermal product with or without penetration enhancement technology should be capable of producing therapeutically relevant plasma and tissue concentrations of a drug or its active metabolite(s). Development of a drug for transdermal delivery has generally followed its development and approval for some other route of administration. Although development of a new drug initially for administration by the transdermal route is by no means unlikely, the clinical pharmacological issues for most transdermal drug products relate to potential change in drug pharmacokinetics and pharmacological effect when the route of administration and the rate of delivery of a drug are changed.

A. Pharmacokinetic Issues

Development of a transdermal product frequently involves a change in drug delivery from that of an oral immediate-release formulation (e.g., clonidine) to a type of controlled-release formulation. The continuous, potentially zero-order delivery of a drug from a transdermal system throughout the period of application may be one of its principal advantages. Transdermal delivery systems also allow the opportunity to avoid metabolic pathways associated with oral or sublingual administration that effectively deactivate a drug before entry into the systemic circulation. These benefits are associated with the clinical pharmacological challenge of redefining the bioavailability and pharmacokinetics of a transdermally delivered drug in comparison with the other routes of administration employed for the drug. These challenges are in many ways comparable with those confronted by the conversion of an immediate- to a controlled-release oral drug delivery system. Issues of dose dumping, variable rate of delivery, fluctuation at steady state, time to reach peak concentration, and multiple concentration maxima are common to both controlled-release and transdermal formulations. Just as development of an oral controlled-release formulation raises concern about site of absorption from the gastrointestinal tract, so too does development of a transdermal formulation give rise to concern related to site-of-application effects on formulation performance. These variables include application site effects, such as locus on the body, skin disease, or irritation under the site of application; hair pattern under the application site; and potentially numerous other local factors that may be capable of disturbing the input of drug from the transdermal system (perspiration, temperature, motion).

Conversion of a formulation delivered by another route of administration to a transdermal formulation also raises issues related to congruity in metabolic paths between the nontransdermal and the transdermal routes. For some drugs, congruity is not an issue, owing to lack of metabolism or to formation of only inactive metabolites. For other drugs, metabolism changes depending on the route of administration. For example, the ratio of glyceryl trinitrate (GTN) to either the 1,3- or 1,2-dinitrate metabolites varies depending on the route of administration (10). Because both dinitrate metabolites of GTN may possess clinical activity, this incongruity suggests that the pharmacological activity of GTN may not be comparable between different routes of administration. Difference in the ratio of enantiomers of a racemate may also occur when a drug is changed from another route of administration to transdermal administration, depending on whether the enantiomers are actively and differentially metabolized in either or both routes. Other pharmacokinetic variables and issues, such as protein binding, induction, and end-product inhibition of a specific metabolic pathway may differ depending on the route of administration.

Whatever pharmacokinetic issues apply to the conversion from one route of administration to the transdermal route arise again with the addition of penetration enhancement methods to a currently existing transdermal product. Primary pharmacokinetic and bioavailability parameters may require redefinition, and metabolic pathways affecting the production of potentially active metabolites or the ratio between enantiomers of a chiral drug may need to be reexplored.

B. Pharmacodynamic Issues

Change from another route of administration to transdermal administration may change the pharmacological effect profile of the drug. Change in the time course of a pharmacodynamic concentration–effect relation can occur with development of a transdermal formulation. If change occurs in important metabolite or enantiomer patterns, the apparent concentration–effect relation may also change. Consequently, documentation of a relation between drug concentration in an accessible fluid, such as plasma or blood, and a pharmacological effect of interest will facilitate the development of a transdermal formulation with or without penetration enhancement methodology. Concerns associated with development of a transdermal product are similar to those arising with conversion of immediate- to controlled-release oral formulations. Some of these latter concerns have been addressed in recent workshops and publications (11,12). Assuming an E_{max} model relation, or some variant thereof, exists between drug concentration and effect, it is apparent that the development of a transdermal formulation, by which a drug can be administered comparably with an intravenous infusion, versus an orally administered immediate-release product, for example, may result in substantial change in the time course of pharmacological effect of the drug. When coupled with changes in enantiomer ratios of a chiral drug or changes in parent drug/ metabolite ratios for drugs with active metabolites, pharmacological effect may certainly change when converting a drug from an oral immediate-release to a transdermal formulation. Recent clinical experience with transdermal nitroglycerin products suggests that continuous administration of a drug by the transdermal route also raises issues of tachyphylaxis and clinical tolerance (13).

Therefore, addition of penetration enhancement methods to a new transdermal product or a previously approved transdermal product without an enhancer may require not only review and reevaluation of the effect time profile, but also reevaluation of the primary relation between pharmacological effect and concentration. Reevaluation of the latter rests on the possibility that the primary concentration–effect relation may change in the presence of an enhancer, whereas reevaluation of the latter is based on the possibility that even if the primary concentration–effect relation is undisturbed, the time course of the effect may be affected.

III. METHODS OF ENHANCEMENT

The skin is a structurally and functionally complex, multilayered organ. It is composed of outer epidermis and inner dermis. The outermost layer of epidermis, the stratum corneum, is formed by continuous differentiation of adjacent viable epidermis. Anatomically, the stratum corneum is a coherent multilaminated membrane, 15–30 µm thick, consisting of lipids and proteins arranged in a complex interlocking structure, similar to bricks and mortar. The stratum corneum is poorly permeable, especially to water-soluble compounds. It is breached by hair follicles and sweat ducts that can provide parallel diffusion or shunt pathways. Below the stratum corneum is the viable epidermis, which can be characterized as an aqueous gel. The viable epidermis is not thought to present a significant barrier to drug penetration (14), except when highly lipophilic drugs are applied or when the stratum corneum is damaged.

Because the stratum corneum is the dominant rate-limiting barrier of skin, transdermal research has focused on facilitating drug transport across this barrier. The vehicle component of a dermatological formulation, as well as a drug's physicochemical characteristics, can significantly influence drug penetration through the skin. In addition, the physical nature of the dermatological product influences drug penetration characteristics. For example, some transdermal delivery systems produce a state of occlusion, whereas creams apparently do not, and ointments produce only partial occlusion. Both chemical and physical methods have been employed to increase drug penetration through skin.

A. Chemical Methods of Enhancement

The primary objective in developing a transdermal system with chemical penetration enhancers has been to identify compounds that significantly enhance drug penetration through the epidermis, but that do not severely irritate or damage the skin. As reviewed by Barry (1), chemical permeation enhancers should be safe and nontoxic under conditions of use, pharmacologically inert, nonirritating, and nonallergic (15). Ideally, the penetration effect should be immediate. Moreover, its duration of action should be predictable and reversible, so that skin reverts to its normal integrity and barrier property when the penetrant is removed. Finally, the ideal enhancer should be chemically and physically compatible with a wide range of drugs and pharmaceutical adjutants and should be cosmetically acceptable.

Chemical penetration enhancer increase skin permeability by reversibility damaging or by altering the physicochemical nature of the stratum corneum to reduce its diffusional resistance. Changes in the physicochemical nature of the skin can be achieved by increasing the thermodynamic activity of the drug in a vehicle, by using a penetration enhancer as a cosolvent. Alcohols generally extract polar stratum corneum lipids and increase partitioning for certain drugs. Ethanol has been used as an enhancer–cosolvent in estrogen patches to increase drug penetration (7).

Chemical penetration enhancers also can increase skin permeability by increasing the partition coefficient of the drug into the skin. Increased partitioning of drug can occur by modifying polar, nonpolar, and a combination of polar and non-polar physicochemical pathways (7,8). The polar pathways may be altered chemically by protein conformational change or by solvent swelling. The nonpolar pathway may be altered by modifying rigidity of the lipid structure and fluidization of the crystalline matrix of the stratum corneum. As an example, fatty acid enhancers increase the fluidity of the lipid portion of the stratum corneum to promote absorption of certain drugs (16,17). Some binary-vehicle penetration enhancers act on both polar and nonpolar pathways by altering the multilaminate pathway for penetrants. Enhancers can also increase drug diffusivity in the stratum corneum by dissolving the skin lipids or by denaturing skin proteins.

The choice of a chemical enhancer will have a significant influence on product design and development. The basis structural characteristics of protein conformation and swelling, and lipid structure and fluidity should be assessed to understand the interactions of chemical penetration enhancers with the skin. Chemical agents that maximally interact with the stratum corneum and minimally with viable tissues are desirable.

Despite physicochemical and other methods for increasing the rate of entry of drug into the skin, in some transdermal formulations, the ultimate rate-limiting step for transdermal delivery is the release of drug from the vehicle to the skin surface. This release can be influenced by several factors, including solubility and concentration of the drug, replenishment of drug at the skin–vehicle interface, and partitioning of the drug out of the vehicle into the skin (3). Penetration of the drug from a given vehicle can be increased by presenting the drug in solution, which represents a higher level of thermodynamic activity.

B. Physical Methods of Enhancement

Iontophoresis and ultrasound (phonophoresis or sonophoresis) techniques are physical methods used to enhance percutaneous penetration of various therapeutic agents. In iontophoresis, a small current is used to move large charged drug molecules through the skin. Research is underway to regulate rate of drug delivery (steady state of pulsating) through the skin by controlling the delivery of the electrical current. One of the greatest challenges and opportunities in the area of iontophoretic drug delivery is to provide the correct dose of insulin to diabetics.

A major concern with the use of iontophoresis is that the device may cause painful destruction of the skin with high-current settings. High-quality electrodes with adequate skin adhesion, uniform current distribution, and well-controlled ionic properties are essential to the safe use of this method. The mechanism of transdermal penetration by this technology is still unclear.

IV. REGULATORY CONSIDERATIONS

A. New Drug Applications

1. Efficacy

As with other formulation changes that result in a change in rate of drug delivery (e.g., oral controlled-release formulations), application of penetration enhancement technology to a transdermal formulation may change not only the time course of a known concentration–effect relation, but also the time course of clinical effects. Thus, when penetration enhancement technology is developed for a drug previously administered by the oral route or for a previously existing transdermal formulation, consideration would be given to defining the effect of the change in the plasma-concentration time curve on the pharmacological-effect time curve. In considering this issue as part of the development of a controlled-release formulation, the Food and Drug Administration (FDA) and academic scientists suggested that, under certain circumstances, clinical trials for the conversion of an immediate- to a controlled-release formulation might not be required. Clinical trials would generally be required in the following circumstances: (a) substantial interdose fluctuation for the immediate-release product; (b) bioinequivalence in extent of bioavailability between the conventional and controlled-release products; (c) unpredictable relation between serum concentrations of the controlled-release drug and its therapeutic–toxic effect; and (d) evidence or irreversible toxicity or pharmacodynamic tolerance. Presumably, many of these concerns and conclusions apply to the development of a transdermal product with a formulation enhancer. Unless a drug were creating its effect at concentrations close to maximum effect, it is difficult to imagine that change in rate of drug delivery might not affect the time course of the pharmacological effect.

Development of a controlled-release formulation generally focuses on issues of change in rate of drug absorption. Penetration enhancement methods are also capable of changing the extent of drug absorption, not only in comparison with a transdermal product without penetration enhancement, but also in comparison with administration of the drug by a nontransdermal route. As noted previously, penetration enhancement methods may also change routes of metabolism and enantiomer ratios. For these various reasons, clinical trial data for efficacy may be necessary in the development of a transdermal formulation that includes penetration enhancement technology. Specific recommendations for the pharmacokinetic and biopharmaceutical data relevant to a new drug or new dosage form have been defined in an FDA guideline entitled *Guidelines for the Format and Content of the Human Pharmacokinetics and Bioavailability Section of an NDA*. Further information concerning NDA efficacy documentation for a new transdermal formulation with penetration enhancement technology may also be obtained from the applicable reviewing division in the Center for Drug Evaluation and Research at FDA.

2. Safety

Introduction of penetration enhancement technology also calls for an additional need to document safety in a New Drug Application (NDA). In a sense, these requirements are comparable with those associated with development of a combination product, for which safety of each component alone (the drug and the penetration enhancer) and combined must be evaluated. In addition, penetration enhancement methods usually increase the permeation not only of the drug, but of formulation excipients and of themselves as well. In spite of being excellent penetration enhancers in a transdermal system, many vehicles are limited because of deleterious effect of skin (e.g., dimethyl sulfoxide; DMSO). Dimethyl sulfoxide is a powerful solvent and increases drug penetration, but, at the same time, it damages the biochemical and structural integrity of the skin (1).

Local effects related to skin damage, irritation, and allergenicity are important, particularly if the transdermal system might be applied repeatedly to a single site before full recovery occurs. These effects should be evaluated to understand general toxicological implications, especially in terms of irritation potential. Irritation from transdermal drug products appears to be strongly influenced by the degree of skin occlusion imparted by the product. It is related to stratum corneum hydration and decreased diffusional resistance to formulation components. Chemical enhancers should be evaluated for irritancy potential under conditions of long-term occlusion. Development of computer simulation models with the use of solubility parameters to predict drug–vehicle–skin interactions and flux rate may aid in optimal selection of an enhancer (18). Physical methods for enhancing drug penetration raise different types of concerns that include destruction of the stratum corneum with high-current settings and general skin irritation. These safety concerns will generally require special consideration during development and evaluation of iontophoretic and ultrasound penetration enhancers.

B. Abbreviated New Drug Applications

A generic formulation in the United States must be pharmaceutically equivalent to the pioneer product, according to the following criteria: (a) the active ingredient is the same; (b) the strength of the active ingredient is the same; (c) it is the same type of dosage form; (d) the formulation is intended for the same route of administration; (e) the formulation is generally labeled for the same conditions of use. For some products, there may also be a requirement that excipients be qualitatively or quantitatively comparable between the pioneer and generic formulation. Earlier discussions at the agency suggested that several factors might be considered important in the determination of pharmaceutical equivalence of a transdermal formulation. These factors included mechanism of release of the product from the transdermal system, drug content in the system, and active surface area of the system. More recently, scientists in the Center for Drug Evaluation and Research have suggested that perhaps none of these factors are particularly pertinent to a definition of pharmaceutical equivalence, and that the determination for each transdermal–drug system should be made on a case-by-case basis. For some transdermal systems (e.g., transdermal nitroglycerin), the current position at the agency is that all systems are pharmaceutically equivalent and, if found to be bioequivalent, may be judged therapeutically equivalent as well.

Currently, the agency also tentatively concluded that transdermal formulations containing chemical penetration enhancement methods will not be considered pharmaceutically equivalent to transdermal formulations lacking chemical enhancers. The agency has not decided whether the chemical enhancer used in each transdermal formulation must be the same to achieve a determination of pharmaceutical equivalence. No judgments have yet been made for products containing physical methods of penetration enhancement. The general basis for these judgments is that enhancement technology imposes a sufficiently significant change in formulation, such that pharmaceutical equivalence can no longer be justified, just as an oral product, containing an absorption enhancer that allowed a lower labeled dose, would likely not be considered pharmaceutically equivalent to an oral formulation without the enhancer.

Documentation of bioequivalence of pharmaceutically equivalent dosage forms is necessary to achieve a determination by FDA of therapeutic equivalence. For drugs approved after 1962, documentation of bioequivalence is almost invariably based on performance of an in vivo bioequivalence study with statistical comparison of test and reference pharmacokinetic parameters derived from relevant concentration time curves. Given that delivery of drug by the transdermal route may add additional variance to pharmacokinetic parameters that assess rate and extent of absorption, and in view of the presence of a possible requirement to measure active metabolites or enantiomers, documentation of bioequivalence of transdermal formulations may be especially challenging. The agency is now considering various ways to address these additional changes. To the extent that addition of penetration enhancement technology may promote more consistent and less variable drug absorption across the skin, documentation of bioequivalence of pharmaceutically equivalent dosage forms containing penetration enhancers may become less difficult.

V. CONCLUSIONS

Penetration enhancement technology is an exciting and challenging development that may increase significantly the number of drugs available for transdermal administration. Careful attention to biopharmaceutical, pharmacokinetic, and pharmacodynamic issues will be necessary to assess the effect of a specific enhancement method. Regulatory concerns relative to these scientific disciplines will focus on pharmacokinetic and pharmacodynamic effects of the enhancer alone, the drug alone, and the drug and enhancer in combination. Because a penetration enhancer may promote absorption of other excipients and of itself, certain pharmacokinetic and pharmacodynamic concerns may extend to excipients and the enhancer itself. A summary of specific concerns relative to a penetration enhancer addressed in this article include the following:

1. Mechanism of action
   Primary mechanism
   Duration
   Specificity for enhancement (drug versus excipients)
2. Biopharmaceutics and pharmacokinetics
   Enhancer (fate of enhancer in the body)
   Drug with and without enhancer
   Excipients and enhancer
3. Efficacy
   Alteration in time course and shape of drug and metabolite concentration–
      effect relation
4. Safety
   Alteration in time course and shape of drug and metabolite concentration–
      toxic effect relations
   Local change and reversibility
   Excipient effects

   Careful planning and consideration of the various factors and their potential effects and interactions will facilitate the drug development process and subsequent agency review. General and specific requirements for development of transdermal formulations with penetration enhancers should be reviewed regulatory scientists in the appropriate reviewing division in the Center for Drug Evaluation and Research.

REFERENCES

1. Barry, B. W. Properties that influence percutaneous absorption. In *Dermatological Formulations, Percutaneous Absorption*. Barry, B. W. (ed.). Marcel Dekker, New York, pp. 127–233 (1983).
2. Cooper, E. R. Vehicle effects on skin penetration. In *Percutaneous Absorption*. Bronaugh, R. L. and Maibach, H. I. (eds.). Marcel Dekker, New York, pp. 525–530 (1985).

3. Gummer, C. L. Vehicles as penetration enhancers. In *Percutaneous Absorption*. Bronaugh, R. L. and Maibach, H. I. (eds.). Marcel Dekker, New York, pp. 561–570 (1985).

4. Chien, Y. W. Development concepts and practice in TTS. In *Transdermal Controlled Systemic Medications*. Chien, Y. W. (ed.). Marcel Dekker, New York, pp. 25–82 (1987).

5. Cooper, E. R. Alterations in skin permeability. In *Transdermal Controlled Systemic Medications*. Chien, Y. E. (ed.). Marcel Dekker, New York, pp. 83–91 (1987).

6. Cooper, E. R. and Berner, B. Penetration enhancers. In *Transdermal Delivery of Drugs*, Vol. 2. Kydonieus, A. F. and Berner, B. (eds.). CRC Press, Boca Raton, pp. 57–62 (1987).

7. Walters, K. A. Penetration enhancers and their use in transdermal therapeutic systems. In *Transdermal Drug Delivery*. Hadgraft, J. and Guy, R. H. (eds.). Marcel Dekker, New York, pp. 197–246 (1989).

8. Rolf, D. Chemical and physical methods of enhancing transdermal drug delivery. *Pharm. Technol.* Sept. *12*:131–140 (1988).

9. Pfister, W. R. and Hsieh, D. S. T. Permeation enhancers compatible with transdermal drug delivery systems. *Pharm. Technol.* Sept. *14*:132–138 (1990).

10. Williams, R. L., Thakker, K. M., John, V., Lin, E. T., Liang-Gee, W., and Benet, L. Z. Nitroglycerin absorption from transdermal systems: Formulation effects and metabolite concentrations. *Pharm. Res.* 8:744–749 (1991).

11. Shah, V. P., Flynn, G. L., Guy, R. H., Maibach, H. I., Schaefer, H., Skelly, J. P., Wester, R. C., and Yacobi, A. In-vivo percutaneous penetration/absorption. *Int. J. Pharm.* 74:1–8 (1991).

12. Skelly, J. P., Amidon, G. L., Barr, W. H., Benet, L. Z., Carter, J. E., Robinson, J. R., Shah, V. P., and Yacobi, A. In-vitro and in-vivo testing and correlation of oral controlled/modified release dosage forms. *Pharm. Res.* 7:975–982 (1990).

13. Steering Committee, Transdermal Nitroglycerin Cooperative Study. Acute and chronic antianginal efficacy of continuous twenty-four-hour application of transdermal nitroglycerin. *Am. J. Cardiol.* 68:1263–1273 (1991).

14. Scheuplein, R. J. Mechanisms of percutaneous absorption II: Transient diffusion and the relative importance of various rate of skin penetration. *J. Invest. Dermatol.* 48:79–88 (1967).

15. Kat, M. and Poulsen, B. J. In *Handbook of Experimental Pharmacology*, Vol. 28, Part 1. Brodie, B. B. and Gillette, J. (eds.). Springer-Verlag, New York, p. 108 (1971).

16. Knutson, K., Potts, R. O., Guzek, D. B., Golden, G. M., McKie, J. E., Lambert, W. J., and Higuchi, W. I. Macro- and molecular physical-chemical considerations in understanding drug transport in the stratum corneum. *J. Controlled Release* 2(10):67–87 (1985).

17. Potts, R. C. Physical characterization of the stratum corneum: The relationship of mechanical and barrier properties to lipid and protein structure. *Transdermal Drug Delivery*. Hadgraft, J. and Guy, R. H. Marcel Dekker, New York, pp. 23–58 (1989).

18. Sloan, K. B., Koch, S. A. M., Silvers, K. G., and Fowlers, F. L. Use of solubility parameters of drug and vehicle to predict flux through skin. *J. Invest. Dermatol.* 87:244–252 (1986).

Index